Interpersonal Nursing for Mental Health

Jan Horsfall, RN, MA, PhD, is a senior lecturer in the School of Nursing at the University of Western Sydney, in Macarthur, Australia

Cynthia Stuhlmiller, BSN, MS, DNSC, is a Professor of Mental Health Nursing at Flinders University in Australia.

Simon Champ, BA (fine arts), Grad Dip (painting), is a freelance mental health activist and a lecturer, as well as an artist, living in Sydney, Australia.

Interpersonal Nursing for Mental Health

Jan Horsfall, RN, MA, PhD and
Cynthia Stuhlmiller, BSN, MS, DNSc
with Simon Champ, BA, grad. dip.

 Springer Publishing Company

Springer Publishing Company, Inc.
536 Broadway
New York, NY 10012-3955

Acquisition Editor: Ruth Chasek
Production Editor: Matt Fenton
Cover design by Susan Hauley

02 03 04 05 / 5 4 3 2

Library of Congress Cataloging-in-Publication data:

Horsfall, Jan.
    Interpersonal nursing for mental health / Jan Horsfall, Cynthia Stuhlmiler,
with Simon Champ
        p.cm.
    Includes index
    ISBN 0-8261-1415-6
        1. Psychiatric nurses.   2. Nurse and patient. I. Stuhlmiller, Cynthia M., 1956–
II. Champ, Simon. III. Title.
    RC440 .H65 2001
    610.73'68-dc21   2001020175

Printed in the United States of America by Maple-Vail

First published in Australia 2000 by
MacLennan & Petty Pty Limited
Suite 405, 154 Bunnerong Road, Eastgardens, Sydney NSW 2036, Australia
©2000 MacLennan & Petty Pty Limited

Contents

Mental Health Nursing Practice

Dedications

To the patients who are/were the only people who could teach us what we needed to know and understand. JH & CS

In commemoration of Hildegard E. Peplau (1909–1999), the grandmother of interpersonal psychiatric/mental health nursing. CS & JH

To future generations who will experience a mental illness, in the hope that their journeys will become easier. SC, JH, CS

Acknowledgments

To Keith Hughes, the mainstay of my personal and academic life. To all members of the Division of Nursing, University of Western Sydney Macarthur for the continuance of an effective teaching and administrative milieu conducive to writing. JH

To Gregory Helgeson for his enduring patience, love, support and understanding. To Ma Stuhlmiller for her ongoing inspiration and guidance. To Reta Creegan for challenging me to commit my views. CS

To Tania Alexander who shared in my understanding of living with a mental illness and finding meaning in the experience. To my family who were always there for me, encouraging and inspiring. SC

'The issue in psychiatry has been too often confused by starting from a fixed list of symptoms instead of from the study of those whose characteristic reactions are denied validity in their society.' p. 258

Ruth Benedict, *Patterns of Culture,* 1989 [orig 1934].

'The nursing process is educative and therapeutic when nurse and patient can come to know and to respect each other, as persons who are alike, and yet, different, as persons who share in the solution of problems.' p. 9

'The kind of person each nurse becomes makes a sub-stantial difference to what each patient will learn as he is nursed throughout his experience with illness.' p. x

Hildegard E Peplau, *Interpersonal Relations in Nursing:
A Conceptual Frame of Reference for Psychodynamic Nursing,* 1952

Theory and Practice Underpinnings

1

Ourselves as mental health nurses, consumers and teachers

Introduction

This chapter is a brief introduction to ourselves as individuals with life experiences that have influenced our understanding of what it is to be human in westernized countries at the beginning of the twenty first century. Along with our cultural background, these experiences and emergent world views have shaped our understandings of mental health, mental illness, nursing and mental health nursing.

Since we have written a mental health nursing textbook from an interpersonal perspective, we consider that our beliefs, values and attitudes underpin—or certainly impinge upon—both theory and practice. In this we do not consider ourselves to be unique. The way that any author understands people, work, health, illness, madness and nursing inevitably leads to textual emphases, omissions and the imparting of some human prejudices. That is, personal beliefs seep into terminology, theoretical frameworks and suggested nursing actions in mental health texts, regardless of the awareness of writers or readers.

From an educational perspective, we consider that unacknowledged belief systems built into texts are not necessarily helpful in preparing students for undergraduate clinical placements, for sensitive mental health nursing or for critical thinking in practice after graduation. Whether educators or authors are conscious of these processes or not, students may take the ideas and schemas in texts (and in the lecture hall and tutorial class) at face value. We have therefore decided to be open and speak a little about ourselves as people and how we believe this relates to our appreciation of mental health nursing practice and consumer recovery within contemporary health services. In other words, we will attempt to make some of our beliefs and prejudices transparent, rather than hide them behind taken-for-granted textbook formats and technical language.

Why write another mental health nursing text?

There are at least four broad answers to this question. First, the majority of mental health nursing textbooks are too comprehensive for the needs of most undergraduate nursing students. Many nursing students read no more than 25 per cent of their prescribed mental health nursing textbooks during their undergraduate nursing course. The comprehensiveness of the texts have advantages for many academics. However, the detail of breadth and depth can be a disadvantage from the perspective of the average busy undergraduate nursing student who will experience at least one mental health nursing placement, but who does not expect (accurately, or not) to be working with people with a mental illness. In relation to finding interesting or relevant material, many learners consider that the mental health information they seek is often hidden within non-nursing detail that is not necessarily clear or logical to the uninitiated.

Second, most mental health nursing textbooks are set out along medical lines. While this is a logical and simple structure for authors and specialist practitioners, the undergraduate student has not yet heard of the DSM (*Diagnostic and Statistical Manual of Mental Disorders*), let alone internalized the psychiatric classification system. Furthermore, once the psychiatric nomenclature has been mastered, the student is unwittingly taking in a medical view of people living with a mental illness and about mental health nursing. The focus on definitions of psychiatric disorders, lists of symptoms, technical terms for human phenomena and hypothetical, and at times obscure, biological etiologies begins to dehumanize people with those diagnoses and distance students from patients even before they have met.

The third reason to write another, but hopefully different, mental health nursing text is related to the mental health system's common marginalization of the consumer and the nurse, who are both central participants in mental health service outcomes. Consumer and nurse contributions do not feature prominently in mental health policy, service development, or clinical practice publications. Many contemporary mainstream mental health nursing texts seem to endorse this sidelining by presenting an overview of nursing theorists and their work, but without connecting these ideas to nursing practice when working with people with a specific set of life difficulties related to a mental illness. Often medical and psychological theories and ideologies are privileged in the texts, indicating on a number of levels that nursing is theoretically and practically less important than the older and higher status psychiatric disciplines.

A final hope is to contribute to the contemporary mental health nursing (journal-based) dialogue about the foundations of, and intentions of, mental health nursing. In this discussion, some authors encourage students and clinicians to thoroughly learn their neurochemistry and expect exciting developments of new classes of better designed and more efficient and effective psychotropic medications. Other authors take the view that the primary nursing focus is on the needs and distress of the person experiencing a psychosis, depression or anxiety disorder; and that the administration of medication and observation of its effects is also the business of nursing, but of a second order. This is the perspective that the three contributors to this text take. We wish to encourage mental health nursing to reclaim its place within nursing philosophy (patient-centered caring and respect), nursing theory (interpersonal nursing and a health orientation), and nursing practice (the therapeutic relationship, working with client strengths, enhancing activities of daily living). Hence, our broader aim is to re-humanize mental health nursing at the beginning of the 21st century.

Ideology

The notion in the above discussion that belief systems are built into approaches to mental illness is described by the term 'ideology.' Our aim in this textbook is to critique some mainstream psychiatric ideas and propose some ideologies that are promoted less, possibly because they do not fit well with medical and societal views about psychiatric disorders, biology and 'wonder drugs.'

A general definition of ideology is that it constitutes 'a total system of thought and emotion and attitude to the world, to society and to [humankind]' (Mitchell 1979: 100). Ideology in the present context is used in the sense that a set of ideas in the form of an attitudinal and emotional package or bundle is handed across to the reader once a major idea among the set is presented. For example, terms such as 'scientific evidence,' 'proof' and 'objective research,' are part of a scientific ideological package, which in westernized societies conveys the notion that the ideas presented in this package are more rigorously tested, are valued more highly than other types of knowledge, and are most likely to be correct.

Mainstream psychiatric ideology is characterized by the three following features: individualism, ignoring the practical context of the person's life, and a focus on the present. Western individualism is an ideological assumption built into the foundations of the discipline of psychiatry and this is one aspect of psychiatry that is rarely commented upon in nursing, medical or psychology texts. In medicine it is an individual who is ill or has a disease and should be treated—not a couple or a family. At one level this is obviously true. However, a resolute focus on the diagnosed patient ignores the societal, political or economic factors that may have contributed to the person becoming or remaining mentally ill. Just focusing on the patient as a person separate from her or his family, neighbors or workplace, ignores practical, emotional, interpersonal and religious aspects of other people around the person who may interact helpfully or detrimentally with him or her.

At the economic and political levels this focus on the individual ignores the fact that unemployment is the greatest predictor of mental illness in westernized societies, for both men and women and across all age groups. In Australia at present, 36 per cent of unemployed men and 32 per cent of unemployed women (Australian Bureau of Statistics, 1998: 24) have a diagnosable affective, anxiety, or substance abuse disorder. This does not mean that unemployment *causes* mental illness any more than genes simply cause mental illness. It does mean, both theoretically and clinically, that when the psychiatrically diagnosed person has an income below poverty level and lives outside mainstream 'productive' society, changing these factors is commonly considered to be less important in the person's recovery than adherence to psychotropic medication.

Mainstream psychiatric and psychological ideology is primarily concerned with the present; that is, the medical symptoms that the psychiatrist perceives the patient is displaying or experiencing now. In this scenario, sometimes even the near future—the living circumstances to which a patient will return—is not given adequate attention. Significant troubling past experiences are also deemed to be comparatively unimportant. A consequence for patients and nurses is that it may seem that the mental illness has mysteriously taken over the patient for no apparent reason. Where does this leave the young man who was expected not to cry and has never been able to grieve the loss of his father, who died while he was at primary school? How does this affect the young woman survivor of childhood sexual assault who has been withdrawn and too afraid to tell anyone about the rape?

About the authors

Jan Horsfall

I would like to outline some aspects of my life experiences that are relevant to my beliefs about mental illness and mental health nursing. My beginnings were Australian, provincial and ordinary, and I had never heard about mad people or asylums until I applied to become a trainee nurse in a psychiatric hospital at the age of 20. Before that I had been a laboratory assistant for four years and my best matriculation subjects were mathematics, physics and chemistry.

Oakley Hospital (in Auckland, New Zealand), where I trained to be a psychiatric nurse in the mid-1960s, was large, urban and sex segregated (the female nurses worked primarily with women). When I went for the interview, the only motive I was aware of was that the job would be 'different'—which it was! Until then I had been testing and measuring things in small laboratories (for example, rubber, plastics, blood and urine). My passion was reading lots of interesting and absorbing European novels that involved characters and places that were totally outside my world. I left my South Australian family home at the age of 19 to go to New Zealand—where I knew nobody—to begin what I expected to be a journey to Europe. In rural South Australia at the time, this was an odd thing to do: most of the people I went to primary and high school with during the 1950s have lived their whole life in, or near, Adelaide.

During my three-year training, a registered psychiatric nurse (RPN) and I became key nursing proponents for the establishment of a 'therapeutic milieu' in the admission ward at the hospital. A psychiatrist who had returned from the UK brought back these ideas deriving from Wilfred Bion and Harry Stack Sullivan; he asked us if we were interested in starting up a totally new approach to working with patients in one of the admission wards where my colleague was the charge nurse (nurse unit manager equivalent). This is where I gained both group work experience and the beginnings of an understanding of an interpersonal approach to working therapeutically with people with a mental illness. The other RPN and I were among a small group of nurses at the hospital who seemed (in retrospect) to work, reflect upon and discuss approaches to patients rather more as if we had a vocation than a job. We put much energy, time and enthusiasm into planning, reviewing and improving upon the effectiveness of the milieu and the power of the group work.

About a year later, the matron simultaneously sent us both to the locked ward for dangerous newly admitted patients and severely disturbed long-term patients—again as charge and relieving charge nurse. Here, apart from the newly admitted patients, many people did not respond readily to medication and the majority had been patients for many months, years or decades. The idea of the therapeutic milieu inspired us to try different approaches with this clientele, too. The work was both exciting and challenging.

We organized easels, water paints and brushes for each of the single rooms that were used for the extremely distressed or physically dangerous patients. We developed a seclusion gradient with the knowledge of the psychiatrist. After a comprehensive nursing assessment of each new patient, we would spend time listening to and talking with the women in the rooms, even though the sign on the door stated that between two and six nurses should attend when the door was opened. There were no assaults or suicides, and no more 'escapes' than before. We also introduced personal clothing, refused to serve meals without knives and forks and took difficult young clients out for a run before breakfast (before this became known as jogging). There was a wonderful RPN who provided occupational therapy for these patients in a nearby building; and the other nursing staff were supportive of our general orientation and participated according to their level of interest and confidence.

This occurred over a nine-month period and apparently became problematic for the medical superintendent. I was not yet registered as a psychiatric nurse and he targeted me as a 'ringleader' (which was either untrue, or something that I was doing without noticing my own leadership), threatened me with organizing a failure in my final hospital exams and put pressure on me to leave, which I did some months later. As a consequence of that coercion (probably illegal), I stayed away from nursing for a number of years. I was also the only person who gained an honors result in the psychiatry subject in the state psychiatric nursing registration examination that year.

After I left New Zealand, I traveled with a woman friend for four years in Mediterranean, Middle Eastern and West African countries. This provided me with daily excitement in relation to diverse cultures, languages and customs very different from my own. As a white minority of two, especially in Africa and the Middle East, we learned to manage high levels of personal visibility on the one hand and the arbitrary decision making of authority figures regarding such necessities as visas and public transport on the other. This immersion in other societies was so intense that I am sure it affected the way I understand the breadth of 'normal' human possibilities as well as the imagination I am able to bring to bear when working with people experiencing severe distress.

My reading time increased. Among other ideas I immersed myself in during those times were the 'anti-psychiatry' writings of Laing (e.g., Laing & Esterton, 1964). After returning to Australia and settling in Sydney in the mid-1970s, I studied sociology for four years full-time at university. This allowed me to develop a meaningful intellectual framework for understanding the world I was living in.

Having registered as a psychiatric nurse, I later worked in a large psychiatric hospital in Adelaide; with troubled adolescent girls in London; and with aged patients in Toronto. When I arrived in Sydney in 1976 I worked as a psychiatric nurse in a private clinic. This turned out to be the second really exciting psychiatric setting I worked in. The clients were mixed regarding age, status and psychiatric diagnosis, and I found that I worked competently with people across the social spectrum, including those who were much older than myself, with higher levels of education than myself, or with more wealth. Here, my one-to-one counseling skills were strengthened, since the more holistic milieu approaches had become unfashionable.

In this setting I confirmed my earlier hospital experiences that indicated that interactions and interventions carried out by different nurses had a different impact on some patients. This does not mean that one nurse's nursing is necessarily better than another's, but that the personality, life experiences and subtleties within an individual nurse are unique and have different effects on each unique patient's efforts to come to grips with and deal with their circumstances.

The third and last significant position regarding my practice development was that of a community psychiatric nurse in provincial New South Wales. At one level, this was most like the work in the original training hospital in that it was incredibly diverse and we had to become mental health service Jills- (and Jacks) of-all-trades, as there were very few experts at hand and no psychiatrist was attached to the adult team. In this setting I was able to work intensely with a range of people over a short or medium length time frame. Again, I participated in clients' internal struggles and learned from them what actions, inaction, questions, responses or types of silence enabled them to find their own healing steps to take them forward as people able to activate something more constructive in their lives.

It was incredibly broadening at both the ideas and practice level, because the center took community health seriously and I had to teach myself about health, wellness, community work, secondary prevention, health education and family therapy. Each member of the multidisciplinary team, as counselors and case managers, had a high level of independence regarding the way we worked with clients, but we had the opportunity to discuss complex clinical issues with peers from different disciplines at weekly 'case' meetings.

Most of the clients I worked with were self-referred, some came from general medical practitioners and a minority from psychiatrists with whom I had built up a professional relationship. During this time, I tried to work with persons on their difficulties, and I did not think, plan, work or write in terms of psychiatric diagnoses. The theme that slowly emerged across a range of these adult clients was that of abuse—mostly child abuse. This lead to my awareness of child abuse, sexual assault and neglect as common precursors to adult mental illness, emotional distress and/or relationship problems.

Two theoretical postgraduate degrees emerged directly out of my experience as a clinician. The first was most obviously inspired by my work in community health. After I became an academic in the mid-1980s I took a master's degree in which I developed a multi-factorial and multi-level theory about why some men in our society perpetrate violence against their partner. The question I asked myself was: why do some men hurt, damage and at times eventually kill a woman whom they claim to love? From my perspective, this was important since the great majority of published literature about this type of violence within the family at that time focused on the victims. It seemed to me that focusing on the targets of the violence could offer no insight into the causes of the violence, or strategies to prevent it from becoming even more prevalent. The work was published as *The presence of the past. Male violence in the family* in 1991 and was reprinted in 1994 because a Canadian university ordered a large number of copies, presumably as a prescribed text in a course.

In the early 1990s I worked on a PhD and attempted to answer the question that emerged for me at various times during the 1970s and 1980s: why was psychiatric treatment unhelpful and at times damaging to people it claimed to have the specialist expertise to treat? To answer this question, I explored the history of European psychiatry, drew on concepts from the history and philosophy of science, utilized unconscious defense mechanisms as tools for analysis of psychiatric texts and considered feminist critiques of psychiatry, psychoanalysis and psychology. The work focused on depression and used sociological ideas to critique mainstream psychiatry and psychology for claiming to explain the psychiatrically disturbed individuals in isolation from their interpersonal relationships, gender, culture and socioeconomic status. Some of the ideas from that exploration will emerge in the present work.

Cynthia Stuhlmiller

When I was growing up in Hamburg, New York, one of our neighbors behaved in a most bizarre way, chanting out the window and sometimes becoming so violently upset that she was taken to the psychiatric hospital for long periods of time. I became quite fascinated and curious, spending hours trying to decipher her chants and spying to figure out what was going on. We were given the explanation that she was 'sick in the head,' told she was harmless, but to give her respect and stay away.

As a serious child, I often found myself feeling bad and taking sides with the underdog in any situation. Through music, sports, odd jobs, school, and other activities, I developed confidence and a generally optimistic outlook on life. By the time I entered college, I had many interests and selecting a major meant narrowing my focus. I held out as long as possible. I had volunteered as a Red Cross Candy Striper, visiting patients and replenishing bedside water jugs. I had also worked in a nursing home, attending to the lonely, depressed and confused, bringing my youthful enthusiasm and cheer, while providing hygiene and comfort measures. Even now, I look back at that work as some of the most important and rewarding of my life.

The connection between biology and psychology became illuminated in nursing school when I observed pituitary gland surgery being conducted under hypnosis, without any other form of anaesthesia. From that moment on, I had an enduring respect for the power of the mind and positive attitudes as well as the ability of the human psyche to mediate physiology.

As a new graduate nurse in charge of a medical surgical ward, I became concerned about the large numbers of patients who became isolated and disturbed following invasive surgical procedures. Many of these patients were older and after several days of restricted bed rest, few visitors, and only the brief interactions with medical staff, became agitated, disoriented, and even hallucinated as a result of sensory deprivation combined with the lingering effects of general anaesthesia. With limited opportunity to interact owing to demands of other high acuity patients, I would call for a psychiatric consultation, saying, 'I believe this person needs a chat and some extra support.' The typical consultant response was, 'Give them a Valium®, I'll check in with them tomorrow.' With the arrival of tomorrow, the person would surely be less anxious due to the medication, but more often sedated and thus no longer a staff 'management' problem. The opportunity to address the person's real concerns had been lost.

It was baffling to see the pride staff took in the physiological success of their procedures, while the outcomes were often socially and psychologically devastating to the patient. Yes, their bodies may have been patched up perfectly, but 'so what' for the person who didn't want to live or had overwhelming angst about how they were going to manage with their new condition. With these concerns, I entered graduate school in 1978 at Russell Sage College in Troy, New York to study for my master's degree in psychiatric/mental health nursing so that I could dedicate time to these ignored and unexplored areas of health.

During the course of graduate school, I studied interpersonal mental health nursing and read the works of Peplau (1952), Sullivan, Arieti, Laing, Goffman, Szasz, Freud and others. I worked in several different psychiatric facilities, including a one-year placement at the Veterans Administration Hospital, New York. Among other things, I ran group sessions with veterans in the day treatment center. In listening to stories of war, I noticed a marked difference between Korean, World War II, and Vietnam veterans as they recounted their experiences. For example, World War II veterans described their participation in war as a source of pride, joy and camaraderie—they had fought in a war that was strongly endorsed, valued and esteemed by society. Whereas for soldiers of Vietnam, shame and guilt prevailed— after all, they had lost the war. I came to realize the role of society in shaping people's interpretations of their experiences and the impact these interpretations had on the veterans' ability to live with and accept what, by civilian standards, would have been considered to be acts of inhumanity on a mass scale.

At the completion of graduate studies in 1981, I moved to Menlo Park, California to take a position as a clinical nurse specialist (CNC equivalent in Australia) for an in-patient treatment program that was being developed for Vietnam veterans. While waiting for the position to eventuate, I worked a short stint on a ward in which Ken Kesey had been a nursing assistant when he wrote *One flew over the cuckoo's nest*. Many of the same staff and patients were still there. It felt surreal to be involved in planning 'cutting edge' treatment for Vietnam veterans while working under the archaic conditions and mentality of yesteryear.

My work with the Vietnam veterans program spanned more than a decade. As a founding staff member, I had freedom to develop and test a variety of strategies and approaches. Overall, the program was based on the principles of a therapeutic community where all staff and patients took part in day-to-day decision making and activities. With a young and energetic staff and patient population and few rules or restrictions on program development or patient length of stay, we operated as a close-knit group that worked and played together. Fond memories include camping expeditions, treetop challenge courses, ski trips, invitations to Washington, DC and the White House to show off our choral group, as well as the ongoing treatment groups of Vietnam focus, cognitive therapy, creative expression, anger management, substance abuse, parenting, and art therapy. Because of the unpopularity of the Vietnam War, the rejection of the returning soldiers and the subsequent prevalence of mental health problems and suicide, this program quickly became a sociopolitical icon for absolution of national guilt. By the time I resigned in 1992, the program had grown to 120 beds and was awarded the distinction of National Center for Post-Traumatic Stress Disorder.

The 1980s were an exciting time in America to be a mental health nurse working with people exposed to extreme stress situations. With the Vietnam veterans gaining recognition for their plight, the diagnosis of post-traumatic stress disorder came out in the 1981 *Diagnostic and Statistical Manual of Mental Disorders*—the official book of psychiatric classifications. This new diagnosis drew together a variety of clinicians, researchers and theoreticians from around the world in their effort to help populations affected by war, disaster, mass murder, and other catastrophic events. The diagnosis quickly became widely used because of global communication, and offered a means to formalize and legitimize suffering that had long been unacknowledged. At the time, I thought this might be an important step toward healing.

With an interest in learning more about stressful collective events and their psychological impact on people, I became involved in volunteer work for the American Red Cross Disaster Action Team. I also began doctoral studies at the University of California, San Francisco (UCSF), School of Nursing, to pursue formal investigation of disaster response. As a condition for entry into the doctoral program, community service was required. I volunteered for one year in a program called Soteria House, a residential treatment center for people with schizophrenia. The treatment consisted entirely of person-to-person interaction based on acceptance, respect, tolerance, commitment, and a positive expectation of recovery. No medications were used or hierarchical structures imposed. I have been witness to many occasions of improvement and recovery.

During my study at UCSF, I became interested in the work of Arron Antonovsky who, like me, was interested in studying how people managed to stay well despite horrific circumstances. Coursework with Richard Lazarus, known as the grandfather of stress and coping research, provided a framework for my investigations. Of the nursing faculty, Susan Gortner and Afaf Meleis helped consolidate my thinking about the importance of the philosophy of science and the development of nursing theory. Patricia Benner (see Benner, 1984), my research supervisor, not only taught me the value and significance of capturing people's lived experience, but instilled in me a deep pride and appreciation of what it is to be a nurse.

My study of the rescue workers following the 1989 San Francisco Loma Prieta earthquake (Stuhlmiller, 1992) began my critique of the effects of psychiatric diagnosis in defining the life experiences of others. I became increasingly annoyed by the growing popularity of the methods of professionals who rushed in to define experiences as 'traumatic,' prescribing counseling rather than applying a humanistic perspective that would respect and foster people's own restorative capabilities.

Following my doctoral studies, I taught clinical nursing at the University of San Franciso. While taking students to both public and private health care facilities, I noticed the role that economics plays in mental health care. In the USA, if one has money, a diagnosis of multiple personality can result in private therapy with the utmost empathy. If one is without private insurance and experiences similar distress, a diagnosis of schizophrenia will result in a quick discharge to the streets with a bag of tranquilizers.

In 1993, I received a Fulbright award to teach and conduct research in Tromsø, Norway. There, I gained a further appreciation of culture and its impact on mental health as I discovered ways of interpreting experiences that, in America, would have been considered to be a disorder but, to Norwegians, were just a fact of life. This experience further galvanized my concerns about medicalization and the effect it has on a person's sense of self. Living in Tromsø gave me an insight into a rich local philosophical view of nature and people that stands in sharp contrast to the American attitudes of conquering nature, reverence for technology and belief in the 'quick fix.'

With this background of experiences, I bring to this book a strong perspective on the power of connection (nursing home and medical surgical experiences), the power of body and mind (hypnosis), the power of creating meaning (Vietnam and disaster work), the power of positive expectations (Soteria House), the power of economics (work as a clinical instructor), and the power of culture (Norway and diagnostic labeling). My belief is that the nurse enlists these powers for the sake of returning them to the persons who have been cut off from them or have lost their way. My involvement in this book is in response to the erosion and marginalization of caring and connecting practices that I have witnessed over the course of my career. There can never be a replacement for human-to-human touch, involvement, concern, hope, comfort and understanding, and their powerful impact on health and healing. My words are an effort to keep alive this mission, and pass along pride in and recognition of the importance of nursing.

Simon Champ

Diagnosed with schizophrenia in my early twenties, I became concerned with the injustice, stigma and neglect of people who experience a mental illness in our society. Since 1982 I have been involved in lobbying and education about mental health issues.

I was a founding member of the Schizophrenia Fellowship of NSW which was established in 1985. I served on the National Community Advisory Group on mental health, advising the Commonwealth government on mental health issues from 1993 to 1997. I was the inaugural chair of the Australian Mental Health Consumer Network, serving as chair from 1996 to 1998.

Currently I am a director of Sane Australia and represent the Australian Mental Health Consumer Network on the Mental Health Council of Australia. I am a frequent speaker on mental health issues at conferences and regional events in Australia. I have been involved in many education projects that have included working with high school students, doctors, nurses, police officers, and many other groups who want to learn more about mental health issues.

I have done much work with the media and starred in Anne Deveson's 1991 documentary *Spinning out*. Most recently, I have been included in an anthology of consumer writings entitled *From the ashes of experience. Reflections on madness, survival and growth*, edited by Phil Barker, Peter Campbell and Ben Davidson.

I have a degree and postgraduate qualifications in fine art from Sydney College of the Arts, Sydney University, where I trained in painting. My interest in creativity and spirituality helps balance my life as a mental health consumer activist.

Living with schizophrenia has changed my life in many ways. The form of schizophrenia that I have seems to recur often. Until this last 18 months, even with constant compliance with medications, I had never been in remission for longer than 10 months. In periods of remission I often reflect on the experience of psychosis and remission, trying to integrate them into my life and find meaning in the experience.

Writing, keeping diaries and making art have been a valuable means to help me draw meaning from the experience of having mental illness. Sharing my writing and art with others can sometimes help others better understand issues for those with a mental illness. It also politicizes the personal—in representing my reality as an artist and writer with a psychiatric disability I try to give voice to personal realities that are often misrepresented or stereotyped by other groups in society who talk about people who, like me, have a psychiatric disability. Traditionally, mental health consumers have been talked about, our realities and lives described for us, our own voices suppressed, turned into case studies or ignored in the interest of the dominant paradigm. As people who have experienced a mental illness, part of our struggle for human rights is our right to represent our concerns in forums and debates. An extension of that is the hope that the education of mental health professionals will include consumer insights and lived experience presented by consumers themselves.

It was interesting to be asked to contribute to a nursing textbook, for it is in this form that traditionally much of the 'colonization' of consumer experience and expression has occurred. I do not use the language and forms of nursing texts or academia and it was a challenge to see how my work could be integrated into the whole text. That, perhaps, is the problem for people who experience mental illness—trying to fit. Some of us are looking for alternative ways to maintain the authenticity of our voices.

Aims of this textbook

The aims of this textbook are:
- to present more information than is usual, from specific consumer perspectives
- to help diminish nurse stereotyping of consumers by psychiatric diagnosis
- to alert students to some ethical dilemmas in mental health service provision
- to raise awareness about consumer rights and human rights
- to remind readers that consumers and nurses are people with a common humanity
- to explore the person and behaviors of the nurse, as well as those of the consumer
- to improve understandings of interactions that create consumer and nurse distress
- to introduce undergraduate students to mental health nursing practice principles
- to focus on what nurses can do
- to encourage student interest in the workings of human societies
- to highlight some issues regarding contemporary mental illness and health
- to assist in developing a greater understanding of distressed behavior in order to increase the likelihood of compassionate nursing care.

Some final comments about the book

Because we did not intend to write a lengthy textbook, some issues have been omitted, covered briefly or discussed only once. One strategy that we used to reduce repetition was to emphasize certain nursing strategies, consumer experiences, factors or issues in one chapter that are also relevant in at least one more of the clinically focused chapters. The following topics are important and are woven through the lives of many people with a mental illness; these issues require nursing awareness, understanding, consideration and appropriate actions.

- Child abuse or neglect constitute traumatic experiences that increase vulnerability.
- Consumer self-esteem should be maintained or enhanced.
- Ethnicity and cultural factors permeate nurses' and consumers' lives.
- Financial factors are significant in relation to many people's survival.
- Holistic nursing assessment is the foundation for effective nursing care.
- Holistic safety is central to a nurse's duty of care.
- Hope.
- Making a personal connection with the patient.
- Negative labeling or stereotyping of consumers is always unhelpful.
- Seeking meaning with the consumer in distress and psychosis.
- Substance abuse is often a concomitant of a mental illness.
- Therapeutic milieu.
- Unconscious defense mechanisms.

We acknowledge the diverse needs of undergraduate students and hope that this book will be helpful to different readers in different ways. Individuals may well find that certain sections become more meaningful in the light of specific clinical experiences, therefore we would like to think that some RNs will read the book during their early months and years of practice in mental health settings.

References

American Psychiatric Association, 1994, *Diagnostic and statistical manual of mental disorders (DSM-IV)*. APA, Washington.

Australian Bureau of Statistics, 1998, *Mental health and well-being profile of adults. Australia 1997*. AGPS, Canberra.

Barker, P., Campbell, P. & Davidson, B. (eds)., 1999, *From the ashes of experience. Reflections on madness, survival and growth*. Whurr, London.

Benner, P., 1984, *From novice to expert. Excellence and power in clinical nursing practice*. Addison-Wesley, Menlo Park, Calif.

Horsfall, J., 1991, *The presence of the past. Male violence in the family*. Allen & Unwin, Sydney, Australia.

Kesey, K. 1962, *One flew over the cuckoo's nest*. Viking, New York.

Laing, R. D. & Esterton, A., 1964, *Sanity, madness and the family*. Tavistock, London.

Mitchell, G. (ed.), 1979, *A new dictionary of sociology*. Routledge & Kegan Paul, London.

Peplau, H.,1952, *Interpersonal relations in nursing*. G. P. Putnam's Sons, New York.

Stuhlmiller, C.. 1992, An interpretive study of appraisal and coping of rescue workers in an earthquake disaster. The Cypress collapse. *Dissertation Abstracts International*, 52, 09B p. 4671. (University Microfilms No. 9205240.)

2

Student/nurse self-awareness and therapeutic interaction

Key concepts
in this
chapter:

■ advocacy ■ assertiveness ■ caring
■ consumer personhood ■ empathy
■ ethical mental health nursing practice
■ facilitative/therapeutic communication
■ hope ■ human rights ■ listening
■ reflection on mental health nursing
practice ■ therapeutic use of self

Introduction

This chapter focuses on therapeutic communication, empathy, assertiveness and advocacy, since these are the foundations of ethical mental health nursing practice. To support healing in others, it is necessary for students and RNs to explore attitudes, feelings and behaviors. This is because the capacity to communicate facilitatively, use self, and develop therapeutic relationships with consumers depends on who you are, your attitudes, personality and how you behave. Consequently, your cultural background, age, sex and life experience—your whole self—contribute to your ability to communicate effectively and develop an effective professional relationship with consumers of mental health services.

The importance of reflection in mental health nursing practice

Literature on reflective mental health nursing practice emerged in the early 1980s, particularly from educators exploring their assumptions about learning, teaching and knowledge in connection with what they did in the classroom. By the late 1980s nurse educators were writing about reflecting on their practice; and clinical teachers and nurse academics were preparing students for reflecting on practice during student clinical practicum and as practitioners thereafter. Reflective practice aims to encourage professional and personal development at a pace and depth appropriate to the individual and to lessen the theory–practice gap.

Reflection is:

> The process of internally examining and exploring an issue of concern, triggered by an experience, which creates and clarifies meaning in terms of self, and which results in a changed conceptual perspective (Boyd & Fales cited in Palmer et al., 1994: 13).

The aims of reflective practice are to learn from clinical experience, direct one's own learning, explore successful and unsuccessful nursing actions, view an event from different perspectives, name and analyze feelings and thoughts during the event, and to improve practice as a result of these processes (Palmer et al. 1994).

Reflective questions

Explore the following questions.

- Does your family reflect the mainstream, or a minority, culture?
- How do you think your cultural background influences your attitude to others?
- At your school, were some children recipients of ethnicity-based comments?
- In your university course, are (or were) there students who are physically isolated?

Discuss these questions with a friend; ask other nursing students. What are your feelings about these experiences now? What consequences might some answers have for your ability to provide high-quality care to all patients?

Facilitative communication skills for mental health nurses

Virtually all mental health nursing texts investigate communication skills, since they are the foundations for 'what nurses do' in mental health and other specialties. When communication strategies are outlined, to some eyes they look simple, like common sense—something that anybody could do. As is often the case, looks are deceiving. Communicating effectively is not always easy, because in the clinical setting you are required to put these skills into practice on the run. Some communication skills will be comparatively easy because you have been using them for much of your life already; others will be very challenging because your family has (unconsciously) not enabled you to use them and/or they are a bit scary, because you cannot predict what reply you will get. If they were as simple as they appear to be, our society would probably not need mental health nurses, counselors, psychologists, or any other psychotherapists.

The following are 12 fundamental facilitative communication skills.

1. *Active listening* requires you to offer your undivided attention to another person. To do this, you must ignore your personal concerns at that time. Listening involves absorbing an overall picture of what the speaker is saying and recognizing the feelings that are expressed directly and indirectly. Active listening also means controlling your urge to interrupt as well as conveying your intent to understand the essence of the person's message.
2. *Clarifying* what the other person has said involves asking questions to determine the gist of the message or facts the person is trying to convey.
3. *Paraphrasing* is re-stating key points made by the person. You should do this in your own words, but ensure that what you say is clear and recognizably close enough to the meaning that has been conveyed.
4. *Checking perceptions* involves asking whether an assumption you have made, or a conclusion you have drawn, fits with the other person's view.

Listening, clarifying, paraphrasing and checking perceptions all fit into a cluster of therapeutic communication strategies that are underpinned by emotionally supportive inquiry into aspects of the consumer's world. These actions involve finding out from the consumer what is happening to them. The two broad aims for these and the following skills are to establish rapport and gain information from the consumer for ongoing assessment purposes, so that you have a common ground on which to begin building a therapeutic relationship.

Active exercise

Being listened to can be a special and useful experience. If you are a listener already, then you will be aware that your listening can affect the behavior and viewpoint of the person you listen to.

When you are next on a bus, talking to a neighbor or having lunch with another student, listen to this one person for five minutes without doing anything more than encouraging them to go on.

- Did you notice anything about the speaker, their response or how they spoke?
- What were the differences between listening and a normal conversation?

Tune into a conversation that you have today and notice what you are doing when you are *not* listening to the speaker.

- What were you thinking or doing?
- How do you normally excuse yourself from listening to another person? What could you say to yourself to justify not listening?

Watch someone who is in conversation with you tomorrow and work out if they are listening to the subtleties of what you are saying. How do you know that the person did not really want to hear about the details of what you were saying?

The second cluster of therapeutic communication strategies involves you sending some of your understandings back to the speaker.

5. *Reflecting conversation content* involves sending back to the speaker enough detail about what they said to show that you have understood.

6. *Reflecting feelings* involves naming feelings that the speaker has revealed. This should not be done too early. If you name the wrong feeling it jolts the dialogue and you have to reconnect at a supportive level.
7. *Using silence* involves staying with the silence and the person, and not filling the space because of your own anxiety. Staying with silence allows the speaker to feel attended to. Silence gives the person the chance to sort out words and gives you time to think about what you are doing, too.

This third cluster of facilitative communication skills is less exploratory, less tentative and a bit more confronting. The skills involve you taking more of a lead and declaring your considered understanding of the conversation. Consequently, sensitive confidence is required.

8. *Pinpointing* is verbalizing what you have noticed or heard that the person may not have openly stated; for example, 'Given the brief comment you made about your partner's views, it seems that you may not see eye-to-eye on this.'
9. *Confronting* at the information level is addressing inconsistencies between what the person says and what the facts appear to be. At the interpretive level, confronting is commenting on an observed but unexpressed feeling; for example, the person may look uncomfortable, but has not said anything about it.
10. *Interpersonal feedback* involves providing clear information about your own response to the person's behavior, or other people's responses that you have noticed when the person behaves in a specific way.

The following two therapeutic communication skills emerge from complex cognitive and emotional syntheses that serve to pull an interaction with a consumer together, or to set out an agreed-upon understanding for the purpose of collaboratively moving on to some different issues.

11. *Linking* is the nurse's uncovering of connections between consumer events and feelings, or behaviors and consequences. This joining together of experience and reaction helps the consumer make more sense of what has happened to them.

12. *Summarizing* is pulling together main points, insights or agreements that emerged in conversation. This shows what you have achieved together.

These 12 therapeutic communication strategies are the fundamental communication interventions used by RNs in mental health and other settings. Most mental health nursing texts outline these beginning counselling skills (see, for example, Kneisl, 1996, McDonald, 1996, Stuart, 1998). These communication strategies are often difficult to separate; and they overlap considerably in practice. Some RNs expert in mental health may not use these words to describe what they do, but are likely to draw on most, if not all, of the strategies.

Facilitative communication skills form the foundations of negotiation and counseling. Some 'do nots' can be added to these: do not speak for others; do not tell anyone how they feel; do not tell anyone how they should feel; do not tell someone what you think their problem is; do not assume something is true about the person until you have asked; do not give advice. Some reinforcing 'do's' include: listen; show an interest in the person and what they are saying; assume that the speaker is knowledgeable about herself or himself; deal with what is important to the consumer; understand that emotional healing is a complex process, not simple information or logic. The development of advanced counseling skills often involves further education, including supervision, training, reflection, reading, conceptualizing, peer discussion and/or courses.

The importance of processing our own emotions

Processing our own emotions makes working with others' emotions possible. To draw on and improve the skills discussed above, you use emotional, creative, spiritual, intellectual and social aspects of your personality. This is what makes mental health nursing flexible and transportable on the one hand, and personally rewarding or confronting on the other.

One aim of mental health nursing is to *be with* people who are panicking, miserable or afraid. As with facilitative communication skills, being with someone sounds easy. Don't we do this at home, at university, in sports, when we're out having fun? Yes, we are in the ordinary sense of those words. When we expect an RN in a mental health setting to be with a consumer, we mean to be with them emotionally, to concentrate on them and their concerns, to throw a human lifeline at times of fear, despair or relief.

Simon Champ: consumer story and reflection

Spaces

Just as music is made of silence as well as sound, the spaces between notes are as important as the notes themselves, fine nursing is a balance between action and non-action.

The spaces between interventions with a consumer may be as important to healing as your presence as a nurse. Healing takes time and, particularly when it is the mind that is in transition, space to allow change to unfold is essential.

There is a pressure in our society to do, to be seen to be active. To turn the beds, organize the patient, get out and about. Nurses often seem uncomfortable with silence and simply really being with someone. It is one of the skills that must be the hardest to teach, to help nurses learn how to be fully with someone. With them in their grief, with them in their anger or loneliness or even their joy. To listen to the message of another's reality even when it is unspoken. To learn about those spaces in another that cannot always be conveyed in words, that perhaps do not arise in conversation but only become apparent in silence and with time.

So often nurses rush to fill spaces and silence, forgetting that their very presence may be speaking a language of its own. So often nurses' conversation can be a distraction from confronting the reality of a consumer's life, if the nurse is personally uncomfortable with what the consumer is really experiencing.

To understand what it is to be present, to really be with a person is not easy but consumers, especially if they are experiencing a psychosis, will soon tell if you are not really present in an interaction with them. Even as we speak with someone our voice can betray our mind drifting to other concerns. Even with the camouflage of words, the nurse's eyes will reflect a distance between them and a consumer, as their mind is distracted. Yes it is the being with a person that is so essential to good nursing but so hard to teach, for so much of that skill is with the unspoken and non-action.

Acceptance of the person and their feelings is an essential aspect of being with a consumer in the mental health sense (Peplau, 1989). You are unable to be emotionally supportive of another person, if you are wishing (or telling them) that they should stop crying, that they must speak, that things aren't so bad. If we are more concerned about our own fears, then we will not be able to be with a highly distressed person in a therapeutically caring way. There is a connection between our ability to accept someone else's emotional disturbance and our capacity to accept ourselves and our own distress. To provide a basic level of psychic safety and security for consumers, we need a sense of security within ourselves (Walsh, 1994). This is not an entirely teachable skill, as its development requires a commitment to ongoing personal exploration and emotional development.

Reflective questions

Useful reflective questions to ask yourself on clinical practicum include: What role should I have taken up? What role did I assume? Did I feel comfortable? What did I do? What did others do? Did anything improve for the patient or for me? Did I learn anything new and useful? (Palmer et al., 1994). Other questions that may reach deeper levels of reflection include: Did my attitude or expectations affect the situation? Were my nursing actions thought through beforehand or did I just react? Did I draw on any theoretical assumptions? Were there ethical consequences of my actions or inaction? Are there organizational issues involved in this situation?

Remember the last time you were with someone who was upset and crying. Did you

■ Say that they would be alright?
■ Try to perk them up by telling a funny story?
■ Think that there was something seriously wrong with the person?
■ Tell them about something worse that happened to you?
■ Leave the room or go out as quickly as you could?
■ Say that crying never got anyone anywhere?

—continued

—continued

Think about your main response and those listed above. Ask yourself

- Would any of those responses help the person deal with his or her distress?
- Were your actions motivated by your needs, or those of the person crying?

Mental health nursing, more than other specialties, increases your exposure to people in distress. One main challenge to nurses in all settings is to manage anxiety, which is commonplace in human interactions. It is essential to develop the ability to bear our own and other people's anxiety. Peplau (1989) considers that recognizing anxiety, naming anxiety and connecting anxiety to experience is one of the major issues for most consumers of mental health services. She also explains that if the nurse does not own and manage her or his own anxiety, the consumer is likely to tune into the nurse's anxiety, which impedes the consumer's progress.

In mental health settings, nurses have to bear their own and others' sadness. Living in contemporary society inevitably involves emotional loss, ensuing grief and doing something to relieve the pain. Provided that the nurse has not been prevented from grieving for complex family or social reasons, then recovery from a death or separation is highly likely to enhance emotional growth in the long term. Our own experience and resolution of loss and grief may provide us with inner knowledge relevant to other people's grief. If we have not processed our feelings of distress, then other people's loss and misery is likely to be unbearable. In that case we will be unable to be with the people who are sad or depressed in supportive and helpful ways.

Reflective questions

Sometimes a situation in the clinical setting can bring to mind surprising memories from the past. These feelings are often associated with loss or pain experienced by the student earlier in life. Alicia, an undergraduate nursing student, was not behaving in a satisfactory manner in her clinical placement, and it seemed that something was wrong. On speaking with Alicia, the clinical teacher found that she was distressed by working with people with a developmental disability. Alicia felt resentful about the fact that the disabled residents were alive but her own father was not, as he had died suddenly of an illness when she was young.

Consider the following questions.

- Have you experienced the death of a close family member? What after-effects remain from that loss?
- Are there secrets in your family that affect you and your siblings?
- Do you have any connection with a person who suffers from an addiction? How has that person's behaviors affected your life?
- Are you closely associated with a person who has a long-term mental illness? Does this color your view of consumers, mental health nurses or psychiatrists?

These are common experiences within families. It is likely that major family events will have consequences for all members, but these are most significant for people intending to work in the health or welfare sectors.

Keeping a journal

If anything emotionally significant has happened in your family, you could keep a private journal and write about the events, what went wrong for you then and what feelings you have now about the event(s) and the people involved. What coping mechanisms did you use to 'get through' that period in your life? This is one way of

—continued

—continued

beginning to process painful experiences, to help slowly free yourself from unresolved losses that may affect inter-actions with others at the present time.

When you feel motivated, buy an exercise book specif-ically to keep as a journal for reflective practice. A common sense way of setting out the journal is to use the left-hand side to describe the event, interactions or practice issue you wish to explore; and the right-hand pages for reflection on and analysis of emotions and thoughts arising from that situation. It is better to write up the journal on the day the issue arises and it is helpful to write as much actual conversational dialogue as possible (Palmer et al., 1994). Balance positive and negative entries, although the latter may produce more potential for practice change potential.

You could document a clinical event that is important, strong feelings you have about a patient, any nagging doubts you have about an interaction. You can reflect on these as you write them down, and later on. To analyze the events you could, for example, consider whether the person reminded you of someone else; if the emotion is related to events in your private life; whether you identi-fied with, felt repelled by, or had some other gut reaction to the consumer.

Another important aspect of human experience that nurses in mental health need to be able to face and deal with is conflict between people and conflict within oneself. Often in classrooms students say that conflict in families is 'bad.' Con-flict in families and other groups is inevitable, and perhaps the absence of conflict could be considered more worrying and unhealthy.

In general, people learn about conflict within their families. If your family was silent about disagreements, then you may have difficulty naming the problem through lack of role models and experience. If a parent used verbal or emotional violence to cover over conflict or to stop some family members from having their views heard and their needs met, then you too are likely to have difficulty facing conflict because you may be afraid that it will end in violence and remain unresolved. Another classical way of not dealing constructively with conflict is for one parent to be aggressive about the matter. The other parent, out of intimidation or lack of support or resources, remains silent and 'gives in' to the dominator whose conduct is invariably selfish and immature. In contemporary society, another major method for conflict avoidance is that one or both parents use alcohol (or other drugs), possibly culminating in an absence from the household, violence, or 'sleeping it off.' All of these patterns involve not dealing with the conflict or the issues at the heart of it; and they set the stage for further conflict, resentment, or other more damaging behaviors.

Facing conflict and working through it is not common in our society. That is why mediation between warring nations is required; and within nations there are bodies to arbitrate on legal or industrial matters between neighbors, competing businesses, unions and employers, aggrieved employees, or within families.

The first action to be taken in relation to conflict is to be able to acknowledge that there are different needs, viewpoints and interests. If neither party denies this, then you are off to a good start. If we are interested in having a satisfying life and do not want to attempt to avoid conflict by resorting to aggression, passivity or alcohol, then we will have to practice managing conflict with our friends, partners, classmates, teachers, and so on. Constructive strategies that emerge from these experiences will be helpful for nursing in mental health: you may learn what not to do, for a start!

An overall requirement in mental health nursing is to explore your own emotional history, especially with regard to significant events in your life. An honest appraisal of your own strengths and limitations is helpful for both you and consumers. Lindow (1993: 27) characterizes the most helpful psychiatric ward that she was ever in in the following way: 'The staff do not have all the answers . . . The patient is just as likely . . . to find a solution to one of the problems.'

Facilitative communication and therapeutic relationships depend on your ability to balance a healthy acceptance of self with the professional responsibility for personal development by working through issues involving your own anxiety, depression and aggression, to enable you to work with consumers in safe and competent ways. Self acceptance and ego management are necessary processes. This means that you accept your age, culture, personality and development as they are, without putting yourself down for not being an 'expert.' The nurse in mental health needs to develop a balance between self-confidence and humility in the face of other people's pain and experiences. Because mental health nurses work with people in extreme states of distress, none of us have the 'answers' to consumers' difficulties (Arthur, 1999). It is more important for nurses to ask a few focused questions of consumers in a non-interrogatory way and attend closely to their responses (Wadsworth & Epstein, 1997). Facilitative communication involves offering minimal advice to people, even when you are asked. In the mental health setting, generally it is more appropriate to listen, support and inform consumers, rather than advise.

Sex, gender and sexuality are an aspect of daily interactions. Every student or new RN has something unique to offer consumers. Your uniqueness arises in part from your personal background, and includes your cultural heritage, understandings you have gained from life experience and ways you manage gender, sex differences and sexual orientation.

Just as sex is one of the most recognizable aspects of a baby at birth, so sex in later life is often the most important thing about you from many people's perspective, whether you think that this should be so or not. Sex is to do with being male or female. Gender is associated with social and cultural norms and expectations that are superimposed on the more straightforward aspects of being male or female. Loring and Powell (1988) have shown that even experienced clinicians alter psychiatric diagnoses on the grounds of sex or ethnicity. This is an example of stereotyping others on the basis of one's own personal beliefs about men, women, or certain ethnic groups. Sex and gender relations will feed into every consumer's experience of treatment in a mental health setting and most likely into their expectations of you as a nurse.

Discussion questions

Hardly anybody says they hold sexist views these days, so to truthfully explore our own stereotypes about men and women requires some hard work.

Discuss the following in same-sex pairs in a nursing tutorial session.

- What are the 'manly' men you know like?
- What are the 'womanly' women you know like?

Discuss the same questions shortly afterwards in mixed-sex pairs in a nursing tutorial.

- Did you notice yourself saying or doing anything differently this time?
- Do you think the other person would have said what they said in exactly the same way to the same-sex partner?

Discuss the following questions in a larger group.

- Why do you think so many women want to be nurses?
- Why do you think that so few men want to be nurses?
- What do these answers tell you about your expectations of women?
- What do these answers tell you about your expectations of men?
- What do they indicate about your view of nurses and nursing?

Therapeutic use of self

The easiest therapeutic use a nurse can make of self is to *represent reality*. Experienced mental health professionals may forget the significance of this (Champ, 1998) but many consumers are hospitalized precisely because a psychiatrist deems that their sense of reality is disturbed. Theoreticians may discuss the concept of reality and question its existence; however, when working with people experiencing a psychosis, it is vital that the daily activities we consider 'normal' are reinforced. Interacting with consumers to involve them in an ongoing awareness of the wider world is important. These processes include orienting the consumer to your name, status, intentions and role. Nurses should encourage or assist the person with some of the rituals that structure our days, such as eating meals, having a tea or coffee, maintaining a basic level of hygiene, wearing clothes. It is helpful to talk about ordinary events happening outside the unit, such as news, sports, music, or specific subjects related to the consumer's interests, or your own (Heller 1996).

A primary aim of the therapeutic use of self is to *connect with the consumer* in a range of ways, from ordinary conversation, through routine organization-driven tasks (such as filling in forms or taking the person from A to B), to intimate and intense consumer-focused explorations. Nursing efforts to develop rapport and trust involve an investment of time, and repeated contact is valued by the consumer (Rogers et al., 1993). To develop rapport and trust, you have to reach out to the person. Mostly in ordinary social interaction, if one person reaches out, we expect the other to respond. In a mental health setting you are not reaching out primarily so that the other person will respond to you, but in order to make therapeutic contact because the other person is having difficulties.

If the consumer cannot respond to your efforts, or responds negatively to your attempts, *this is not due to your failure as a person, a student, or as a nurse.* It is probably due to the consumer's inner turmoil or distractions. Do not take consumer non-response or rejection personally. You will need to try again later.

Because each consumer is unique, it will be helpful if you can *develop a range of interacting possibilities*. This means trying to say the same thing in a range of ways. It means being very quiet at times and being conversational and up-front at other times. On occasion, you will need to take charge of some intimate aspects of a person's daily living; in other situations, you will need to step back and patiently encourage a consumer, who is slow and having trouble concentrating, to do the same things for herself or himself. The broader your repertoire of ways to talk, behave and negotiate, the more chances you have to effectively connect with different consumers. Because of ongoing but interrupted interactions with consumers, nurses have to manage a range of relationships in the clinical setting: therapeutic, formal, brief, neighborly, fun, casual, intense. Making the transition from the level of intense emotional sharing to ordinary casual greetings can be challenging for nurses (cf. Barker et al., 1999).

One way of considering how to extend different aspects of yourself to broaden your communicative repertoire is to use a

Jungian framework. Jung (1978) considers that there are four major activities of the mind that are relevant to communication style, problem solving, decision making, dealing with conflict and management of change; all of which are required in mental health nursing. These four domains are cognition (thinking), emotions (feelings), sensing (related to the five senses) and intuiting (having 'a hunch').

Keeping a journal

This exercise can be carried out by yourself in a journal or on a big sheet of paper. Late in the afternoon one day this week when you are not too tired or too busy, reflect on your day in the following ways.

- *What did I think today?*
- *What did I feel today?*
- *What did I see, touch, hear, smell, taste today?*
- *Did I have any memorable but unsure perceptions or feelings about someone or an interaction today?*

It is possible that you will write more down under one heading than another.

   Think about people that you find interesting, exciting, or are attracted to:

- *If you are a thinker, are other people's words and ideas exciting?*
- *If every day is a day full of feelings, are you attracted to others who feel a lot too?*
- *If you are a person of action and live through the body, do you find thinkers foreign or interesting?*
- *If you often feel sad, do you find people who are physically active uplifting?*
- *If your head is full of thoughts, are people with roller coaster emotions attractive?*

Among consumers in mental health settings, you will find thinkers, feelers, sensers and intuiters. If you develop your abilities in all of these domains you will have easier access to a broader range of people over time.

Nursing in mental health also requires the gentle *art of being patient*. People who seek mental health services are just like us as people. However, the life difficulties associated with living with a mental illness are complex and for many consumers these have been long-term. Given consumer distress and the interpersonal difficulties that arise because of this, the use of therapeutic communication skills once or a few times over days or weeks will not fix things up. Because the consequences of living with a mental illness are often profound and interfere with many activities of daily living, we as nurses must teach ourselves to recognize small positive consumer changes. When little improvements are evident, it is important to let the consumer know (Yoder & Rode, 1990), as they are probably still experiencing inner turmoil and have a limited understanding of how their behavior appears to others. Patience and perseverance in the face of small gains are necessary mental health nursing talents.

Management of your self is not only about a balance of self-acceptance and self-challenge. At a more complex level, the personal capacity to feel, recognize and *allow other people's anxiety, depression and aggression to pass through you* is a powerful way of using self therapeutically. This involves using yourself as an emotionally aware person and staying with other people's tension, distress or pain. Ritter (1997: 20–21) describes this as *not* having an 'aim to mend, resolve or correct, but to hold in suspension opposing forces.' Such an emotional staying with the person allows tension to build inside them, which demands a release. Generally for students and new RNs, using this process is not appropriate when working with people in an actively psychotic state or with those who are vulnerable to self-harming actions.

Applying this emotional pressure aims to allow the consumer to talk about things that are bothering them, that in ordinary social circumstances they would withhold. These are the 'opposing forces' within a person: to behave in the usual self-suppressing way, or to take a risk and speak about what is troubling. It is this sort of self-censoring that is invariably related to people's anxiety disorders, depression and a multitude of relationship and life difficulties. This staying with the consumer's emotional processing begins with the straightforward skill of listening. The challenge to most nurses in these situations is to stop from rushing into the silence or the tension, to break it. Breaking the tension provides relief for you, but it does not help the other person to acknowledge their troubled feelings or thoughts. Supporting consumers through such difficult passages may assist them to uncover meaning in their experiences and trials. All people try at times to find meaning in life events and this can be particularly helpful for those whose world has been turned upside-down by mental illness.

The holding of the person's tension in suspension is likely to result in a deeper level of discussion. As this staying with the tension encourages consumer risk taking, it also involves you stepping into the unknown. Such *emotional risk taking* has to be sincere on your behalf. If you do not want to hear that the consumer hates her or his child, if you cannot bear information about sexual assault, if you are afraid that the consumer is afraid of killing himself or herself, then this is not a process for you, at this stage. Risk taking is a bit like making a home visit to an unknown person: you can never know what might emerge. This is the excitement of mental health nursing: you take one small interpersonal risk and another emotional risk may emerge. If you do not take the first step, the second with its healing potential will not occur. Often consumer 'secrets' are not major disclosures like those suggested above, but worries that any of us might have, about a disagreement with someone, a troubling thought or an uncomfortable feeling, which seems overwhelming when left inside, but ordinary and harmless enough when expressed and discussed in the open. But, nurses must be a little prepared for a range of possible consumer reactions to our own communication strategies (Romme, 1996).

Implicit and explicit messages to consumers

As we assess consumers, so they determine how safe they feel with us (Horsfall, 1993). Often this is by intuition, listening, watching and working out how they feel in interaction with us. *Congruence* is one mode of nurse behavior which is likely to be picked up by consumers. Basically, congruence means behaving in ways that fit with what you say. A second element of congruence is that your emotions match your words. At another level, congruence is part of role modeling acceptable behavior, effective communication and the appropriate expression of your personal opinions and feelings (Beech & Norman, 1995).

Finding out how *reliable* you are is an obvious way for consumers to ascertain how safe they feel with you. This non-verbal level of security is a foundational factor for trust and the initiation of a potentially therapeutic relationship. Being reliable relates to doing what you say you will, or re-negotiating arrangements caused by unpredictable events. It also means not making promises—preferably at all—that you may be unable to fulfill, due to unforeseeable events. Honesty is a vital aspect of your commitment to reliability and ethical practice. This means being honest both with yourself and the consumer. Thoughtful honesty sends a range of positive messages to consumers who may have perceived limited openness in some health professionals with whom they had interacted previously (Romme, 1996).

When you train yourself to be alert to small changes in animation, facial expression, speaking, ease of movement, interaction with others, or ability to attend to personal hygiene, you are *recognizing signs of improvement and, hence, of hope*. Champ (1998: 57) believes that 'people facing psychiatric disabilities can flower with hope. Hope is an essential ingredient for recovery.' A level of realistic expectation of improvement is fundamental because it is an unspoken ingredient of human life. Garrett (1998: 49) echoes this view: 'hope . . . is an essential imaginative ingredient in overcoming anorexia.' Hope is especially important for people diagnosed with a mental illness, as frequently they have been given explicit or implicit messages that they are not their 'usual' self any more and that the condition lasts forever. It is crucial that nursing students do not confuse unrealistic statements like 'there's always a light at the end of the tunnel' with the need for consumers to feel interest, interpersonal warmth and support (Melbourne Consumer Consultants' Group, 1997) to keep their inner sense of hope alive. Personal meaning and hope are likely to be connected.

It is unethical and unacceptable for health professionals to predict a 'life sentence' for a person by using a medical label that has negative connotations and is socially stigmatizing. This perpetuates the stereotyping of a person on the presumed grounds that all people with diagnosis X will display behaviors

A, B and C, with an inevitable outcome of Z. At the very least, the psychiatric diagnosis can be named and explained a little, and the person told that we do not fully understand these illnesses, that professionals and consumers can work together using a range of strategies over time to see what can be achieved, and that there is a range of drugs that may help. To undermine another person by saying or implying that their situation is without hope is inhumane and unprofessional.

Communicating caring is an important part of the messages you send to consumers. Consumers feel and value caring from nurses. Among 475 mental health service users who commented on the quality of nursing care in response to a questionnaire that was part of a research project, 59 per cent were satisfied or very satisfied—this being the highest percentage for any professional group. These respondents characterized good nursing practice as caring (Rogers et al., 1993). In another small-scale qualitative research project, Beech and Norman (1995) found that 'communicating caring' included the largest number of positive mental health consumer experiences; and its absince attracted the highest number of negative comments. Subcomponents of nurses' communication of caring include being available, listening and helping people examine their communication, offering support and encouragement (hope), and explaining nursing actions. According to this study, most examples of poor nursing involved consumers' observations that nurses did not respond helpfully to their worries, were insensitive to their feelings and preferred to gather in the office rather than talk with them (Beech & Norman 1995).

Finding the middle ground between rescuing and avoiding is very important in your interactions with consumers. Rescuing is jumping in to play the guardian angel or savior role. The message sent by the nurse to the consumer is: I know best, I can fix things for you and I can make it better. Rescuing is a bit like being too controlling. Ultimately, attempting to rescue a consumer is related to your needs, not their actual needs.

Avoidance tends to send the following messages to consumers: you are unworthy, I don't like you, I don't want to waste my time on you. This behavior also reveals something about the nurse: I don't know what to do, I'm scared, I haven't got the skills required to make contact with you. Avoidance sends negative messages to the consumer about the nurse, as it is experienced as indifference or hostility.

Reflective questions

Many nurses become nurses in order to help people and this is a worthy orientation. Society will always need people to help others. But, this desire to help can get out of balance.

Ask yourself these questions about your response to patients a on clinical practicum.

- Do you find yourself spending more time with some patients than others?
- If you do feel good when you are with them, what is it about them that does this?

Have you heard RNs talk about 'good patients,' those who are 'really nice' and those who are 'no trouble'? On your next clinical placement, talk with a 'good patient.'

- What sort of personality does the patient have?
- What is the patient's cultural background?
- What sex is the patient?

On another day during your next clinical placement, talk with a patient who is described as 'difficult', 'unmanageable' or 'a pain in the bum,' Ask yourself the same questions as above.

- What sort of patient would you call 'difficult'?
- Would you, less than consciously, avoid such a person on a busy day?

Consider how these responses affect your responsibility to do your best to provide good quality nursing care to all consumers, whether you like them or not. Is spending more time with some consumers related to the same sorts of things that encourage you to spend less with others? Do rescuing and avoidance have anything in common?

Some broad principles can be helpful for students and nurses new to mental health to prevent pitfalls such as those mentioned above. These principles include listening to consumers and keeping the well-being of the consumer in mind, both now and for the future. Observe yourself in case you spend too much time with, or you are trying extra hard to fix something up for, a consumer. Preserving the consumer's dignity and allowing her or him as much personal control as possible are also guidelines for relevant and ethically sound nursing care (Perkins & Repper, 1998). Individualized care is contingent on the cultural identification, sexual orientation and age of the consumer. Your own ethnicity, sex, age and values contribute to the possibility of providing compassionate and appropriate nursing care. It is vital to develop flexible communication skills, so that if you feel an interaction has gone too far in one direction, you can negotiate another pathway with the consumer to aim to re-balance it.

Complex mental health nursing skills: empathy and assertiveness

Kalisch (1973) defines empathy as 'the ability to enter into the life of another person, to accurately perceive his [sic] current feelings and their meaning.' This complex process involves drawing on your sense of humanity in the first instance; that is, knowing that people can experience a universal range of emotions. Empathy begins with putting your own needs and concerns aside and being open to the other person's perception of their inner experience.

It is crucial that the recognition of another's distress is an actual awareness, and not the projection of your own distress onto her or him. Empathy is not based on similarities between yourself and the client, or between your experience and theirs. That is more likely to lead to over-identification with the other person, which is never therapeutic (Yegdich, 1999). This is why it is necessary to work through your own personal pain over time, and use clinical supervision or preceptorship to assist in the clarification of the difference between consumer issues and your own. According to Carl Rogers, empathy is 'one of the most delicate and powerful ways we have of using ourselves' (cited in Stuart 1998: 39) within the therapeutic relationship for assisting in consumer healing. Commonly, empathy conveyed by nurses is experienced by the consumer as being important (Rogers et al., 1993). The ingredients in the process may be unclear, but the person involved feels understood at a deep level, and re-connects with their own inner energy for life changes and potential for developing meaning.

Empathy emerges from within an established therapeutic relationship in which the consumer feels safe and aspects of her or his emotional life have been discussed. A precondition for empathy is that in specific interactions, the nurse concentrates on the consumer and what is important to him or her. Empathy is altruistic: the authentic needs of the consumer are the fundamental concern. The emotional aspects of empathy involve stepping into the consumer's emotional shoes; the cognitive aspect of empathy involves a stepping out of the other person's feelings, while retaining an awareness of their power. One consequence of empathy may involve the nurse supporting the other person's exploration of past life experiences. Often the nurse will assist the consumer to re-frame some perceptions in a meaningful way that normalizes the associated feelings and defuses them to some degree. Without either the emotional connection, or the ability of the nurse to verbalize a key aspect of the connection that resonates with the consumer's experience, what occurs is not empathy.

Both empathy and assertiveness are essential for comprehensive mental health service provision (Bowe 1999). Since nurses do not commonly work with consumers in isolation from other people, assertiveness is particularly required to negotiate with other nurses and health professionals.

A basic definition of *assertiveness* is to respectfully and clearly express your views, observations or feelings, without any likely negative consequences or implications for the other person. Assertiveness is distinguished from passivity, which is not speaking your mind, expressing your feelings or asking for what you want; this allows other people to metaphorically walk over you. Communicating assertively is also contrasted with aggressiveness, which involves expressing a strong feeling (usually anger) and taking what you want without regard for other people's sensitivity, integrity or rights. Aggressive and passive communication and behaviors fit together like a hand in a glove and can be seen in many family dynamics. In ordinary social interactions, the aims of an aggressor are to be disrespectful of another, concede minimal rights to that person and get as much as they can for themselves. Passive communication often results in that person not being respected and other people (aggressors) taking advantage of her or him.

Apart from family experience, there are other barriers to behaving as an assertive, thinking, feeling person. Nelson-Jones (1996) outlines some of these impediments. Non-assertive people may believe that they do not have the right to express their opinion, or that their opinion is invalid or that they will upset someone by speaking about their concerns. In general, if the issue bothers you professionally you do have the right to express your viewpoint. False protection of others is no excuse for non-professional silence. Practice is the only sure way of being able to assertively say what you want to. People with a long history of passivity may find that their assertive words don't work because they do not 'feel' assertive to others; this means that ongoing practice is needed to get the words, voice tone and posture together to ensure that the whole message is congruent.

The aim of communicating and behaving assertively is to work in the functional middle ground without diminishing anybody else or behaving unprofessionally. Assertiveness can decrease the likelihood of inappropriate control, indifference, intrusiveness, emotional distance, or savior or avoidance behaviors when working with mental health consumers. A long-term personal and professional commitment to assertive communication is necessary for nurses to effectively advocate for, and with, consumers in difficult situations.

Consumer advocacy and human rights

Nurses need to be skilled facilitative communicators, assertive and empathic, before they can advocate for and with consumers in situations involving dilemmas or conflict of interest (Horsfall, 1998). Advocacy is the moral commitment to respect the autonomy of others and to support or facilitate their self-determination. Nurse advocacy responsibilities include:

- supporting the choices of people with intact decision-making ability
- informing consumers about diagnosis, medication and treatment options

■ ensuring that the information is comprehensible
■ discussing the likely consequences of each option
■ supporting consumer choice by facilitating expression of concerns, values, interests and priorities
■ minimizing ethical conflict by acknowledging different view-points and mediating at an early stage (Taylor, 1996: 564–6).

As well as advocating for consumer-focused individual choice between options, nurses have broader responsibilities. These other areas of advocacy include:

■ informing and educating consumers about their civil and human rights
■ developing, implementing and evaluating service policy to prevent consumer rights infringements
■ monitoring mental health settings vis-á-vis consumer rights neglect or abuse
■ ensuring consumers have sufficient clear information to give informed consent to specific treatments
■ speaking out to maintain safe working conditions when budgets are cut
■ questioning service providers who draw on stereotypes or diagnostic labels rather than individual assessment (Keglovits & Meder, 1996: 208).

Perkins and Repper (1998) consider that the best advocate for people who live with a mental illness is themselves. This is so. However, when a person is hospitalized, they are especially vulnerable and perhaps most in need of professional advocacy on their behalf, at least in the early days after admission. To provide relevant care under these circumstances, the nurse has to balance a duty of care approach with consumer justice and rights (Bowden, 1995). Mental health nurses are most intimately involved with new patients and are professionally obliged to prevent human rights abuses or neglect and support con-sumers' access to the least restrictive treatment.

Ethical mental health nursing practice

Facilitative communication, assertiveness, negotiation skills and a commitment to advocacy underpin the possibility of ethical mental health nursing practice. Without the interpersonal skills, the ability to present points of view confidently, and an awareness of broad contextual issues, ethical practice is likely to be compromised.

Most discussions of ethics in mental health focus on the individual nurse in relation to an individual consumer. Hence, the character and moral awareness of the nurse feed into ethical decision making (Horsfall, 1998). Wilson (1996) outlines nursing competencies required for ethical reasoning. These include the ability to recognize dilemmas, options and their consequences; make clinical judgments; prioritize professional ethics over personal values if they conflict; and draw on personal strength and commitment to carry ethical decisions through to action. Ethical decisions often have consequences that go beyond an individual.

The nurse uses ethical reasoning within professional relationships. Professional relationships differ from social relationships primarily in that that the former are one-sided, with the nurse expending more energy to explore consumer issues with an orientation towards recovery. 'It becomes the ethical responsibility of the nurse to ensure that any personal needs, concerns, and desires of the nurse [are] handled outside the therapeutic relationship' (Arnold, 1996: 233). This is a relationship for the consumer, focusing on health-related issues.

Caring is a requirement for effective mental health nursing, but if it is non-professional (i.e., carried to extremes), the nurse may become overwhelmed by the concerns of the consumer. A broader stance is also needed whereby the nurse retains an ongoing awareness of consumer perspectives and concerns regarding social justice. Caring and justice perspectives are complementary and both are necessary for ethical mental health nursing practice. Another way of stating this is that there can be tensions between an ethic of care and consumer autonomy interests. In trying to address these tensions, Perkins and Repper (1998: 48) say that 'as the oppression of people who experience serious mental health problems will undoubtedly continue until they enjoy full rights as citizens, we feel it is important to start from a civil rights perspective.' Such a view supports the centrality of advocacy for ethical mental health nursing practice.

The consumer–nurse relationship itself is embedded within complex organizational structures which do not necessarily actively support ethical practice. Budget cuts, insufficient nursing employees, higher consumer acuity, and contradictory health and hospital policies place nurses in the middle of a management—consumer sandwich. This location can thwart nursing efforts to advocate for and with consumers and to follow through with actions arising from ethical decision making. In some health services, the medical hierarchy expects nurses to carry out medical orders and act on behalf of doctors (Liaschenko 1995), to the detriment of the professional judgment and autonomy of the nurse. Also, if administrators expect nurses to unquestioningly carry out their instructions, this can doubly impede the possibility of ethical practice. However, if nurses work with and for consumers in mental health settings, then such a professional alliance has significant therapeutic, ethical and advocacy potential to support, or to negotiate, change if the rights of consumers are compromised.

References

Arnold, E. 1996, A pathway for healing. Therapeutic relationships. In: V. Carson & E. Arnold (eds), *Mental health nursing. The nurse–patient journey*. W.B. Saunders, Philadelphia.

Arthur, D. 1999, Assessing nursing students' basic communication and interviewing skills. The development and testing of a rating scale. *Journal of Advanced Nursing*, 29(3): 658–65.

Barker, P., Jackson, S. & Stevenson, C. 1999, The need for psychiatric nursing. Towards a multidimensional theory of caring. *Nursing Inquiry*, 6(2): 103–11.

Beech, P. & Norman, I. 1995, Patients' perceptions of the quality of psychiatric nursing care. Findings from a small-scale descriptive study. *Journal of Clinical Nursing*, 4: 117–23.

Bowden, P. 1995, The ethics of nursing care and the 'ethic of care.' *Nursing Inquiry*, 2(1): 10–21.

Bowe, R. 1999, *Shared skills. The identification of core competencies for mental health professionals who work in community mental health teams*. The Surrey & Chichester Education Consortium, Guildford, UK.

Champ, S. 1998, A most precious thread. *Australian and New Zealand Journal of Mental Health Nursing*, 7(2): 54–9.

Garrett, C. 1998, *Beyond anorexia*. Cambridge University Press, Cambridge.

Heller, T. 1996, Doing being human. Reflective practice in mental health work. In: T. Heller, J. Reynolds, R. Gomm, R. Muston & S. Pattison (eds), *Mental health matters. A reader*. Macmillan, Houndmills, UK.

Horsfall, J. 1993, Ask and adequately inform. RPN responsibilities. In: Royal Melbourne Institute of Technology (RMIT), *Proceedings. Psychiatric nursing conference*. RMIT, Melbourne.

Horsfall, J. 1998, Structural impediments to effective communication. *Australian and New Zealand Journal of Mental Health Nursing*, 7(2): 74–90.

Jung, C. 1978, In: A. Storr (ed.), *Selected writings*. Fontana, London.

Kalisch, B. 1973, What is empathy? *American Journal of Nursing*, 73: 1548.

Keglovits, J. & Meder, M. 1996, Advocacy, client rights, and legal issues. In: H. Wilson, & C. Kneisl (eds), *Psychiatric nursing*, 5th edn. Addison-Wesley, Menlo Park, Calif.

Kneisl, C. 1996, Therapeutic communication. In: H. Wilson & C. Kneisl (eds), *Psychiatric nursing*, 5th edn. Addison-Wesley, Menlo Park, Calif.

Liaschenko, J. 1995, Ethics in the work of acting for patients. *Advances in Nursing Science*, 18: 1–12.

Lindow, V. 1993, A service user's view. In: H. Wright & M. Giddey (eds), *Mental health nursing*. Chapman & Hall, London.

Loring, M. & Powell, B. 1988, Gender, race and DSM-III. A study of the objectivity of psychiatric diagnostic behavior. *Journal of Health and Social Behavior*, 29: 1–22.

McDonald, F. 1996, Principles of communication. In: K. Fortinash & P. Holoday-Worrett (eds), *Psychiatric mental health nursing*. Mosby, St Louis.

Melbourne Consumer Consultants' Group (MCCG). 1997, *Do you mind? The ultimate exit survey. Survivors of psychiatric services speak out*. MCCG, Melbourne.

Nelson-Jones, R. 1996, *Human relationship skills. Training and self-help*, 3rd edn. Harcourt Brace, Sydney.

Palmer, A., Burns, S. & Bulman, C. (eds). 1994, *Reflective practice in nursing. The growth of the professional practitioner*. Blackwell, Oxford.

Peplau, H. 1989, In: A. O'Toole & S. Welt (eds), *Interpersonal theory in nursing practice. Selected works of Hildegard Peplau*. Springer, New York.

Perkins, R. & Repper, J. 1998, *Dilemmas in community mental health practice. Choice or control*. Radcliffe Medical Press, Abingdon, UK.

Ritter, S. 1997, An overview of interpersonal approaches to communication between nurses and people with mental health problems. Keynote address presented to 23rd Annual Conference of The Australian & New Zealand College of Mental Health Nurses. (Proceedings on disc.) Adelaide.

Rogers, A., Pilgrim, D. & Lacey, R. 1993, *Experiencing psychiatry. Users' views of services*. Macmillan, Houndmills, UK.

Romme, M. 1996, Rehabilitating voice-hearers. In: T. Heller, J. Reynolds, R. Gomm, R. Muston & S. Pattison (eds), *Mental health matters. A reader*. Macmillan, Houndmills, UK.

Stuart, G. 1998, Therapeutic nurse–patient relationship. In: G. Stuart & M. Laraia (eds) *Stuart & Sundeen's principles and practices of psychiatric nursing*, 6th edn. Mosby, St Louis.

Taylor, C. 1996, Ethical issues in psychiatric- mental health nursing. In: S. Lego (ed.), *Psychiatric nursing. A comprehensive reference*, 2nd edn. Lippincott, Philadelphia.

Wadsworth, Y. & Epstein, M. 1997, *'Building in' dialogue between users and staff in acute mental health services*. Action Research Issues Centre, Melbourne.

Walsh, K. 1994, Ontology and the nurse–patient relationship in psychiatric nursing. *Australian and New Zealand Journal of Mental Health Nursing*, 3(4): 113–18.

Wilson, H. 1996, Ethical reasoning. In: H. Wilson & C. Kneisl (eds), *Psychiatric nursing*, 5th edn. Addison-Wesley, Menlo Park, Calif.

Yegdich, T. 1999, On the phenomenology of empathy in nursing. Empathy or sympathy? *Journal of Advanced Nursing*, 31(1): 83–93.

Yoder, S. & Rode, M. 1990, How are you doing? Patient evaluations of nursing actions. *Journal of Psychosocial Nursing*, 10: 26–30.

3
Psychiatric models, consumers and mental health nursing

Key concepts
in this
chapter:

■ behavioral model
■ class and mental illness
■ cognitive model ■ consumer-focused care
■ critique of mainstream psychiatric models
■ ethnicity and mental illness
■ holism ■ medical model
■ political awareness and nurses
■ sex or gender and mental illness

Introduction

In order to fulfill obligations for ethical mental health nursing practice, the previous chapter proposed that nursing students and RNs have a responsibility to develop a knowledge base deriving from mental health service consumers. Traditionally students of mental health nursing have been immersed in knowledge arising from psychiatry topped up with nursing and/or psychology—the mix or emphasis depending on the curriculum and the era.

Before delineating some consumer expectations of nurses and mental health services, this chapter outlines, then critiques, prevailing ideas promoted by mainstream psychiatry. Medicine does have theoretical and practice knowledge relevant to improving consumer mental health, but until the present time these have been over-emphasized at the expense of both consumer concerns and nursing theory and practice. The time is overdue for mental health nursing to validate and draw on consumer expertise, and offer this knowledge equal space and value vis-à-vis psychiatry and psychology.

Mainstream psychiatric models

The three predominant models in present day psychiatric theory and practice are the medical model, behavioral model, and the cognitive model. At times two or three are drawn upon for treatment purposes. Frequently, one or more underpin nurses' understanding of the causes of mental illness.

Medical model propositions

- The study and treatment of madness is a medical specialty, i.e., psychiatry.
- Madness is a mental illness and is therefore like all other illnesses.
- The cause of mental illness is organic (bodily, somatic, physical).
- The central nervous system and brain are the sites of physical malfunction.
- Genes or heredity is the underlying cause of mental illness.
- Brain structure and blood flow are implicated in mental illness.
- Mental illness is precipitated by neurotransmitter imbalance.
- Medical treatment, as with other illness, is somatic; that is, mostly medication (see Wilson 1996 and other authors for further information on this model).

Behavioral model propositions

- Human beings are complex animals, different from others by degree, not kind.
- People can be best understood by their behaviors or actions.
- Behaviors are observable, describable and indisputable.
- Mental illness symptoms, as revealed by behaviors, are the treatment focus.
- The cause of behaviors is, to a large extent, irrelevant to treatment.
- Past experiences of a person with a mental illness are irrelevant.
- Problematic behaviors can be changed by reinforcing positive behaviors.
- Behaviors can be changed by punishing (or not rewarding) negative acts (see Wilson 1996 and other authors for further information on this model).

Cognitive model propositions

- Thoughts and beliefs (cognition) are humans' defining characteristics.
- All mental illness involves distorted thinking that is irrational, or wrong.
- People who experience life difficulties also often have distorted thinking.
- People's thinking (not events or interactions) causes emotional distress.
- Cognitive therapy aims to change negative thinking and irrational beliefs.
- The client and nurse explore the client's view of self and the world to ascertain which habitual thoughts, expectations and beliefs are problematic.
- The client learns to recognize the problematic (often automatic) thoughts.
- The client disputes own negative thoughts and practices positive thinking (see Stuart 1998a and other authors for further information on this model).

Each of these three models can make a positive contribution to an RN's conceptualization of and interventions with people living with a mental illness. In this chapter the focus is more on a critique of some of their assumptions or propositions, since uncritical information deriving from the models is readily available to students in psychiatric, psychology and mental health nursing textbooks. During the last 40 years, medicine has monopolized knowledge generation in psychiatry and, according to consumers, it has not always focused on them as people or on their expressed needs (Lindow, 1993).

Another reason for critiquing the models and proposing other perspectives is that the prevailing models do not actively support the positive effects that nurse engagement can make to enhance consumer well-being. Furthermore, they do not offer clues as to how a nurse should communicate or develop a professional relationship to achieve therapeutic consumer outcomes.

The aetiological claims of psychiatry

Contemporary cornerstones of psychiatry hark back to the last third of the nineteenth century. By then, psychiatry had a beginning bank of effective tranquilizing drugs, two of which remain (albeit rarely) in use today. Chloral hydrate was invented in 1869 and paraldehyde in 1882. Koch discovered micro-organisms in 1876 and X-rays were invented in 1895. The syphilis spirochaete was discovered in 1894, alongside the growing awareness that it was associated with sexual adventurism and resulted in what was called general paralysis of the insane—the tertiary phase of untreated syphilis in which psychiatric symptoms are evident (Horsfall, 1997a).

These bastions of psychiatry: a belief in physical causes of madness, technological imaging to reveal these physical causes and medication to sedate the person, are still with us. A focus on the brain preceded even these tendencies. By the 1830s an eminent psychiatrist named Griesinger had concluded that the brain alone is the seat of madness. The expectations at the turn of the nineteenth century that certain areas of the brain would determine certain types of psychiatric symptoms possibly remained on the research agenda at the turn of the twentieth century (Horsfall, 1997b). Present day positron emission tomography (PET scans) of cerebral structures are claimed by some researchers to provide imaging evidence that ventricular enlargement causes schizophrenia. The data are contradictory, the sample sizes are small, the logic dubious and the claims do not necessarily adhere to facts (Dawson, 1997).

Genetic causation of psychiatric conditions also has a lengthy history. The first empirical data that aimed to show that madness was inherited were collected by Kallman between 1893 and 1902. He subsequently claimed to have proven that schizophrenia is hereditary, even though it was not named as such until 1911 and a definitive diagnostic definition was not forthcoming for some time afterwards. His view of schizophrenia was that sufferers included people of the 'lowest type' and 'maladjusted cranks.' An influential researcher, Kallman left Germany to establish the first genetics research institute in the USA (Horsfall, 1997b).

At the outset it was likely—contrary to claims of scientific objectivity—that the search for genetic causation of psychiatric disorders was tainted by a confusion between being mad and being poor. Also the late nineteenth century belief in the 'superiority' of north-western European races and the concern of the eugenics movement to eradicate people because of their physical or mental 'inferiority' fed into the human sciences of the era. Those who followed the Eugenicist, considered that some families were deteriorating, as each generation emerged, along a path to madness and that society would be better off without them. These beliefs, along with those of European racial superiority, continued at least until World War Two.

Studies seeking to show the genetic transmission of schizophrenia, bipolar disorder and depression (at least) continue to be well funded. Some of the flaws evident in Kallman's first data remained for decades. A clear definition of a disorder is required to ensure that what the researchers are diagnosing is the specific condition, not some social peculiarities or another disorder. Different definitions produce different estimations of genetic heritability. The looser the definition, the higher the claimed rates of genetic transmission (Horsfall, 1997b).

If schizophrenia is merely genetic, then 100 per cent of pairs of monozygotic twins (raised in either the same or different environment) would be either schizophrenic or not schizophrenic. This is not the case. Furthermore, re-examination by scientists in the 1970s, 1980s and 1990s, of seminal research into genetics and schizophrenia has revealed inadequate sampling techniques, poor methods and the misinterpretation of data (Dawson, 1997).

Neurotransmitter causes of schizophrenia and other psychiatric conditions have a more recent history than that of genetics. The dopamine hypothesis for schizophrenia causation emerged in the mid-1960s and retained scientific credibility for more than three decades, in the face of mounting evidence and coherent arguments by a minority of researchers against the claim. Contemporary critics of this hypothesis include Carlsson—one of its former proponents (Dawson, 1997). A belief that an excess, or insufficiency, of one neurotransmitter at the synapse can cause a complex syndrome like schizophrenia is simplistic. The most profound problem with such a schema is the assumption that one neurotransmitter works alone and consistently at all sites, under all bodily circumstances. Another major flaw is the idea that electrochemical transmission from one nerve cell to another could translate exactly into the complex experience of hallucinations and/or delusions. Dopamine, as one example, stimulates the hypothalamus, which is involved in the fine regulation of hormones that have a range of diverse effects throughout the body (Krupnick 1996).

Psychiatric ideologies and their consequences

These medical models of psychiatric aetiology—brain structure, genes and neurotransmitters—have all been absorbed by mental health nursing texts, curricula and clinicians (Hall, 1996), regardless of the era of education. Alone, or in combination with each other, these hypothetical psychiatric explanatory frameworks could be described as biological reductionism (Horsfall, 1997b). This means that the complexity and subtlety of humans and our minds have been theoretically reduced to specific body systems, and the wholeness of a person in their social and cultural context is forgotten.

These claims have become more enshrined in psychiatric orthodoxy by later revisions of the American Psychiatric Association's (APA) *Diagnostic and Statistical Manual of Mental Disorders* (DSM). This internationally endorsed psychiatric reference book claims to be empirically based and a-theoretical. It is really neither. The assumptive theory is that of the faulty material (physical) body of the person with a psychiatric diagnosis. The primary mode of treatment for psychiatric conditions is medication. Psychiatrists diagnose according to the DSM and treat with medication manufactured by international pharmaceutical companies. Increasingly, drug companies provide prescribing doctors with 'scientific' information and even promote general medical practitioner awareness of new or not well recognized 'diseases' (e.g., high cholesterol, or panic attacks) for which they have a specific medication (Moynihan, 1998).

If psychotropic drugs were 80 per cent effective for 90 per cent of consumers, then perhaps this would be of little concern. This is not the case. In previous decades, drugs in the

antipsychotic class of medication were known as major tranquilizers: title change notwithstanding, the primary action of
this group of drugs is still tranquilization. The drugs are much
more effective in reducing combativeness, hyperactivity and
tension (74%, 73% and 71% effective), than they are in providing relief from hallucinations or delusions (58% and 48% effective respectively) (Dawson, 1997).

This simple medical medication model can be ultimately disempowering for nurses and consumers. Both are dependent on
the psychiatrist for a diagnosis and on the pharmacist to fill the
prescription. If nurses believe that drugs are *the* treatment, this
can easily result in nurses having a primarily surveillance role
on behalf of doctors and drug companies—ensuring adherence
to the drug and monitoring side-effects. An unquestioning belief
in drug cures and an undue focus on symptom reduction can
also distance nurses from consumers and their daily life concerns (Hall, 1996); and this may leave both parties waiting for
the medication to have effects beyond those that are likely
(Horsfall, 1997a).

Chafetz et al. (1998) take a balanced position. They state that
second generation psychotropic medications are more effective
and safer than earlier drugs. They see nurses in mental health
as having to be well informed about the positive and negative
effects of medication. However, nursing care plans 'involve far
more than psychopharmacology (as drug effects are frequently
... disappointing), we also need psychosocial skills to ...
support, manage illness, and prevent relapse' (ibid.:10).
Humans are experiencing, socially interacting and adapting
creatures. Experience is not predetermined by genes and sorted
out by neurotransmitters. Our lives and the lives of consumers
are much more complex than that.

Lego (1992) briefly discusses a consumer called John. His
medical diagnosis was that of 'endogenous depression'—which
means that the psychiatrist considered his mood disorder came
from inside him, rather than as a response to some experiences
in the outer world. During a drug trial he described the effects
of the medication as feeling as though they dragged him up and
out of a quagmire. He was actually taking a placebo! If the belief
in a new drug can contribute to a mood lift and precipitate more
positive thinking, then the provision of appropriate support and
hope in themselves may influence mood and well-being. It is

possible that emotion may affect neurotransmitters positively or negatively in ways as powerful as the assumed effect of medication on neurotransmitters and subsequent behavior, mood or thoughts.

As well as reducing the human person to physical fragments such as cerebral lobes and ventricles, genes and neurotransmitters, this view of ourselves and consumers ignores a broad range of social circumstances. Excluded aspects of our lives include:

- the quality of the air, water, food and levels of artificial toxins
- the limits imposed by global and national economics determining, for example, whether or not you have to struggle to stay alive in the midst of famine
- income limitations; for example, if you are a member of a family in which there has been three generations of unemployment
- the political and historical circumstances in your country of birth, which may be quietly oppressive, openly brutal or reasonably benevolent.

We are whole people and we are connected to our ecological, economic and political environments—whether we think so or not. Materialist medicine assumes that we consist of the sum of our separate bodily systems. Part of our environment is internal, but it is external too.

For each person it is a matter of serendipity (luck) whether, for example, you are born in this or another century, born African, Asian or European or with a mixed lineage, or that you live in a northern, southern or equatorial country. We have no choice in this, and the vast majority of parents do not either. As individuals, chance also determines our sex, original nationality, class, ethnicity, cultural and religious affiliation. We are born into these circumstances. You may notice too that these very characteristics are those that form the basis of sexism or equality, racism or pluralism, religious bigotry or acceptance, cultural intolerance or multiculturalism. Living with very limited opportunities is known to influence health negatively (Horsfall, 1998).

These macro-social givens—sex, class, ethnicity, religion and culture—have ramifications within our families, in classrooms, on the streets and at work. Consequences arise from comparative advantage and disadvantage at birth and their impact as you grow up; these include: how sexism is acted out in your family and your school; how racism is revealed or hidden in the classroom and the neighborhood; and if religion is a force for social justice, or social control. This involves other people's treatment of you and your family members and vice versa. These interactions between people contribute significantly to our social, moral and cognitive development, and therefore to our potential for mental health or difficulties (Horsfall 1997a). Institutionalized (commonplace, but not necessarily visible) sexism, racism, as well as viewing poor people as inferior and members of some religious groups as alien, affect people's sense of personal rights and social responsibilities, self-esteem and competence in our social world.

As well as ignoring these social facts of life, mainstream psychiatry marginalizes a range of more subtle human qualities, such as our emotions, spiritual needs, beliefs and attitudes. Emotions may be played down in our society, spirituality may have become impoverished or commodified, and our beliefs in fairness and equality may be ignored or manipulated by politicians. But denying or diminishing these human qualities does not mean that they are not important to consumers and providers of health services (Horsfall, 1997b).

In an exploration of mental illness, Hacking (in Borch-Jacobsen 1999) considers that for people to become mentally ill, there must be a social niche which supports this possibility. He outlines five factors that are necessary for a person to be deemed mentally ill.

- The consequences of the illness must include actions that are socially unacceptable, odd or deviant.
- Specific deviant behavior must be listed as symptoms in pre-existing illness classification systems.
- The deviant behaviors must coincide with the negative side of behavioral polarities; for example, emotionality as opposed to self-control, doom and gloom in contrast to optimism, and chaotic ideas as opposed to rational self-expression.
- The illness must provide unconscious relief from circumstances experienced as impossible, even if the illness itself creates further problems or disabilities in the longer term.

■ There must be a social system that deems the illness to not be the 'fault' of or amenable to the free will of the sufferer; that is, it is caused by genes, a biochemical imbalance, a spell being cast, and so on.

These five factors encourage the consideration of complex social, psychological and biological interactions, rather than simple biological or psychological reductionism.

Mainstream psychology

The discipline of psychology also has its roots in European philosophy and science, but the psychology that we recognize emerged in the late nineteenth century, and is therefore younger than western medicine. Psychology could be defined as the study of the nature, functions and workings of the human mind. Such a discipline sounds relevant to our lives; however, for many contemporary students it does not fulfill its implicit promise of developing skills to understand ourselves and others.

Contemporary psychology offers a cognitive and behavioral complement to the physical approach of medicine. Like medicine, as the discipline evolved, it ceased to consider the person as a whole and developed segmented strands of study that different academics or researchers pursued. Students may study, for example, cognitive psychology, behavioral psychology, abnormal psychology, neuropsychology, experimental psychology, or community psychology. The knowledge in the sub-domains of the discipline has limited conceptual or practical connection with that developed and discussed in other strands.

Overall, mainstream psychology has reduced people to separate bits, such as cognition, perception and behavior. Apart from consisting of disconnected areas of knowledge, psychology too omits the political, economic and social environment of the people whose cognition (for example) is studied or treated. The experiential aspects of being a person with a particular sex, class, ethnicity, age and sexual orientation is also ignored. Similarly, the qualities that we probably do not share with animals (for both medicine and psychology frequently refer to animal analogies), such as spirituality, soul, emotional complexity and unconscious processes, fall outside present-day mainstream knowledge development in psychology (Dawson, 1996b, Horsfall, 1997b).

How do psychiatry and psychology affect mental health nursing?

Mental health nursing emerged as an occupation well after psychiatry and psychology were established disciplines. Psychiatry had won an ideological struggle in a number of European countries as well as the USA in the mid-to-late-nineteenth century to legally and professionally be in charge of the treatment of the insane. Consequently, psychiatric nursing developed under the economic, political and practical patronage of psychiatry (Horsfall, 1997a).

Particularly in recent decades, mental health nursing has inherited an extensive body of knowledge from psychiatry. This includes psychiatric aetiological hypotheses, the international classification systems which organize these disorders into categories and the cluster of symptoms that distinguish one psychiatric diagnosis from another. These constitute the knowledge foundations of mental health nursing in most textbooks written in English (Horsfall, 1998).

In the practice domain, psychiatrists expect nurses to ensure that consumers take their medication, to assist with electroconvulsive treatment (ECT), to observe designated at-risk patients at all times, to adhere to seclusion protocols and to institute community treatment orders. In each of these regimens, the psychiatrist decides (with or without consultation) whether or not to 'prescribe' the 'treatment,' but it is nurses who implement, maintain, monitor and document these processes, along with consumers who attempt to manage the consequences. Medicating, ECT, community treatment orders (Perkins & Repper, 1998), 'special observation' and seclusion are not viewed positively by many consumers. However, with regard to medication, nurses are obliged to teach themselves and consumers about dose in relation to body mass and ethnicity; to consider the timing of daily or weekly medication; to be aware of synergistic or antagonistic drug interactions; and to ascertain individual difficulties associated with specific medication side effects.

Psychology also has a range of therapeutic modalities to offer. These have been taken up by some mental health nurses in the hospital and in the community. Methods deriving from cognitive, behavioral, gestalt, psychodynamic and humanistic models have assisted nurses to work constructively with many consumers. Although helpful, these counseling styles have their limitations, not the least being their lack of consideration of the consumers' actual ongoing personal, practical and economic circumstances (Dawson, 1996a, Hopton, 1995, Horsfall, 1997b).

Mental health nursing, in order to offer effective care to consumers, and to complement (or provide an alternative to) medicine and psychology, has to reclaim or invigorate its nursing base. Given the above critique of psychiatry and clinical psychology, mental health nursing needs to strain towards holism, humanism and an awareness of political inequalities (Hall, 1996) which constrain consumer opportunities and nursing effectiveness.

Holism embraces the environmental, cultural, social, family, emotional and spiritual aspects of a person's life. It is a perspective that considers the person to be an integrated organic and functional whole, greater than the sum of her or his physical, emotional, behavioral and spiritual attributes. The unity of body, mind, spirit and soul in holism is congruent with a humanistic belief system.

Humanism in nursing expresses respect, hope and caring through the interpersonal therapeutic relationship. It is a philosophical view that places humans at the center of our concerns. Humanism values each individual person and embodies the belief that all people are capable of good and self healing, given sufficient interpersonal support. Each individual is considered to be ultimately responsible for their actions and inaction. All people are deemed to be able to choose responsibly when given the opportunity and to have the potential to solve their own problems.

The *political perspective* supports consumers' human rights and challenges prejudice, inequality and injustice associated with sexism, ethnocentrism and heterosexism at the interpersonal and macro-social levels. Because this orientation is political and economic, it differs from the individual internal focus of humanism and the more spiritual and ecological facets of holism involved in viewing the world as an integrated entity.

A more holistic perspective is necessary for nursing to fulfill its brief to improve the well-being of consumers of mental health services. Stuart (1998b), for example, articulates a mental health nursing model that integrates the biological, psychological, sociocultural, environmental and legal–ethical aspects of patient care. She considers consumers' responses to stress—in the context of social, economic and personal resources which act as buffers—and deems these to be the focus of psychiatric nursing care. This reveals a debt to the humanism of Peplau (1952) who saw nursing as working with human responses to illness in the belief that each person has their own internal potential for healing, recovery or a dignified death. In highlighting the differences between medicine and nursing, Stuart (1998b) considers that mental health nursing needs to be concerned about patients' vulnerability, their adaptive or non-adaptive coping mechanisms and the provision of care. Hall (1996) believes that mental health nursing could relinquish medical diagnosis as a special focus and work with the personal needs of consumers. Hummelvoll and Barbosa da Silva (1994) similarly consider that because medicine reduces people to their physical body, it is therefore inadequate for mental health nurses aiming to understand people who live with a mental illness.

Consumers: The raison d'être of nursing

Along with other critical mental health nurses, Horsfall (1997a) argues that many nurses and consumers are disenfranchised by mainstream mental health nursing as it is practiced and documented in Australia, the United Kingdom and the United States of America. Mental health nurses would not have jobs without state health departments and private hospitals, or without the people who live with a mental illness and seek assistance at the hospitals and community health centers in which nurses work. It seems that the allegiance of nurses has often been more with employers in the past. Perhaps it is time for nurses to ally ourselves more closely with consumers and their needs and concerns.

Nevertheless, mental health nurses often manage to provide a valued and caring service to consumers in the face of serious constraints, such as staff shortages, consumer acuity, high patient turnover and rigid administrative or medical protocols. In their study of approximately 500 consumers in the UK, for example, Rogers et al. (1993)—none of whom is a nurse—found that mental health nurses were by far the most helpful professionals, and psychiatrists the least helpful. This is heartening evidence, since nurses are most advantaged in their access to consumers, but simultaneously are the least advantaged workers when budget cuts (evident in Australia, North America and the UK) produce conditions (such as those just mentioned) that create high levels of stress for nurses and consumers.

As mental health nurses, we can explore the lives of consumers of mental health services, regardless of medical diagnosis. Potential service users are commonly afraid of 'going mad,' feel isolated, have lost certainty in their lives, are emotionally distressed and their self-esteem is low (Leete, 1987, Lindow, 1993, McGuiness & Wadsworth, 1991, for example). To be therapeutic, nursing must offer consumers realistic reassurance and information, opportunities to connect with understanding people—consumers and professionals, a sense of being able to survive, a safe environment to express and normalize feelings, and support the use of their personal strengths. Consumers have been saying for over a decade that health professionals do not provide these resources frequently enough.

Humelvoll and Barbosa da Silva (1994) include the following concepts in their *holistic* psychiatric nursing model.

- Open mindedness. This personal quality begins before the nurse meets a prospective consumer.
- Mutual responsibilities. Whether in hospital or at home, the nurse has to clarify each party's expectations of the other.
- Authentic interest. This is a social and emotional endeavor on behalf of the nurse to make contact with and be present with the consumer.
- Equality. To achieve this, the nurse's attitude is respectful and interactions aim for a partnership that is, or will become, as equal as possible.
- Work with consumer values. The consumer's interests, aims and sense of meaning make up the framework within which they live and these need to be honored by the nurse.

- ■ Hope. Hope provides a sense of being able to endure and go forward. It is an essential ingredient if survival, goals and plans are to be achievable.
- ■ Self-esteem. To maintain and enhance the consumers' sense of worth and competence, their concerns, strengths and skills should be acknowledged and drawn on.

These cornerstones for holistic and humanistic mental health nursing provide challenges and potential rewards for nurses and would greatly improve the quality of care received by most consumers of mental health services. However, to increase its comprehensiveness and effectiveness, nursing in mental health must increase its commitment to advocacy, defending consumer rights and working to prevent illness. Such an orientation entails different expectations of mental health nurses. In his critique of humanistic nursing claims, Hopton (1995) insists that caring is an inadequate basis for effective mental health service provision. Health promotion and health education—outside the one-to-one therapeutic relationship framework—are now essential aspects of mental health nursing. Hopton (1995: 342) says that nurses 'can only fulfill these roles if they are engaged in practical political activity to challenge social injustice.' In other words, health promotion and health education require nurses to enter the broader political domain outside the therapeutic relationship and the hospital.

Structured consumer life contexts

Horsfall (1998) has critiqued the mainstream mental health disciplines for ignoring or side-lining macro-social life structures. The key concepts to be addressed are class, ethnicity and sex.

Class

There is ample evidence from a series of epidemiological studies undertaken in the USA over at least a 60-year time frame that lower socioeconomic class is strongly associated with high rates of mental illness and physical illness. In the USA, Holzer et al. (1986) estimated that any person in poverty was 2.86 times more likely to experience a psychiatric disorder than anybody above the poverty line. Recent Australian data gleaned from

10,600 representative respondents, found that only those in full-time work had rates of anxiety disorders and depressive disorders lower than the rates for the population as a whole (Australian Bureau of Statistics [ABS] 1998: 24). In other words, people who are unemployed, 'not in the labor force,' or in part-time work have higher than average rates of anxiety and depression. Another indirect way of estimating class is level of education. Again, people who have post-school qualifications are the only group who have lower anxiety and depression rates than the average Australian (ABS 1998: 26). (These Australian data did not include information regarding schizophrenia as the rate is less than one per cent of the population.)

This does not mean that having a middle level income or a good education prevents anxiety, depression or schizophrenia, but they increase the level of personal resources which in turn decrease the level of the harshness of the daily struggle for money to buy food, rent and power. Another way of saying this is that money and education provide material, practical and emotional buffers.

Ethnicity

In the UK, Pilgrim and Rogers (1993) observe that African-Caribbean and Irish immigrants have higher rates of psychiatric hospitalization than other minority groups. Kutchins and Kirk (1997) in the USA indicate that Black patients have higher diagnosis rates for schizophrenia, paranoid personality disorder and lower rates of mood disorder diagnoses. Ethnic affiliation and lower socioeconomic class effects are likely to overlap. Hence, higher hospitalization rates may relate more to structured economic inequalities for many members of specific ethnic minority groups across a range of 'developed' countries. In the USA, Asians, Afro Americans, Hispanic and indigenous peoples have higher rates of public hospital use in comparison to Euro Americans, who are more frequently treated in community and private facilities. This is just as likely to be related to class as culture.

Perhaps surprisingly, in Australia the prevalence of mental illness in people born outside Australia is lower than that for those born in the country (ABS, 1998: 27). Citing different sources, Easthope and Julian (1996) found, especially within economically disadvantaged groups, increased rates of psychiatric hospitalization for depression and higher rates of schizophrenia among immigrants from non-English speaking backgrounds.

Psychiatric research in westernized nations traditionally ignores or minimizes class differences (Kutchins & Kirk 1997); focused studies of specific ethnic sub-groups that take financial status into account are not common either. It is quite likely that the higher levels of mental health in some immigrants indicate the level of income, opportunity and a health-welfare safety net not available in their country of origin. On the other hand, higher rates of mental illness among some immigrants may derive from culture shock, loss of extended family, alienation from mainstream society due to poor language skills, or from trauma associated with war, oppression, or torture. It is not that certain ethnic groups are more prone to mental illness, but that their life history is one of violence, tragedy and loss, or of first-generation immigrants struggling to adapt to a host nation with alien values, traditions and ways of life.

Sex

Ethnicity affects overlap with sex as well as class. Busfield (1996) notes higher hospitalization levels for people with Afro-Caribbean cultural affiliation in the UK and higher rates of diagnosis of schizophrenia and substance-induced psychoses, and considers these to be related to institutionalized racism in society at large and within the health professions. Diagnostic biases may indicate European psychiatrists' fear of Black male violence and their consequent attribution of inappropriate suspiciousness and dangerousness to Black men.

The recent Australian study (ABS 1998) has shown that when the most common psychiatric difficulties are considered—anxiety, depression, alcohol and substance-abuse disorders—the rates of mental illness for men and women are virtually equal at just over 18 per cent for both sexes. This means that to be female is not to be inherently vulnerable to mental illness, as psychiatric textbooks indicated for most of the twentieth century. Likewise, to be male is not the same as being sane, as texts and male psychiatrists have unconsciously assumed over the same period of time. As human beings, we all have the potential to express emotional disturbance in ways that are consistent with contemporary definitions of mental illness. Patterns of expressions of distress do differ noticeably by gender. Men predominate in diagnoses of alcohol abuse, substance abuse, antisocial personality disorder and avoidant personality disorder. Women predominate in diagnoses of depression, anxiety disorders, borderline personality disorder and dependent personality disorder (Horsfall, 1994).

Class, ethnicity and sex are factors that structure the lives of both consumers and providers of mental health services. If, as nurses, we focus only on the behaviors and emotions of individual consumers we may ignore important macro-social aspects of consumers' lives. If we are only aware of individual distress, specific psychiatric diagnoses and psychotropic medication, then we may miss issues that consumers have in common as a group. Then, mental health nurses can be merely accepting of poverty, inequality and homelessness, and focus on medication, pseudo rehabilitation and one-to-one counselling (Horsfall, 1998). These are political issues, and poverty, homelessness and unemployment are not conducive to anybody's mental health.

What consumers say they want

Consumer critiques of mainstream mental health services have tended to focus on the absence of the humanistic and holistic approaches, but this is not entirely the case. Consumer groups that organize around survivorship (Perkins & Repper, 1998) tend to have a more macro-social and political agenda that may include an antipathy to psychiatry and the medication industry, along with a focus on the eradication of racism, sexism and demands for more employment opportunities.

The following points are a synthesis of some ideas set out by Leete (1987), Lindow (1993), McGuiness and Wadsworth (1991), Melbourne Consumer Consultants' Group (1997) and Yoder and Rode (1990), but not only from these sources. Consumer voices predominate in the first four of these publications.

Consumer expectations of mental health service providers include:

- To be safe—emotionally, physically, sexually, spiritually—in hospital and in the community
- To have positive relationships with other consumers
- To have positive relationships with health workers
- To work in an authentic decision-making partnership
- To be empowered to be in charge of their own lives and choices
- To know about and be able to join established self-help and peer support groups
- To have their culture, religion and sexual orientation accepted
- To be respected as an equal, valued and unique person
- To be listened to and taken seriously
- To have a sense of hopefulness about them and their future conveyed
- To receive comprehensible and appropriate information and explanations
- To have actual access to 24-hour crisis services
- To not be stigmatized by health professionals, lawyers and the public
- To have access to good quality community services
- To negotiate in the selection of their case manager (or primary nurse, or key worker), especially if difficulties have been experienced
- To have access in all settings to advocacy resources—including for complaints procedures
- For there to be real support and/or treatment options, including those that are not mainstream, and to be able to choose between them
- To have opportunities to feed back information into responsive service policies
- To have equal access to a choice of affordable, functional housing
- To have appropriate vocational rehabilitation, along with supported, flexible and transitional employment opportunities.

These reasonable and straightforward consumer expectations are congruent with the intentions of *humanistic and holistic* mental health nursing as outlined by Humelvoll and Barbosa da Silva (1994), for example. The first ten of these 20 requests should be comparatively easy to achieve. To offer such care depends on the nurse expanding her or his self-awareness, using effective communication skills, having a genuine interest in other people and developing an understanding of the possible effects of classism, racism and sexism on the lived experience of consumers and health professionals. Without this last orientation, it may be impossible to provide truly humanistic care.

Consumer requests outlined in the second half of the above summary address issues associated with political inequalities. Consequently, these are more difficult to achieve. The need to expand specialist mental health and generic health and welfare service provisions to cater to the range of legitimate needs of consumers around the clock requires money, political will and persevering lobbyists. Even expectations which seem simple, like the choice of case manager (or primary nurse) would—if actually available—translate into uncharacteristic service flexibility. Ultimately this would have workforce implications if, for example, even only 20 per cent of consumers requested a case manager of the same sex and ethnic background.

Likewise, to receive non-stigmatizing services from non-stigmatizing professionals sounds simple. But the acculturation that many health workers have experienced within their profession and within services, indoctrinates them into a prevailing culture that associates certain diagnoses with poor outcomes or considers certain types of people to be 'problem patients.' Political will, money for retraining and restructuring would be needed to develop good quality services that are non-stigmatizing for all consumers. Such political change cannot be achieved by individual nurses, but would require an alliance of consumers, nurses, other health professionals, community development organizations, social justice groups, health policy makers and administrators.

What nurses can do

The available consumer literature has the potential to inform all mental health workers how to improve our professional relationships and provide more relevant care. Mental health nurses need to take such information into account, consider the consumer requests that are more important in their particular service and pursue those that are central to nursing practice. As well as the previous synthesis of consumer requests, the following is a brief overview of practice-related issues that are pertinent to mental health nurses in particular.

- Establish an egalitarian relationship. Some consumers have commented on a 'them and us' perception of the approach of many nurses towards consumers (McGuiness & Wadsworth, 1991).
- Offer structured, flexible and relevant hospital programs (Leete, 1987).
- Do things with consumers. One advantage that nurses often have is to be able to work with a consumer on something the consumer chooses and this helps develop rapport and the therapeutic relationship.
- Recognize consumers' strengths and limitations (Leete, 1987). It is vital that consumers continue to use their intact skills, but it is also important that nurse expectations are realistic and people are not set up to fail by attempting to do something that is beyond them at the time.
- Give specific positive feedback on even small progress made and good things done by individual consumers (Yoder & Rode, 1990).
- Validate user self-expertise. As educated nurses, we have expertise that can be relevant to consumers, but we must not forget that the person who knows the consumer's values and needs best is the consumer (Fung & Fry, 1999).
- Offer consumers time and opportunities to share their worries.
- Set up regular relaxed but focused nurse-led group therapy to facilitate open problem-solving, to offer mutual support and sharing in a safe and structured environment (Leete, 1987).
- Provide information about recovery and empowerment (Champ, 1998). Sometimes consumers are given a psychiatric diagnosis that feels like a death sentence. What they need to know about are strategies that might help them out of their present desperate situation.
- Nurses need to be knowledgeable about psychiatric diagnoses, medication and treatment effects and options. Consumers ask nurses to realize that going through a psychotic

episode, bearing a psychiatric diagnosis, taking psychotropic medication and receiving electro-convulsive treatment can cause psychological harm (Lindow, 1993).

■ Stigma may well be part of that damage. The Melbourne Consumer Consultants' Group (1997) relates stigma to the health professionals' collective delusion that they are 100 per cent mentally well and consumers are 100 per cent mentally ill and are therefore inferior, other, different. Exploration of our values and biases is one way to begin to prevent ourselves from falling into this trap.

■ In community settings, it is important for nurses to know the signs that indicate that the particular person may be becoming unwell. Nurses can also help consumers recognize some of these signs that indicate that the person is on the slippery slope heading towards another episode, and work out together whom to contact and how to get help if such experiences recur.

■ Consider the possibility that people who are mental ill may be more at risk in our society from our collective fears about madness, rather than from their actual psychotic experiences (Horsfall, 1997b).

References

American Psychiatric Association. 1994, *Diagnostic and statistical manual of mental disorders (DSM-IV)*. APA, Washington.

Australian Bureau of Statistics. 1998, *Mental health and wellbeing profile of adults. Australia 1997*. AGPS, Canberra.

Borch-Jacobsen, M. 1999, What made Albert run. Review of mad travellers: Reflections on the reality of transient mental illnesses by Ian Hacking. In: *London Review of Books*, 21(11): 9–10.

Busfield, J. 1996, *Men, women and madness. Understanding gender and mental disorder*. Macmillan, Houndmills, UK.

Chafetz, L., Bride, G. & Lego, S. 1998, Merging the CNS and NP roles in advanced psychiatric nursing. Pro and con. In: A. Burgess (ed.), *Advanced practice psychiatric nursing*. Appleton & Lange, Stamford, USA.

Champ, S. 1998, A most precious thread. *Australian and New Zealand Journal of Mental Health Nursing*, 7(2): 54–9.

Dawson, P. 1996a, Humans, not biological processes. *Journal of Psychosocial Nursing and Health Services*, 34(12): 31–3.

Dawson, P. 1996b, The impact of biological psychiatry on psychiatric nursing. *Journal of Psychosocial Nursing and Health Services*, 34(8): 28–33.

Dawson, P. 1997, A reply to Kevin Gourney's 'Schizophrenia: a review of the contemporary literature and implications for mental health nursing theory, practice and education'. *Journal of Psychiatric and Mental Health Nursing*, 4: 1–7.

Easthope, G. & Julian, R. 1996, Mental health and ethnicity. In: M. Clinton & S. Nelson (eds), *Mental health and nursing practice*. Prentice Hall, Sydney.

Fung, C. & Fry, A. 1999, The role of community mental health nurses in educating clients and families about schizophrenia. *Australian and New Zealand Journal of Mental Health Nursing*, 8(4): 162–75.

Hall, B. 1996, The psychiatric model. A critical analysis of its undermining effects on nursing in chronic mental illness. *Advances in Nursing Science*, 18(3): 16–26.

Holzer, C., Shea, B., Swanson, J., Leaf, P., Myers, J., George L., Weissman, L. & Bednarski, P. 1986, The increased risk for specific psychiatric disorders among persons of low socioeconomic status. *The American Journal of Social Psychiatry*, 1(4): 259–71.

Hopton, J. 1995, The 'political correctness' debate and caring in psychiatric nursing. *Nurse Education Today*, 15: 341–5.

Horsfall, J. 1997a, Psychiatric nursing. Epistemological contradictions. *Advances in Nursing Science*, 20(1): 56–65.

Horsfall, J. 1997b, Some consequences of the psychiatric dis-integration of the body, mind and soul. In: J. Lawler (ed.), *The body in nursing. A collection of views*. Churchill Livingstone, Melbourne.

Horsfall, J. 1994, *Social constructions in women's mental health*. University of New England Press, Armidale, NSW.

Horsfall, J. 1998, Mainstream approaches to mental health and illness. An emphasis on individuals and a de-emphasis of inequalities. *Health*, 2(2): 217–31.

Hummelvoll, J. & Barbosa da Silva, A. 1994, A holistic-existential model for psychiatric nursing. *Perspectives in Psychiatric Care*, 30(2): 7–14.

Krupnick, S. 1996, General nursing roles in psychopharmacology. In: S. Lego (ed.), *Psychiatric nursing. A comprehensive reference*, 2nd edn. Lippincott, Philadelphia.

Kutchins, H. & Kirk, S. 1997, *Making us crazy. DSM: The psychiatric Bible and the creation of mental disorders*. The Free Press, New York.

Leete, E. 1987, The treatment of schizophrenia. A patient's perspective. *Hospital and Community Psychiatry*, 38(5): 486–91.

Lego, S. 1992, Biological psychiatry and psychiatric nursing in America. *Archives of Psychiatric Nursing*, VI(3): 147–50.

Lindow, V. 1993, A service user's view. In: H. Wright & M. Giddey (eds), *Mental health nursing*. Chapman & Hall, London.

McGuiness, M. & Wadsworth, Y. 1991, *Understanding anytime. A consumer evaluation of an acute psychiatric hospital*. Victoria Mental Illness Awareness Council, Melbourne.

Melbourne Consumer Consultants' Group. 1997, *Do you mind? . . . The ultimate exit survey. Survivors of psychiatric services speak out*. MCCG, Melbourne.

Moynihan, R. 1998, *Too much medicine?* ABC Books, Sydney.

Peplau, H. 1952, *Interpersonal relations in nursing*. GP Putnam, New York.

Perkins, R. & Repper, J. 1998, *Dilemmas in community mental health practice. Choice or control*. Radcliffe Press, Abingdon, UK.

Pilgrim, D. & Rogers, A. 1993, *A sociology of mental health and illness*. Open University Press, Buckingham, UK.

Rogers, A., Pilgrim, D. & Lacey, R. 1993, *Experiencing psychiatry. Users' views of services*. Macmillan, London.

Stuart, G. 1998a, Cognitive behavioral therapy. In: G. Stuart & M. Laraia (eds), *Stuart & Sundeen's principles and practice of psychiatric nursing*, 6th edn. Mosby, St Louis.

Stuart, G. 1998b, The Stuart stress adaptation model of psychiatric nursing care. In: G. Stuart & M. Laraia (eds), *Stuart & Sundeen's principles and practice of psychiatric nursing*, 6th edn. Mosby, St Louis.

Wilson, H. 1996, Philosophy and theories for interdisciplinary psychiatric care. In: H. Wilson & C. Kneisl (eds), *Psychiatric nursing*, 5th edn. Addison-Wesley, Menlo Park, Calif.

Yoder, S. & Rode, M. 1990, How are you doing? Patient evaluations of nursing actions. *Journal of Psychosocial Nursing and Health Services*, 28(10): 26–30.

4
Watch your language: psychobabble and other rhetoric

Key concepts
of this
chapter:

- controlling language
- gender and psychiatry ■ labeling
- patient, service user, survivor, consumer
- psychiatric terms ■ professional jargon
- terminology that has changed with time
- words that join and distance

Introduction

Each profession has its own jargon that determines how thoughts, ideas and events are understood and people responded to. Words are particularly powerful in mental health nursing because they are used to define the perceptions and reality of people's experiences. Words, associated gestures and the actions of the nurse also convey power, authority and knowledge that are laden with social, cultural and political meaning. Mental health nurses work in an environment in which their everyday language maintains the values and norms of mental health services (Tilley, 1997).

This chapter aims to highlight how words and professional terminology convey meanings that exert power and influence over people and their experiences. Some words and expressions that reflect the changing and prevailing values and attitudes that have shaped notions of mental health and illness and guided care will be examined. While not a complete or exhaustive review, the examination has been divided into sections:

1. an evolution of psychiatric terms
2. gender issues

3. the language of control
4. terms that distance or join people.

The significance of language cannot be underestimated. Words can be used as helpful tools of validation and understanding and as weapons that can create deep and lasting harm. As Peplau wrote in 1966, 'language influences thought and not the other way around, so what talking to the patient helps to do is correct or influence the language usage of the patient, therefore the thinking of the patient' (quoted in Welt & O'Toole 1989: 258). The nurse who is aware of and sensitive to language and its powerful effects on mental health will choose his or her words carefully and resist jargonistic conventions that can lead to misunderstanding.

Evolution of psychiatric terms

From madness to mental illness

In Europe during the Middle Ages and the Renaissance (until approximately the sixteenth century) people who displayed unusual or deviant behavior were believed to be possessed by the devil or evil spirits. Such people were left to fend for themselves by-and-large or placed on boats called ships of fools to drift along the rivers of their region. During the seventeenth and eighteenth centuries, large numbers of mentally ill people were provided with very basic food and shelter in workhouses along with criminals and poor people. Thus, the ABCs of community response until the nineteenth century were assistance, banishment, and/or confinement (Rosenblatt 1984). In the nineteenth century, asylums built specifically for the mentally ill increased in number and size, particularly in the industrializing nations such as France, Germany and Britain. Many of these large asylums were geographically isolated. In some asylums the insane were placed on display and a small entrance fee could be paid by the public to see this 'entertainment' (ibid.).

The modern era of psychiatric care is credited to have begun in the late 1700s with Pinel in France and Tuke in England who were outraged by the deplorable conditions endured by people confined in institutions. By releasing people from their chains and providing adequate food and clothing, they set out to create a humane environment to protect and provide social support.

During the nineteenth century, laws were passed to put newly professionalizing medical doctors in charge of the insane in these asylums. This slowly transformed the asylums into hospitals or places of treatment, to correspond with the scientific developments of the mid-1800s when madness came to be understood as psychiatric illness (Scull, 1979). Because of the increasing value placed on scientific understanding in this era, doctors became the experts regarding what constitutes sickness, who is ill, and what treatment should be carried out (Illich, 1976).

At the turn of the twentieth century, the work of Freud, Kraepelin, Bleuler and others significantly advanced 'science of the mind' and forever altered the world's view of mental illness (Keltner et al., 1991). The theories and terms coined in this period still stand as some of the most prominent in the field of psychiatry—a domain of exclusive knowledge. Medical explanations of psychiatric illness were further solidified during the 1950s with the use of psychotropic medication (Johnson, 1997). Psychiatrists deemed that chemical imbalances could be restored by pharmacological means, thus making people more controllable and less dangerous. In the 1950s and 1960s, activists came to believe that inhumane conditions found in custodial mental hospitals were contributing to mental illness; and the civil rights movement, along with a faith in psychotropic drugs, led to deinstitutionalization and the establishment of community mental health centers in the USA (Shives, 1998). Other western nations followed and were further motivated by the possibility of reducing expenditure on large hospitals.

From patient to consumer to survivor

In the last 30–40 years, the terms that refer to the people nursed in hospitals have changed. The word *patient* (noun) is the most enduring term used to indicate the person who receives medical treatment and nursing care. Implications that a patient should be *patient* (adjective) or possess *patience*, endurance, be uncomplaining, calm, tolerant and understanding, may also be subliminally associated with the term. However, in western terms, if patience or being patient is related to passivity, submissiveness, resignation, or renders the person susceptible, then being a patient is to be the inferior person in a situation of unequal power.

A patient who receives medical or surgical treatment or suffers from a physiological condition is still commonly seen to have more legitimate health needs than a patient with a psychiatric illness. In an effort to correct the stigmatized position of mental health patients, Carl Rogers introduced the more equal term *client*. This solution not only appeared to help relocate power to the client, it also coincided with the 1960s ideals of deinstitutionalization or provision of treatment for the mentally ill in community outpatient settings. Being the client obtaining a service from a mental health professional implied a contractual agreement between the service provider and the customer or client. The term client was intended to promote more respect and equality, holding both parties responsible for keeping to an agreed-upon treatment.

Other terms emerging from contact with mental health services include *service users, survivors, consumers* and *recipients*. As Perkins and Repper (1998) point out, each label has similarities but also significant distinctions related to their origin. The term service user has been adopted by some users of mental health services (especially in the UK) who are concerned with reform and improvement in services. The term survivor connotes someone who has succeeded in living through the negative aspects of the mental health system. Having survived, their aim is also to contribute to change in political, social and health aspects of living with a mental illness.

The term consumer—similar to client and service user—implies that services are selected, consumed, or used voluntarily. This term is linked to the introduction of general management principles of the 1980s, which have tended to modify the clinical views of services. There are a number of difficulties associated with viewing users of psychiatric services as consumers. For example, they do not necessarily have the same access to clinical knowledge as health care professionals and they frequently don't have an actual choice from among a range of alternatives (Pilgrim & Rogers, 1994).

Because mental health treatment can be involuntarily imposed, the term recipient is used by some to reflect a more accurate position irrespective of choice. Current discussion among consumers indicates a growing dissatisfaction with the term (The Mental Health Services Conference, Hobart, Tasmania, 1998). To consume is to use up, deplete or exhaust, and thus suggests a one-sided relationship that negates a meaningful exchange or transaction between people. A consumer as a customer, shopper, buyer or patron tends to be purchasing material goods, not human services. As acknowledged by many mental health nurses, including Barker (1997a), the naming of people who receive services remains controversial and disputed. Barker (ibid.) admirably attempts to avoid patient, client, user, consumer, or service recipient synonyms and prefers to call service recipients *people*. When there is potential for confusion, he uses the terms people-in-care or person-in-care; which, despite being cumbersome, do provide a more accurate reflection of the relationship between the person and the nurse.

The transformative power of words and their meaning has been under examination in other areas of mental health, such as in situations of extreme stress (Stuhlmiller, 1996). Imagine for a moment that you have been attacked on the street and your wallet has been stolen. Are you a victim or a survivor of the assault? Imagine that you have just been in a multi-vehicle car crash. You are uninjured but a person in one of the other cars has been seriously hurt. Are you experiencing a trauma or a crisis?

These scenarios require some consideration and it is unlikely that a clear answer is forthcoming, even if you have actually experienced such a situation first hand. Your appraisal of the situation will depend on a number of factors. The words you choose for your interpretation, however, carry with them an understanding that will contribute to your overall sense of personal power and future prospects.

To be a survivor is to endure, persist, and come through. To be a victim is to be a casualty and impotent in the face of an external determining event. To be traumatized is to be injured, harmed or adversely affected; whereas a crisis is a turning point that holds the possibility of a range of outcomes including negative and positive (Stuhlmiller, 1996). Caution should be exercised when using the word trauma, particularly if you are assigning the term to someone else's experience. Given the opportunity to explore and select their own terms, people may chose more empowering interpretations that include resiliency, growth or discovery.

From managerial to legaleze terms

In the 1990s, as economic rationalism and the era of managed care began to gain a foothold in many western countries, the term *revenue generating unit* (RGU) began to be used in some arenas to refer to the patient/client. The RGU seems to accurately reflect the values and concerns of business enterprises aimed at providing treatments based on a fee for service and the accompanying predictions of cost containment. This reveals in stark language the fact that business concerns have overridden human concerns and resulted in 'high tech, low touch' practices in the health sector.

Other managerial terms are currently in vogue in clinical settings. Consumers of community mental health care are referred to as *cases* who require case managers to conduct case reviews and attend case management meetings and aggression management courses to ensure that competent and proper control, direction, supervision and administration are provided to the case. The 'caseness' approach exemplifies another means of objectifying the person and reflects the power disparity between the knower and the known (Susko, 1994).

Evidenced-based practice, *best practice*, and *clinical pathways* are management or administrative driven terms and techniques that suggest that only certain forms of knowledge stand as evidence and that people's lives are so predictable that treatment can be ordered and administered through a formula that eliminates sensitive clinical reflection. These terms can be quite insulting to effective, experienced clinicians who may wonder what they had been doing prior to these terms—giving poor or middle-of-the-road care, based on whims? Will the recipients of such treatment follow the prescribed clinical pathway to newly discovered recovery?

Arising in the litigious USA, a patient can be bizarrely referred to as a *plaintiff*, and this phenomenon has fueled an increasing trend for some affluent people to have a doctor and lawyer who are experts on their specific diagnosis. In societies where disability payments can be financially more bountiful than poorly paid work, it is no surprise that financial recompense can become a focus for both patients and professionals. For example, the growing field of traumatology has given rise to expert witnesses who are paid handsomely to claim irreversible damage created by the stress of extreme experiences (Benjamin et al., 1988, Ellard, 1997).

Mental nurse, psychiatric nurse, mental health nurse

In the nineteenth century, keepers of the insane were called *attendants*. They were responsible to the medical superintendents to carry our their orders and maintain the general upkeep of the institution. With the transformation of madness into mental illness, medicine and nursing began to emerge as the surveyors of the mad. In England, the creation of a registry for attendants under the *Lunacy Act 1890*, marks the formal recognition of psychiatric nursing. The title of *mental nurse* was inaugurated in the General Council's Supplementary Registry for Mental Nurses of 1923 in the United Kingdom (Morrall, 1998).

Over the past 50 years, the term mental nurse has been replaced with *psychiatric nurse*. Prominent nurses such as Altschul (1997) still prefer the term mental nurse to psychiatric nurse. She says, 'Mental is not a dirty word; it has a respectable etymology, it refers to the mind. To have a mental disorder is no more shameful than to have a bodily disorder' (ibid.: 12–13).

It is interesting to note how nurses currently refer to themselves. It is often a function of where and when they were trained. For example, there is still a cohort of nurses who have been trained specifically to work with psychiatric patients in institutional settings. They have not been educated as comprehensive nurses and may retain the unfashionable title of psychiatric nurse. Currently, in Australia for example, the term *mental health nurse* is in vogue and the term psychiatric nurse is unfashionable in many settings. Presumably, this development has been aimed at altering the perception of the psychiatric nurse as working exclusively in a psychiatric hospital, and at broadening the brief to include mental health promotion, prevention of mental illness and working with people with less severe forms of mental distress.

Presently, there is much debate about mental health nurse preparation, education, nomenclature and credentialing (The Australian and New Zealand College of Mental Health Nurses chat list, 1999). The *mental health worker* may gain greater acceptance and change mental health service provision as we know it. Preparation for this role would involve basic education for psychiatric work and could dissipate disciplinary boundaries and the focus of care. At the moment, this alternative does not sit well with those committed to the basic tenets of nursing and who believe that the mental health paradigm is far more consistent with nursing than the psychiatric paradigm (see chapter 3). Critical examination of the discourse and focus of mental health nursing can be found among authors such as Barker (1997b), Barker & Reynolds (1996), Dawson (1997a; 1997b), Fursland (1998), Hall (1996) and Horsfall (1997).

Hierarchically authoritative clinical language

Gender and psychiatry

Some recent authors argue that throughout documented history, men are considered to be normative and women aberrant (Hyde, 1991). For example, in the biblical story of Adam and Eve, Eve initiated sin by eating the apple in the Garden of Eden. In Chinese mythology, the yin and yang refer to feminine and masculine characteristics, wherein the yin (feminine) is portrayed as the dark side of nature. Women have also been found to be evil or destructive as witches or agents of the devil (Hays, 1964). From this perspective, men are seen as making and policing societal rules. However, women are expected to follow the norms, but they do not set them (Sharf, 1996). As Horsfall observes (1994: 6), 'When we investigate definitions of normality they turn out to be androcentric [male-centered]; and when we investigate prevailing definitions of masculinities within our society they turn out to be close to the definitions of normality!' These facts play a key role in understanding the ideology that shapes the dominant discourses of medicine, psychiatry, and mental health nursing.

Speedy (1993: 175) asserts that because language is dominated by paternalism, the reality created is paternalistic (fatherly).

> Thus the language of psychiatry (from which psychiatric nurses gain much of their knowledge) is medical, authoritative, male-identified and powerful. It is used to control and regulate women and men in ways that are required for social acceptability in our society.

Chesler (1972) observes that psychiatry reinforces women's inferior position because psychiatry's definition of 'mental health' corresponds to the way in which males think and act. This fact is confirmed through an examination of twentieth century cross-national statistics on gender and psychiatric illness that demonstrate that women have been diagnosed as mentally ill more frequently than men (Delacour & Short, 1992). There are also some medical diagnoses specific to women (Short et al., 1998). An example is dysmenorrhoea (painful menstruation). At one time, women presenting for this condition were considered to be neurotic and the disorder was understood to be the result of improper attitudes toward femininity or non-acceptance of male authority (Speedy, 1993). As noted by Delacour and Short (1992: 19), 'Diagnosis is a social act, occurring within a sociocultural context and at a particular historical moment.' Therefore, medical diagnoses can be viewed as an authoritative social barometer, indicating which behaviors are normal and which are not (Speedy, 1993).

As a reflection of social history, gender traits and differences were considered at one time to be connected to the development of specific defense responses and mental disorders. Men, driven by independence, could develop problems related to the need to be independent. Adler, a neo-Freudian and founder of the school of individual psychology in the early 1900s, believed that the neurotic male perceived himself as possessing the feminine traits of obedience, cowardice and tenderness. To overcome these characteristics, he should attempt to develop defiance, bravery and stoicism (Hinsie & Campbell, 1970). Males are most often diagnosed as anti-social or psychopathic. The psychiatric term narcissism is also associated with the stereotypical egocentric male personality and understood to be a defense against feminine sharing and ego-blurring tendencies.

In many cultures and during many historical periods, women have been socialized to be passive, submissive, and insecure (Short et al., 1998). In European societies, over the last 150 years in particular, women have been considered to have dependent, hysterical (or histrionic) tendencies. Descriptive words associated with females included: soft, suggestible, emotionally labile, excitable, dramatic, sexually provocative or frigid. Psychiatric conditions most commonly attributed to women are depression, anxiety, eating disorders and post-traumatic stress disorder (Sharf, 1996).

Furthermore, until recent decades, women were blamed for personality problems that their children developed as adults (Hinsie & Campbell, 1970) by being either too close and smothering or too cool and distant. Subsequently, theorists have been forced to recognize that either or both parents may be unsupportive, controlling, emotionally neglectful or abusive.

Gender has also been shown to have an impact on the way professionals perceive and respond to patients. Chesler (1972) observed that often women were misdiagnosed because they did not conform to gender role stereotypes held by male doctors and thus received higher rates of psychiatric treatment and hospitalization than men. Gallop (1997) reports that doctors and nurses may agree that a patient is difficult. However, nurses (mostly women) were more likely to consider that patients' problems are related to failed relationships, and nurses will often take responsibility for the patients' lack of improvement and blame themselves for their inability to establish a therapeutic relationship or do more for the patients. On the other hand, doctors (mostly men) explained patient difficulties in terms of the patients' failure to respond to medications or failure to accept the help the doctor has offered them (Gallop & Wynn 1987).

Feminist therapists aim to eliminate sex-biased values and propositions inherent in psychiatry and mental health care. They seek to understand gender, power, and other differences between men and women. They also look for sources of bias in historical developments, sexist use of language and labels, and bias in diagnosis and therapeutic techniques. If mental health nurses can be more aware of the ideologies that shape the dominant language of their practices, they can work toward insuring that both men and women are treated equitably and with human (rather than sexist) understanding.

Control and language

This section aims to explore the terms used to attempt to control other people. The words used are not unique to mental health nursing; in fact they have been honed and enriched over time from multi-disciplinary sources. They are, however, some of the most prevalent words that can be heard in areas where nurses are involved in observing and documenting the behavior of others.

The either/or terms

In mental health settings, people are commonly described as behaving appropriately or inappropriately, being well or unwell, compliant or non-compliant, normal or not normal, possessing or lacking insight, secure or insecure, cooperative or uncooperative. Such dichotomous classifications are out of place in the real world of complex people. Although the either/or terms often only relate to specific behavioral aspects or areas of functioning, the danger is that they come to represent the whole person. The more you get to know about a person, the more likely you will find that either/or descriptions are not useful.

The terms inappropriate or unwell are used too frequently in mental health settings. They are used to describe communication or behaviors deemed to fall outside the norm and thus indicative of a mental illness. The accompanying voice inflection and intonation used by the mental health professional conveys their level of frustration, irritation, or compassion for the individual that they are referring to. Because these terms are merely judgments applied to a wide range of observations, they are vague and not necessarily useful. Such words require clarification, explanation and reflection, otherwise they become value statements that can discount, obscure, or minimize the value of the symbolic meaning expressed by the patient.

Non-compliance is a term that deserves special mention in the field of mental health. To be non-compliant means that the person has decided not to follow the advice or recommended treatment of the professional. However, adhering to an imposed regimen can be antithetical to mental health principles that are aimed at promoting responsibility, choice and independence. Mental health professionals would argue that following treatment plans is in the best interest of the person, yet often the person does not have any input into the plan. To suggest that mental health professionals know what is best for another person is paternalistic and negates the possibility that self-determination promotes self-esteem, control and mental health.

Popular mental health nursing terms

Mental health nurses use the following words to describe the people that they find most challenging to care for: manipulative, argumentative, controlling, defensive, defiant, disruptive, demanding, angry, hostile, aggressive, agitated, attention-seeking, acting out, dysfunctional, treatment resistant, and lacking boundaries.

In a study by Mohr and Noone (1997) more than 4000 entries of nursing notes about psychiatric patients were analyzed for the most commonly used descriptive words. The words were then categorized by a panel of expert psychiatric nurses as either pejorative (negative) or non-pejorative. Manipulative was rated to be the most pejorative word and argumentative, controlling and defiant were the most frequently used. Quiet was rated the least pejorative word, with compliant and appropriate being the most frequently used non-pejorative words.

Mohr and Noone (1997) point out that although some of the words used by nurses actually have multiple meanings, nurses selected the negative connotations for their descriptions. For example, the word manipulative can mean 'to handle with skill,' In the mental health setting, manipulation has negative connotations, when in fact there are two categories of manipulation, adaptive and maladaptive, both of which may be useful forms of coping, depending on who is judging. Therefore being manipulative may be a very effective coping strategy for the person, although not necessarily acceptable to mental health staff or others. Similarly, being argumentative, controlling, defensive, defiant, disruptive, demanding, angry, hostile, aggressive, agitated, attention-seeking and acting out, are all common responses to feelings of powerlessness or lack of control. These behavioral coping efforts, aimed to regain a sense of control or protect a fragile sense of self may or may not be useful. The power to distinguish between adaptive or maladaptive becomes that of the observer who may not have a full understanding of the person's behavioral intent.

In the Mohr and Noone (1997) study, being quiet is judged by psychiatric nurses to be a desirable patient characteristic. However, being quiet could be a response to extreme sadness or loneliness—both causes for concern. Terms used without description, validation, or the backing of comprehensive assessment can lead to ill-construed biases and hasty judgments, to the detriment of patient well-being (Mohr 1999).

Orlando (1972) points out that patients can become distressed when nurses misunderstand their experiences or communications. Therefore, assigning words that denote psychological states from the point of view of the nurse rather than the patient can lead to misunderstandings that reinforce negative patient self-concept or disguise other troublesome feelings. In addition, judgments condensed to single words can prevent gaining a sense of the actual issues that people are struggling to get control over. Verbal and behavioral responses provide help to understand what is going on for a person (see chapter 12). In mental health nursing, behavioral manifestations or symptoms are to be honored for their importance in signaling specific issues requiring attention and help. In the current medical climate, decreased argumentativeness, aggressiveness or demanding behaviors—all considered to be sure signs of improvement and health—may in fact be a result of medication effects, not problem resolution.

Glenister (1997) provides a harsh but realistic critique of the socialization of mental health nurses into the vocabulary and practices of coercion and control. He argues that 'nurse-speak' substitutes notions of care for actions of control, cooperation for conflict, and mental health services for psychiatric surveillance. New graduates become assimilated into the use of jargon and begin to adopt, as part of everyday reality, language that they may have previously viewed as unacceptable. Glenister (1997) advises that the way to stay human as a mental health nurse is to periodically refuse to use the jargon of lecturers, nurse managers and work peers. By disengaging from the familiar everyday ways of expression and exploring from a perspective of strangeness and wonder, the nurse can authentically observe the activities and listen to the language of others and discover the patient concerns that underpin certain actions and speech. Crawford and colleagues (1999) argue that nursing language should be addressed and critiqued in all nurse education and that protocols should be established to improve descriptive accuracy. They suggest that nurses should develop a heightened awareness of the controlling aspects of nursing language through increased opportunities for reflection on practice.

The following exercise may help to sensitize you to the words used by nurses in mental health settings, and their meanings.

Keeping a journal

This exercise can be conducted alone or with other nurses in a clinical setting. In a notebook or on a piece of paper, write down all the key words you hear used by nurses in describing the communication or actions of patients. After you have generated an extensive list that may take several days to compile:

* *Count the frequency of use of each word on any given day.*
* *Look up the dictionary definition of each word. Does the dictionary definition of the word match the meaning intended by the nurse who used it?*
* *Think about how you might determine if there is a discrepancy between the dictionary definition and the word as used by the nurse.*
* *Evaluate the usefulness of each word as it is expressed—how does it open up or close off understanding of the person?*
* *Decide whether there are any words that should be eliminated or be replaced with terms that will more accurately depict observations.*

Labeling

Assigning a diagnosis is a fundamental practice in psychiatry. Diagnoses offer the patient and clinician a mechanism for recognizing and understanding the aspects of experiences that are shared by others. These labels, however, provide shortcuts to knowing people.

As is well known, labels mediate thoughts and determine, at least partially, how people relate and react to the world around them (Whorf, 1956). A label, once assigned to a person, can lead to a number of steps in which social and psychological factors induce or reinforce, in varying ways and to varying degrees, how the person functions in social roles (Link, 1982: 203). If the label is derogatory, individuals begin to incorporate the negative views of themselves based on the unfavorable meanings and associations (Scheff, 1966). Self-effacing labels can create immediate, cumulative and long-lasting damage. For example, children who have grown up with constant criticism very often develop low self-esteem and become overly critical of self and/or others. Chronic mental disease labels also create self-fulfilling prophecies for individuals and families as they try to square the disease label with their expectations for themselves and family members over their lifetime (Hall, 1996).

These prophecies apply to mental health professionals as well. Rosenhan (1973) studied the experiences of eight 'normal' people who were admitted to 12 psychiatric hospitals, claiming that they heard voices (although they did not). Once admitted, they acted in their usual manner and denied hearing voices. The staff inferred all of their behavior to be a result of psychopathology. Consequently, people who were bored and pacing the hallway were reported to be anxious.

People in positions authorized to assign labels to others are powerful. As the arbiters of reality they can therefore describe and prescribe identities and relationships. Anyone using the diagnostic scheme becomes the resident expert, not only on the persons' disease, but also on their life (Hall 1996). A major focus of psychiatry is on diagnosis and cure of disease. Therefore, the links between knowledge and power are firmly planted in science and biomedicine and that is why local, popular, or indigenous beliefs are excluded. This explains why the purported 'objective' discourse around case studies, assessments and medical diagnosis predominate and why the personal, relational and temporal aspects of the individual person's experience of being in crisis are lost (Foucault 1975).

Hall's (1996) critique of the psychiatric model illustrates how medical labels undermine nursing care and have life-eroding effects on people with mental illness who are classified as diseased. She argues that:

1. diagnoses do not consider cultural and self-defined goals or meanings or ingrained patterns of oppression and discrimination
2. positive aspects or strengths of the person are ignored

3. the assumption of certainty and cure is misleading
4. the constricted view of the person leads to stigma, stereotyping and humiliation.

Most seriously, the disease framework creates a pseudo-under-
standing of behavior while creating barriers to actual understanding of the person. When disease dynamics inform the care
plan, understanding the patient as a person is reduced and hierarchical and paternalistic relationships between the nurse (the
healthy one) and the patient (the sick one) are encouraged (ibid.).

Peplau has long argued that the concern for nurses is not the
diagnosis but the person's response to illness. Instead of seeing
symptoms as indicators of disease, nurses would do better to
see them as problem-solving actions that have a highly individual meaning and purpose (Peplau, 1995). In her claim that the
primary responsibility of nurses is advocacy for patients, consideration of their needs, and an interest in the person as having
dignity and worth, she writes, '. . . it would behoove nurses to
give up the notion of a disease such as schizophrenia and to
think exclusively of patients as persons' (ibid.: 2).

Distancing terms

People often use expressions that distinguish one group from
another. 'I am like you: but we are not like them' is an age-old
distinction. 'I am like you' joins people of similar backgrounds
or interests, while 'we are not like them' distances the group
from those who are seen as different.

Civilizations commonly create ways to join some members
and exclude others. For example, one author was raised as an
American Catholic and learned the perceived privileges of such
membership. Catholics would go to heaven if they fulfilled their
obligations of faith; and Russians were anti-American and from
the 'Evil Empire' according to President Reagan. What would
become of people of other religious faiths who would not be
saved—would they all burn in hell? Russians surely must have
the capacity to feel bad when their husbands, wives or children
are killed. What about the Catholic Russians, how could they be
evil and saved at the same time?

Ethnic and religious brainwashing methods of dehumaniza-
tion have been carefully manufactured to promote national

agendas during certain periods in history. Military training is founded on the notion that rank and order must override judgment and reflection. How else could soldiers kill fellow humans unless they were convincingly persuaded that the enemy is a great threat and danger to the welfare of the citizens the soldiers serve. The term 'gook' (referring to a North Vietnamese soldier) became a key dehumanizing word used in the Vietnam War to enable mass murder of North Vietnamese people.

Words used to dehumanize others for the purpose of war are an extreme case. However, on an everyday basis, words are powerful weapons with the same effect of banding people together to create a distinct identity that can been seen as exclusive, removed, or separate from the masses. Words give identity and elicit reactions. Appreciation or disdain are conjured up when words such as the following are mentioned: The Greens (environmental group), Ku Klux Klan (white supremacists), hippies (1960s free spirit life-stylers), vegans (vegetarians who eat no animal products).

People who are different become a topic of conversation and can also become a target of distrust and hate. Schoolyard bullying is generated by identification and exaggeration of a personal characteristic determined to be unpopular. The underdog or object of bullying is viewed as an outcast with or without any peer group affiliation. Occasionally, the outcasts will create their own group, language and special connection, to band against the oppressor.

Name calling is a common means of distancing people according to their perceived worth and adequacy. The name callers may believe that they have special status and are connected to each other through the act of identifying and naming those who are different. At the same time, through the process of discrimination, they distance themselves from the others they have judged as different. There are the 'o' categories of psycho, sicko, wacko and loco (an ethnic twist). There are also words such as crazy, nuts, mental, moron, retard, deranged, demented and insane that are used to describe people seen as different from the norm. Name callers, much like diagnosticians, believe that they possess knowledge that enables them to discriminate between good and bad, or normal and not normal. As a result, pejorative name calling intensifies stress and uncertainty and imposes isolation on the person being named.

Some words are used as terms of endearment. To be considered non-mainstream, off-beat, or eccentric can be complimentary in some circles. To be different is to also be special or distinguished. People with creative talents or insight may possess oddities that capture the attention of others in positive ways.

Much terminology deriving from the psychiatric paradigm is based on the deficit view of the person being labeled, using words that join people around disorders and pathology and, at the same time, distance them from others considered healthy. It is a language of disease and symptom orientation, deviation, impairment, disability, inability, vulnerability, risk and breakdown. Important as it might be to identify problems needing therapeutic attention, separating people from each other based on deficits can lead to isolation and alienation.

Joining language

The language of mental health nursing and specifically salutogenesis (wellness) (see chapter 5) acknowledges that although people are not the same, they have a great deal in common and all possess strengths and abilities. The words used tend to be those that join or bond people through positive commonalities. People have constructive potential, and deficits are viewed as challenges and opportunities that can lead to growth and discovery.

Using words to connect and join individuals requires attending to how people are more alike than unlike. Consider the terms discussed in this chapter from a salutogenic perspective. For example, because all people experience problems but not all people have psychiatric disorders, reference to a person as having a difficulty rather than naming the disorder may promote connection. The diagnosis could be used sparingly or be reserved for the psychiatric record. Perhaps the simple title of nurse is sufficient to identify the person's roles and duties rather than claiming specialization—after all, nursing is a holistic endeavor. While psychiatric terms may provide a short-hand account of people's mental functioning, ordinary language and descriptions are more likely to be understood by everyone.

Reflective questions

Stigma refers to a socially determined state or condition that is considered abnormal, substandard, or associated with disgrace. Stereotyping is a generalization about how members of a particular group or category are believed to look or act. Historically, people with mental illness have been ostracized and separated from others because of fear and perceived differences. Although anti-stigma campaigns and other efforts to break down stereotypes about people with mental illness have been a focus of attention in recent years, progress is slow. Consider the following questions.

＊ Besides people with a mental illness, what other groups are stigmatized or stereotyped?
＊ What labels or words are used to describe these groups?
＊ What effect do these words have on people?
＊ Have you ever been stigmatized or stereotyped? How have you stigmatized or stereotyped others?
＊ Psychiatric diagnoses can be considered a form of stereotype. In what ways can you guard against discrimination and the negative aspects of stereotyping?

Food for thought

Mihordin (1974: 88–89) provides an ironic commentary on the use and interpretation of communication in the mental health setting.

> If a patient says he is ready to leave the hospital and deal with his own affairs, he is actually denying his sickness. If the patient makes something out of what you say that is different than what you intended, remember, they are the ones with the neurotic distortion and delusional thinking. Of course you might feel sad, nervous or not feel like talking, but the patient has neurotic depression, anxiety states, and mutism. If a patient behaves in an unacceptable fashion one day and not the next, you must point out their emotional instability, after all, us normals are consistent every day.

This passage illustrates how the relational context can determine the way in which messages are interpreted. Communication has the possibility of being additionally skewed when the exchange occurs between people of unequal status. The person in the one down position is suspect and less credible than the person in the position of authority. In the mental health setting, the question of authentic communication is further amplified because impaired verbal and behavioral expression is a manifestation of mental illness. The nurse must be careful not to overinterpret messages or jump to conclusions simply because the person has a mental illness.

Notice that the everyday feelings of the professional, such as sadness and nervousness, are assigned the terminology of clinical syndromes—neurotic depression and anxiety state—in the other person. These are words of dysfunction and render the person less than the professional who might have the same feelings.

Mihordin (1974: 88–9) continues:

> Always focus on the patient's problems. Don't look for the normal behavior, anyone can do that and it is a waste of our professional time. Flash your professional credentials often to remind people that you have the upper-hand. Because they are the patients, their achievements do not matter, only their diagnosis which explains everything and cuts down on the time that would be wasted getting to know the person as a unique individual.

The attitude conveyed in this excerpt has no place in the agenda of salutogenic mental *health* nursing. Nursing from a salutogenic perspective propels the nurse to focus on strengths, capabilities, achievements, and personhood. The salutogenic nurse uses words to create commonality and connection. What is possible, what can be done, and how we are similar, are questions used to link people to each other and the world—all are goals of mental health nursing.

References

Altschul, A. 1997, A personal view of psychiatric nursing. In: S. Tilley (ed.), *The mental health nurse. Views of practice and education.* Blackwell Science, London.

The Australian and New Zealand College of Mental Health Nurses chat list, 1999: anzpsych@listbot.com or http://anzpsych@listbot.com. (Homepage for ANZCMHN http://www.healthsci.utas.edu.au/nursing/college)

94 Interpersonal nursing for mental health

Barker, P. 1997a, *Assessment in psychiatric and mental health nursing. In search of the whole person*. Stanley Thornes, Cheltenham, UK.

Barker, P. 1997b, The human science basis of psychiatric nursing. *Journal of Advanced Nursing*, 25(4): 660–7.

Barker P. & Reynolds B. 1996, Rediscovering the proper focus of nursing. A critique of Gournay's position on nursing theory and models. *Journal of Psychiatric and Mental Health Nursing*, 3(1): 75–80.

Benjamin, J., Shieber, A., Levine, K. & Halmosh, A. 1988, The iatrogenic contribution in post-traumatic stress disorders. *Journal of Occupational Health Safety—Australia & New Zealand*, 4(1): 68–73.

Chesler, P. 1972, *Women and madness*. Doubleday, New York.

Crawford, P., Johnson, A., Brown, B. & Nolan, P. 1999, The language of mental health nursing reports. Firing paper bullets? *Journal of Advanced Nursing*, 29(2): 331–40.

Dawson, P. 1997a, Thoughts of a wet mind in a dry season. The rhetoric and ideology of psychiatric nursing. *Nursing Inquiry*, 4: 69–71.

Dawson, P. 1997b, Is anyone out there? Psychiatric nursing meets biological psychiatry. *Nursing Inquiry*, 4: 167–75.

Delacour, S. & Short, S. 1992, Nursing, medicine, and women's health. A discourse analysis. In: G. Gray & R. Pratt (eds), *Issues in Australian nursing 3*. Churchill Livingstone, Melbourne (pp. 41–60).

Ellard, J. 1997, The epidemic of post-traumatic stress disorder. A passing phase? *Medical Journal of Australia*, 166(20): 84–7.

Foucault, M. 1975, *The archaeology of knowledge*. London, Tavistock.

Fursland, E. 1998, Face to face. Philip Barker and Kevin Gournay. *Nursing Times*, 94(24): no page numbers.

Gallop, R. 1997, Caring about the client. The role of gender, empathy and power in the therapeutic process. In: S. Tilley (ed.), *The mental health nurse. Views of practice and education*. Blackwell Science, London.

Gallop, R. & Wynn, F. 1987, The difficult in-patient. Identification and response by staff. *Canadian Journal of Psychiatry*, 32: 211–15.

Glenister, D. 1997, Coercion, control and mental health nursing. In: S. Tilley (ed.), *The mental health nurse. Views of practice and education*. Blackwell Science, London.

Hall, B. 1996, The psychiatric model. A critical analysis of its undermining effects on nursing in chronic mental illness. *Advances in Nursing Science*, 18(3): 16–26.

Hays, H. 1964, *The dangerous sex. The myth of feminine evil*. Putnam, New York.

Hinsie, L. & Campbell, R. 1970, *Psychiatric dictionary*, 4th edn. Oxford University Press, New York.

Horsfall, J. 1994, *Social constructions in women's mental health*. University of New England Press, Armidale, NSW.

Horsfall, J. 1997, Some consequences of the psychiatric dis-integration of the body, mind and soul. In Lawler, J. (ed.), *The body in nursing*. Churchill Livingstone, Melbourne (pp. 177–97).

Hyde, J. 1991, *Half the human experience. The psychology of women*, 4th edn. Heath, Lexington, Mass.

Illich, I. 1976, *Limits to medicine. Medical nemesis. The expropriation of health.* Penguin, Harmondsworth, UK.

Johnson, B. (ed.) 1997, *Psychiatric–mental health nursing. Adaptation and growth*, 4th edn. Lippincott, Philadelphia.

Link, B. 1982, Mental patient, status, work and income. An examination of the effects of a psychiatric label. *American Sociological Review*, 47(2): 202–15.

Keltner, N., Schwecke, L. & Bostrom, C. 1991, *Psychiatric nursing. A psychotherapeutic management approach.* Mosby, St. Louis, Mo.

Mental Health Services Conference, 1998, Consumer comment (Plenary session, September 8). Hobart, Tas.

Mihordin, R., 1974, The nunsuch handbook. *Perspectives of Psychiatric Care*, 12(3): 126–8.

Mohr, W. 1999, Deconstructing the language of psychiatric hospitalization. *Journal of Advanced Nursing*, 29(5): 1052–9.

Mohr, W. & Noone, M. 1997, Deconstructing progress notes in psychiatric settings. *Archives of Psychiatric Nursing*, XI(6): 325–31.

Morrall, P. 1998, *Mental health nursing and social control.* Whurr Publishers, London.

Orlando, I. 1972, *The discipline and teaching of nursing process.* G. P. Putnam's Sons, New York.

Peplau, H. 1995, Another look at schizophrenia from a nursing standpoint. In: C. Anderson (ed.), *Psychiatric nursing 1974–1994. A report on the state of the art.* Mosby, St. Louis, Mo.

Perkins, R. & Repper, J. 1998, Users, survivors, patients, clients. Different words, different meanings. In: *Dilemmas in community mental health practice. Choice or control.* Radcliffe Medical Press, Abington, UK.

Pilgrim, D., & Rogers, A. 1994, *A sociology of mental health and illness.* Open University Press, Buckingham, UK.

Rosenblatt, A. 1984, Concepts of the asylum in the care of the mentally ill. *Hospital and Community Psychiatry*, 35: 244.

Rosenhan, D. 1973, On being sane in insane places. *Science*, 179: 250–7.

Scull, A. 1979, *Museums of madness.* Penguin, Harmondsworth, UK.

Sharf, R. 1996, *Theories of psychotherapy and counseling. Concepts and cases.* Brooks/Cole Publishing Company, Pacific Grove, Calif.

Scheff, T. 1966, *Being mentally ill. A sociological theory.* Aldine Press, Chicago.

Shives, L. 1998, *Basic concepts of psychiatric–mental health nursing*, 4th edn. Lippincott, Philadelphia.

Short, S., Sharman, E. & Speedy, S. 1998, *Sociology for nurses. An Australian introduction*, 2nd edn. MacMillan Publishers, Melbourne, Vic.

Speedy, S. 1993, The search for meaning in caring for mentally ill people. *Australian Journal of Mental Health Nursing*, 2(4): 170–82.

Stuhlmiller, C. 1996, *Rescuers of Cypress: Learning from disaster.* (Book 2 of the International Healthcare Ethics Series.) Peter Lang Publishing, New York.

Susko, M. 1994, Caseness and narrative. Constructing approaches to people who are psychiatrically labelled. Challenging the therapeutic state, part two. Further disquisitions on the mental health system. *Journal of Mind and Behavior*, 15: 87–112.

Tilley, S. 1997, The mental health nurse as a rhetorician. In: S. Tilley (ed.), *The mental health nurse. Views of practice and education.* Blackwell Science, London.

Welt, S. & O'Toole, A. 1989, Hildegard E. Peplau. Observations in brief. *Archives of Psychiatric Nursing*, Vol. III(5): 254–64.

Whorf, B. 1956, Science and linguistics. In: J. Carroll (ed.), *Language, thought and reality. Selected writings of Benjamin Lee Whorf.* MIT Press, Cambridge, Mass (pp. 207–19).

5

Saluting health: the imperative of nursing and mental health nursing

Key concepts
in this
chapter:

- culture ■ disease
- generalized resistance resources (GRRs)
- humanism ■ illness ■ milieu
- pathogenesis ■ salutogenesis
- sense of coherence (SOC)

Introduction

Nursing is the study and practice of caring, assisting, and attending to a person who is sick, disabled or undergoing some life transition, in order to prevent, influence or ameliorate distress and suffering, and facilitate health or well-being. The concepts embedded in this statement provide the foundation from which the imperatives of nursing and mental health nursing are derived. While two paradigms have been influential to nursing—pathogenesis (disease orientation) and salutogenesis (health orientation)—it is argued that the salutogenic perspective is more consistent with the tenets of mental health nursing. To recognize, nurture and honor or 'salute,' the healthy aspects of a person, even in the midst of disease and suffering, is an important nursing focus.

Nursing and medicine: Illness and disease

Have you ever noticed that the words illness, sickness or life transition are used in favor of disease or disorder in definitions of nursing? Have you ever wondered why? These terminological differences help to clarify the disciplinary perspective of nursing as distinct from medicine and other health care disciplines.

Illness is the subjective experience of sickness and involves distress and suffering (*The American Heritage Dictionary* 1982). Disease connotes an abnormal condition of an organism that disrupts or impairs normal physiological functioning (ibid.). It is therefore entirely possible to have a disease but not experience illness, and to feel ill or suffer without having a disease.

Traditionally, nursing courses teach a great deal about diseases, disorders, and the typical physiological and emotional changes that occur in life transitions and developmental changes. After all, most nurses work with people who are undergoing some sort of physiological or emotional health challenge or alteration. This information provides the nurse with the necessary background for understanding causal factors, disease trajectories and general response symptoms.

In turn, the nurse uses this knowledge to launch an investigation into the person's experience of illness to help the person cope. This requires that the nurse enter the subjective world of the person in order to understand their interpretation of the situation and their specific sources of concern, discomfort, distress, suffering and well-being. People experience and interpret their lives according to their own unique blend of biological, psychological, sociological, spiritual and cultural influences. Nurses are thus charged to consider the disease, illness and transition experience in the broad context of the whole person and their total life.

Medicine on the other hand focuses on diagnosing, treating or preventing disease and other damage to the mind and body. In order to identify and treat or eradicate a pathogen or agent causing harm, disruption or disease, medical practitioners search for objective data that will provide confirming evidence for a particular alteration or disease. This concern for cause and effect provides a focus for medicine so that when the identified pathogen is treated or removed, the disease should diminish.

While nursing focuses more on the subjective experience of illness and uses interpersonal methods to alleviate distress and suffering, the primary focus of medicine is on the objective disease or identification and treatment of an abnormality. This is not to say that nurses are not concerned with objective cause and effect relationships of diseases or that doctors are not concerned with the subjective psycho–social–cultural–spiritual aspects of illness, as the overlap is considerable. Ultimately, nursing and medicine each have their own disciplinary focus, along with their respective strengths and limitations.

Medical pathogenesis

Pathogenesis (patho = disease, genesis = origin)—the origin of disease—has long been the central focus of the bio-medical model of western medicine. Isolating and treating disease-causing factors has lead to extraordinary life saving and life altering results. Given this etiological focus on disease, however, our health care system is really a disease care system (Winkelstein, 1972).

The pathogenic paradigm supports the notion that the human organism is one that strives toward balance (homeostasis) and order. When a microbe, vector, chemical, psychological or physical agent upsets homeostasis, neuropsychological, immunological and endocrinological mechanisms function to restore homeostasis. If these mechanisms are inadequate, disease results. Medical intervention is then required to reinforce, enhance or replace the human body's regulatory mechanisms (Antonovsky, 1993).

From the pathogenic perspective, when a person has been exposed to a pathogen this leads to breakdown or a disease with symptoms that create impairment, disability, or a deficit. The person is thereby rendered somewhat helpless in the face of the pathogen. Some symptoms can be dealt with by non-professional traditional methods such as drinking plenty of fluids and resting. More complicated problems require the expertise of medical doctors; and given their extensive education and training about body functioning and pathogenesis, doctors possess specific skills in diagnosis and treatment.

The contributions of medical science are not to be devalued; indeed, few people in western nations would argue against the importance of pathogen detection. Because human conditions are not solely determined by biology but involve a rich interplay of physiological, psychological, social, cultural and spiritual interaction, an exclusive search for biomedical solutions can result in overlooking other important factors that may contribute to the person's health or illness (Antonovsky, 1987).

Within the biomedical perspective, the exploration of coping abilities, strengths and resilience often takes a back seat to the more expedient medical, surgical and pharmaceutical interventions. The effects of lifestyle, environment and social conditions are complicated and involve a broader investigation beyond the scope of conventional medical interventions.

While medical diagnoses may indicate aetiology and point to treatments, they can become shortcuts to defining problems that are much more complex or without a clear-cut cause. The danger is that when experiences are studied from only the pathogenic perspective, idiosyncratic patterns and meanings tend to get lost or are ignored while dominant medical interpretations become entrenched. Lost is the story of the person and the complexities of her or his life that may lead to deeper understanding and knowledge (Antonovsky, 1987).

Pathogenesis and nursing

Traditionally, nurses have been charged with the responsibility to carry out 'the doctor's orders'. Consequently, medical concerns and interventions are often considered paramount to the work of the nurse. To be able to assist and collaborate, nurses must share basic medical knowledge and language with doctors in order to execute treatments as well as communicate them to the consumer.

Consider the environment and routine most nurses find themselves working in. A typical day of an in-patient nurse involves completing task assignments related to medical concerns such as monitoring vital signs, dispensing medications, administering treatments and organizing appointments for diagnostic testing. Assessment, documentation and shift reports are dominated by the medical problem and related treatments. Thus, a significant part of nursing is shaped by medical and pathogenic understandings.

Nurses and consumers alike have adopted the pathogenic orientation in that it is not unusual to hear statements such as, 'I will be with the coronary in bed 5' or 'I am the bipolar in bed 12.' Such reductionist references can be efficient for both the nurse and consumer as a quick way to pinpoint concerns specific to the diagnosis. However, when diagnostic identification begins to define personal identity, little will be noticed beyond the disordered and flawed.

Nursing requires an approach that embraces the concepts of pathology and disease as well as the personal aspects of illness, which include distress, suffering, comfort and understanding. To focus entirely on pathology is to miss the opportunity to have a greater impact on the course of human experience. Care, informed from a nursing perspective, is aimed at not only ameliorating symptoms but also at promoting growth and wellness.

Salutogenesis

Salutogenesis seeks to understand the origins of salutary (healthy) response. This term was coined by Antonovsky (1979, 1987), a medical sociologist who became absorbed by the question of how people manage to stay healthy given their omnipresent exposure to pathogens and stress. Acknowledging that stress is unavoidable and that two people exposed to the same stressor can have varying responses, Antonovsky rejected the hypothesis that health is an absence of stress. Furthermore, Antonovsky thought that the preoccupation with pathogenesis was limiting an all-out search for factors that promote health rather than cause specific diseases.

During a series of research projects, Antonovsky studied what helped people overcome stress. His answer to the question of adaptability became expressed in the mapping sentence definition of generalized resistance resources or GRRs.

Generalized resistance resources (GRRs)

A GRR is a 1. physical   characteristic of an   1. individual
            2. biochemical   2. primary
            3. artifactual-material   group
            4. cognitive   3. subculture
            5. emotional   4. society
            6. valuative-attitudinal
            7. interpersonal-relational
            8. macrosociocultural

that is   1. avoiding   a wide variety of stressors
effective in 2. combating

(Antonovsky, 1979: 103)

According to Antonovsky (1979), life experiences produce generalized resistance resources (GRRs) that are positive ways of responding and adapting to situations. He proposes that the physical and biochemical GRRs include genetic and immune responsiveness to a variety of micro-organisms and stressors. The artifactual-material resources include things such as money, physical strength, shelter, clothing and food. For example, money enables some people to buy specific help that is unavailable to those who cannot afford to do so.

Antonovsky refers to cognitive and emotional resources as knowledge, intelligence and ego identity. Having information can reduce anxiety and uncertainty. A strong sense of personal identity will instill confidence and courage to seek alternatives or adapt constructively.

Valuative-attitudinal characteristics allow a person to formulate coping strategies that are rational, flexible and far-sighted. For example, the attitude 'don't sweat the small stuff' can help to reduce the anxiety of a situation that might otherwise seem large and overwhelming. Interpersonal-relational refers to the person's ability to seek and utilize effective social support. Religious and philosophical beliefs are macrosociocultural GRRs which play a role in helping people withstand or accept unchangeable life circumstances.

Exposure to stress creates a state of tension within the individual which serves as a powerful stimulus that can have negative, neutral or salutary health effects. Successful management of the tension is determined by the adequacy of the available GRRs. If tension is managed effectively, one's ability to deal with stress in subsequent situations may become enhanced. If the stressful demand exceeds the person's GRRs, unmediated tension leads to health breakdown.

Antonovsky (1979) believes that it is not the chemical, physical, microbiological, psychological, social or cultural sources of stress that cause health disruption but rather, the failure to manage the tension created by the stress equates with 'dis-ease' or absence of ease. This idea helps explain the difference between health and health breakdown. Health is both the availability of and ability to successfully utilize personal GRRs and manage the tension, whereas dis-ease results when the GRRs are insufficient or overwhelmed.

Onega (1991) gives examples of specific nursing concerns based on the eight GRRs. She identifies how nurses are directly involved in strengthening each GRR.

1. Physical: evaluating functional ability related to sleep, nutrition and elimination.
2. Biochemical: medication management.
3. Artifactual-material: acquiring needed funds, legal or social work referrals and home visits.
4. Cognitive (knowledge, intelligence and information): education and teaching.
5. Emotional (dynamic yet stable sense of identity): ethical and humanistic concerns such as dignity and respect.
6. Valuative-attitudinal (coping strategies that are rational, flexible and far-sighted): inclusion of the patient in his or her treatment plan and feedback.
7. Interpersonal-relational (social support): the nurse–patient relationship and inclusion of family and significant others in care.
8. Macrosociocultural (religious and philosophical understandings): the person's perceptions and beliefs.

Through assessment, the nurse evaluates the presence or absence of each category of GRR. Nurses use the GRR framework to plan care accordingly. Nursing itself can be considered as a GRR. As care givers, nurses are a direct source of support (Sullivan, 1989). They also arrange to draw upon the talents of other disciplines to supplement and assist. The nurse then uses strategies to strengthen GRRs and/or establish non-existing GRRs (Onega, 1991). If damage, stress or tension is successfully reduced or mitigated by activating the GRRs, a person's sense of coherence will be increased—a concept to be explored in the next section.

Active exercise

According to Antonovsky (1979), specific sources of stress do not cause dis-ease but rather the person's generalized resistance resources have not been sufficient to manage the tension created
—continued

—continued

by the stressor. For example, a person experiencing depression has non-existent or depleted generalized resistance resources (GRRs) that require strengthening. The nurse identifies and helps to reinforce the weakened resistance resource. So, the person with depression may require fortified biochemical resistance as well as emotional and interpersonal-relational support for feelings of worthlessness and loneliness.

Following the example provided by Onega, write down the eight categories of GRRs. Using these categories, assess a person you are caring for in each of these areas. You may find that you do not know enough about the person to make an adequate judgment in some of the categories. Flag those areas for further investigation during your next meeting with the person. Once you have completed the list and identified areas of weakness, write down as many ways as possible that you, the person, and the mental health team can work to strengthen the person's GRRs. Discuss your ideas with the person, their support system, and the team, and together agree upon a fortification plan.

Sense of coherence (SOC)

Antonovsky's interest in GRRs became solidified in a study of women holocaust survivors. He noticed that some of the study participants were actually thriving under objectively difficult conditions. Having lived through the most inconceivable inhuman experiences, these women were healthy. What was the source of their strength, he asked. Through careful examination of a range of possibilities, Antonovsky (1979) found his answer. He named the resource that related most clearly to overall health status, a sense of coherence (SOC). Which, by his definition, is:

> The global orientation that expresses the extent to which one has a pervasive, enduring though dynamic feeling of confidence that one's internal and external environments are predictable and that there is a high probability that things will work out as well as can reasonably be expected. (Antonovsky, 1979: 123).

The three components of a sense of coherence are:

1. comprehensibility
2. manageability
3. meaningfulness.

Comprehensibility refers to the degree to which a person believes that the world is ordered, consistent, structured and clear, and that events and people in the world make sense (Antonovsky, 1979). In translating an exceptional experience such as illness, disability or a symptom into the context of everyday life, people get an overall grasp of the situation and gain strength from understanding it so they can deal with it (Cowley, 1999). ('I understand or comprehend.') The person with a high sense of comprehensibility will understand that things will work out as reasonably as can be expected (Antonovsky, 1979).

Manageability is the extent to which one perceives that there are resources at one's disposal and that they are adequate to meet the demands posed. These include both the resources under the person's own control as well as others such as their spouse, friends, God, history, doctor, and so on (Antonovsky, 1979). ('I can manage.') This concept depends quite closely on the person's physical and practical sense of self-empowerment in coping with their own biology and threats to health (Cowley, 1999).

Meaningfulness relates to the extent to which a person believes that what they are doing is worthwhile, purposeful, and has some significance. People with high commitment to people or projects find meaning in their involvement. ('Something is worth the effort.') The ability to fully participate in the process of shaping future situations provides a sense of meaningfulness. This means discussing symptoms, experiences, treatments and coping mechanisms, in the context of family, friends, personal contacts, and reasons for living (Cowley, 1999).

Promoting a sense of coherence is fundamental to the work of the nurse, particularly in the wake of distressing experiences. Nurses actually explore and strengthen the three dimensions of SOC by:

1. helping the person comprehend what is happening
2. helping them draw on available internal and external resources (GRRs)
3. helping them make sense out of frightening and alienating experiences.

In the roles of educator, resource person, surrogate and counselor, as described by Peplau (1952), the nurse is, in essence, advancing the goals of salutogenesis.

The following excerpt from Simon Champ (1998: 57–8) illuminates how these concepts are central to mental health nursing.

> For me, schizophrenia severely ruptured the relationship that I had enjoyed with myself prior to the illness. My sense of being in the world, my thought processes and, indeed the very way my senses perceived the world would go through involuntary changes. I was plunged at times, into a confusing and frightening world ruled by my own paranoia and delusions. Living with the ever-changing experience of schizophrenia over 23 years has changed my relationship with myself many times and in many ways . . . The nurses I most valued at that time were those who, rather than imposing their reality on me, helped me to explore where reality and well-being might exist for me . . . I have come to see that one does not simply patch up the self one was before developing schizophrenia, but one has to recreate a concept of who one is that integrates the experience of schizophrenia . . . I would like to re-state that the best professionals involved in my care have, like me, opened themselves to the mystery that is schizophrenia. They have gained my trust, sharing and supporting my inner search for meaning and for an understanding of the relationship between myself and my illness.

A shattered sense of personal coherence jumps out of this passage. Simon describes the out-of-control feelings of confusion, fear and ruptured sense of self. He describes recovery in terms of a process or journey of searching, exploring, questioning, recreating, reconciling and integrating 'new concepts into a wider view of self.' He locates the importance of the nurse in dwelling with the frightened and confused person and working toward a discovery of meaning in order to make sense out of the disconnection of self with the world. To explore with Simon 'where reality and well-being might exist for [him],' the nurse must attempt to enter his world to search for clues to help him make sense of, manage, and find meaning in his experience.

In exploring the mystery and uncertainty of people's experience with mental illness, the nurse's personal sense of coherence is also open to challenge. The nurse must maintain a functional level of SOC in order to be helpful and, at the same time, not impose their reality on the other person. To effectively guide and aid others, the nurse must possess a high SOC or be able to convey that life is somewhat predictable and worthwhile. On the other hand, some of the events that befall people are tragic and beyond their control. The nurse's own sense of meaningfulness in life is brought to bear and even challenged when working with people in such extreme circumstances.

The concepts of sense of coherence and generalized resistance resources are intertwined. Having a strong sense of coherence mobilizes the resistance resources at one's disposal. Mobilized resistance resources help mitigate the tension created by the stressors. Effective tension management strengthens the sense of coherence (Antonvosky, 1979). Nurses are resistance resources and set up situations that reinforce the person's sense of coherence or empower the person to uncover or draw on their own sources of strength.

Reflective questions

The three central components that are integral to a sense of coherence are comprehensibility, manageability and meaningfulness. The stronger a person's sense of coherence, the more likely they will be able to maintain or improve health. The mental health nurse helps the patient fortify the generalized resistance resources that are depleted or non-existent which, at the same time, add to the person's overall sense of coherence. After your next one-to-one interaction with a patient, ask yourself the following questions.

- What did I do or say that may have helped the person make sense of their current situation or distress?
- How did I empower the person to identify and draw on personal or outside resources and support to help cope with their current situation or source of distress?
- What did I do or say to promote self-care and meaning in the person's present experience?
- Did anything about the interaction challenge my understanding of the person's experience?

After you identify one specific nursing action that you think may have promoted the person's sense of coherence, answer the following questions.

- Did you notice any changes in the person's affect or behavior following your interaction?
- How might promoting a sense of coherence improve the health status of this person?

Concepts related to sense of coherence

Many other concepts have some connection with that of salutogenesis, such as will to meaning, locus of control, hardiness,
self-efficacy, self-confidence, optimism, resilience, creativity,
positive illusion, and post-traumatic growth. Will to meaning,
locus of control, and hardiness, in particular, will be discussed
here as they have considerable compatibility with the sense of
coherence.

Overall, the literature suggests that people who tend to cope
successfully perceive an untoward event to be a challenge.
Their personalities are characterized by persistence, determination, confidence, an ability to make emotional connections
with others, and acceptance of the limitations of the circumstances when necessary (Tedeschi & Calhoun, 1995). The ability
to make sense out of a situation, along with a positive outlook,
tenacity, flexibility and confidence seem to enable people to
overcome difficult and extreme conditions. Further explanation
of these concepts can equip the nurse with ideas of how to
mobilize a person's resources and strengthen their sense of
coherence.

Seeking meaning in life experiences is an essential theme in
all cultures (Lazarus, 1991). Frankl (1961) described the will to
meaning as a basic human motivation in his investigation of
holocaust survivors. He found that the preservation of self in
such dehumanizing conditions was related to the ability of the
individual to choose. 'Everything can be taken from a man but
one thing: the last of the human freedoms—to choose one's own
way' (Frankl, 1963). The will to live, combined with a search
for meaning in suffering has a powerful impact on coping and
survival.

The everyday work of nurses involves helping people to come
to grips with health problems that are often frightening, traumatic and inexplicable. In an effort to find meaning in living and
facing life struggles, nurses and consumers alike are confronted
with choices related to destiny. Although we are limited by
uncontrollable circumstances, there remains an opportunity to
choose how to respond.

Frankl (1961) describes this 'will to meaning' as a confrontation with the terms of existence. From birth, the person begins
to develop a sense of individual identity, actively searching for

meaning to understand who and what one is in the world (Frankl, 1963). By engaging with the person in this confrontation, the nurse has an opportunity to help the person develop through the process of finding meaning.

People who experience mental illness and distress describe profound existential feelings of uniqueness and isolation that are most often deepened through self or social alienation. Imagine what it is like to feel misunderstood and not valued—to live in a world where you feel disconnected, you don't fit in, or feel controlled by others who send messages suggesting you are evil or not worthy. A person in this situation is seeking validation, understanding, comfort and support in a hostile world where, from their perspective, the evidence is against them.

One important aspect of recovery from mental illness, as underscored previously by Champ (1998), is finding an opportunity to explore the dimensions of experience in physical and emotional safety. Finding meaning in life experiences is a central theme of nursing theory and salutogenic nursing. It is an ongoing process for both the nurse and consumer to confront, learn about and integrate unusual as well as profound life episodes.

Locus of control relates to the extent to which people believe that they have power over the events that happen in their lives (Rotter, 1966). There are two types of control—external and internal—that can be used to understand a person's response to life difficulties. The person who has an external locus of control believes that things outside of themselves such as God, chance and powerful others are responsible for their fate. People with an internal locus of control believe that they can have some direct effect on the things that happen to them. Research studies indicate that those with an internal locus of control tend to cope better in adverse situations because they will act in ways to activate the control that they expect to have. Those with an external locus of control will be more likely to allow others to take charge or let events take their course without attempting to alter them.

Assessing a person's locus of control will help nurses decide the best approach to care. For example, in situations that require health teaching, the nature and level of information given to people should be gauged according to their interest as well as their ability to absorb the material. People with an internal locus of control tend to seek more health information and are more assertive about their treatment (Seeman & Evans, 1962).

The amount of control the person believes they have to determine their outcomes will play a role in the pursuit of health practices including following medical orders, initiation of preventative measures and decision making. In the clinical setting, helping the person become aware of their own capacities and resources, such as self-control over their own actions and feelings, will empower the person to feel confident in responding to future situations (Peplau, 1990). The mental health nurse helps the person gain realistic expectations of their own abilities as well as the situation.

Hardiness is a concept that may also help explain why some people withstand difficult situations better than others. Hardiness consists of the three interacting ingredients of control, commitment and challenge (Kobasa, 1979; Kobasa et al., 1985). People who believe that they have some control over events, who are deeply committed to the people and activities in which they are involved, and accept change as a challenge tend to remain healthier under stress than those who believe that life's activities and social ties lack importance, that they are powerless to shape events, and who experience change as threatening (Sullivan, 1989).

Control is similar to internal locus of control. Commitment is the ability to believe in the truth, importance and interest of who one is and what one is doing (Kobasa, 1982). People with high commitment tend to be involved in work, family and interpersonal relations with an overall sense of purpose. Challenge involves an attitude that considers change to be the norm rather than the exception and that it provides an opportunity to stimulate growth rather than becoming a burden or threat to security. People who welcome challenge are characterized by openness, cognitive flexibility, and a tolerance of ambiguity (Kobasa, 1982: 7–8). The hardy person, despite high stress, will be able to maintain and even improve his or her health status.

Nursing involves helping people to regain a sense of control over what is occurring to them. Hardy people may need minimal support while others may require extra attention to promote hardiness. Although hardiness is a personality trait that usually remains stable, under crisis, hardiness is challenged in all people. The concept of hardiness points the nurse toward exploiting the opportunities for the person to re-establish control, find value in their commitments, and experience success in the challenge of doing so.

Despite the conceptual similarities between the sense of coherence, hardiness, internal locus of control and will to meaning, Antonovsky takes issue with the notion of control as described in these concepts. He believes that the sense of coherence is not dependent upon the controllability of events as much as upon two related factors: that events are comprehensible rather than bewildering; and a sense that events are under some kind of control, though not perhaps one's own (Sullivan, 1993). This differs from Frankl's idea of control, which emphasizes the ability to choose, make decisions, and actively create meaning in one's life, and Rotter's and Kobasa's internal locus of control, which supports the idea that humans are the masters of their own fate. To be hardy, internally controlled and confident is highly valued in western societies; however, in other cultures these responses may be inappropriate, unacceptable or offensive.

Antonovsky (1987) distinguishes between the notion that 'I am in control' and the possibility that 'things are under some kind of control.' For Antonovsky, a sense of coherence may exist in an individual despite the absence of perceived control. A sense of empowerment or participation in shaping one's destiny without the perception of ultimate control is sufficient to foster a sense of coherence. While control and mastery may be thought of as a GRR contributing to a sense of coherence, having a sense of coherence has more to do with the intelligibility and lawfulness of events than the determination of their outcome (Sullivan 1993).

The ability to find meaning, feel a sense of control, sustain commitments, accept challenge, and make sense of and deal with the tension imposed by stress, are resistance resources that have a direct impact on maintaining health. People with mental distress and illness have overwhelmed or depleted their resources to the point of breakdown in health, meaning, and personhood—life's coherence is shattered. Mental health nurses use their knowledge, values, skills and confidence to augment the person's resistance resources and look for salutary factors in the situation to help the person cope successfully.

Conceptual applications

England and Artinian (1996) have identified four interpersonal characteristics of the nurse that will contribute to enhancing a person's sense of coherence. They are:

1. relatedness
2. perceptual accuracy
3. interpersonal competence
4. confidence.

Relatedness pertains to the ability to recognize and energize individuals through their connection to one another. Nurses maintain relatedness through ongoing contact and being concerned enough to find out and meet the needs of the person. This requires perceptual accuracy on the nurse's part and verification from the person in order to understand their sensations, thoughts, feelings and behaviors, and transform them into a meaningful framework for care. Effective communication fosters understanding and validation of the person's experience and reveals their strengths and capabilities. Confident nurses are more able to seek out, recognize and acknowledge other people's abilities. Such acknowledgment and reassurance enables others to recognize and develop their own resources for health and healing (England & Artinian, 1996).

Let's take an imaginary example; Bill, aged 64, was admitted to a mental health unit because of depression following the death of his spouse Betty. The nurse, Greg, notices that Bill is isolated, withdrawn, intermittently agitated and tearful, and is refusing to eat and shower. Greg sits with Bill and offers to help him shower. Although Bill doesn't want to talk or shower, Greg continues to sit with him. After some time, Greg asks Bill to help him understand what he is experiencing. Bill begins to sob and repeat over and over, 'How could she leave me?' Greg sits quietly and allows Bill to express his anger and grief. Greg places a hand on Bill's shoulder and says, 'This must be very difficult for you; tell me about Betty.' Bill begins to reminisce about their 42-year marriage, their children, and the wonderful plans they had made for travel and dining out more frequently after Bill's retirement next year. Greg begins to understand that Bill feels cheated and guilty for not retiring sooner.

Later in the day, Greg returns to find Bill staring at his lunch but not eating. Greg begins to add up the pieces of Bill's story and begins to think, perhaps Bill is refusing food as a means of punishing himself. Greg sits again with Bill and asks, 'When do you think it will be alright for you to eat again?' Bill replies, 'Oh, I don't know . . . it just doesn't seem right.' Greg quickly says in jest, 'You know, this isn't five star dining . . . it might be ok with Betty for you to have something.' Bill, without hesitation, breaks into a smile—as if he is relieved that someone is on to him. In the days that follow, Greg and Bill talk about Betty as well as some of the hobbies that Bill had planned to pursue. Several days later, Greg finds Bill looking at a fishing magazine and he asks Greg if he knows of any good spots to wet a line.

This example illustrates several characteristics of salutogenic nursing. Greg believes that all people possess competencies that will emerge through interpersonal interactions. Greg approaches Bill and sits quietly without demands on Bill to eat or shower. Greg demonstrates respect for Bill by allowing him to control the pace of their interaction and conveys an interest in what Bill is experiencing. As Bill begins to feel that Greg is genuinely concerned, he begins to open up. As Greg learns of Bill's situation, he understands the commitment that Bill has to Betty and feels an empathetic connection of sadness for his loss—a relatedness that Greg expresses verbally and with a hand on the shoulder. Greg listens carefully to Bill's story and considers what relevance it might have to Bill's present situation. Greg adds up his perceptual clues, and uses his interpersonal competence to test out his hunch of how Bill might be expressing his guilt—refusing food. Understanding that feelings of loss, grief, loneliness, despair, frustration, anger and guilt are all part of Bill's complex but meaningful web of depression, Greg realizes that Bill requires time, support and guidance to come to grips with his feelings and make sense of what has happened. Through listening to the story, Greg acts as a sounding board. Through telling the story, Bill begins to integrate his past, present and future. In the meantime, Greg finds ways to engage Bill in activities that cultivate and sustain his interests and capabilities. The focus is on what is possible for Bill, while acknowledging that his feelings and reactions to loss are valid and that his memories are to be honored.

The nurse discovers what personal and material resources are available to the person that can be drawn on to contribute to a sense of coherence so that care can be adjusted accordingly. As a rule, action-oriented activities and experiential education lead to meaningful discovery and involvement in decision making that results in tangible achievement. Repeated activities that demonstrate personal control over outcomes can be used to overcome feelings of powerlessness. Overall, the astute nurse will devise opportunities for people to capitalize on their own strengths and abilities.

Reflective questions

Salutogenic nursing requires the nurse to promote a sense of coherence in the midst of the disconnection created by mental illness. Helping the person find meaning, regain a sense of control, and re-establish personal commitments are the goals of nursing. England and Artinian (1996) believe that there are four characteristics of the nurse that will contribute to this goal being achieved. They are:

1. relatedness
2. perceptual accuracy
3. interpersonal competence (or effective communication)
4. confidence.

Whether you are a beginner or highly experienced, every nurse learns something new about herself or himself in each encounter.

Select a recent interaction you have had with a patient that left you feeling that you had contributed to the person's sense of coherence. Using the four criteria above, examine each aspect of your encounter to discover more about yourself and your skills.

- In what ways or on what levels did you relate or connect to the person?
- What cues did you pick up on about the person, or what was going on that led you to do or say what you did?
- What was the key to successful communication with the person?
- Why did you judge the interaction to be salutogenic?

Add this experience to your mental health nursing repertoire—it will contribute to your own confidence and sense of practice coherence!

Creating a salutogenic milieu

Another important organizing principle that pertains to saluto-genic nursing is the situational environment or context in which nurse–patient interactions occur. The word milieu which means 'middle' in French, and setting or environment in English, is used to describe the people and all other social and physical factors in the environment in which the client interacts (Johnson, 1997).

Despite concerns for humane treatment and improved environmental conditions in late eighteenth century Europe by the proponents of 'moral treatment' such as Pinel in France and Tuke in England, these were overridden by the newly expanding medical profession in the early decades of the nineteenth century (Horsfall, 1997). The idea of using the environment or milieu as a therapeutic tool to promote recovery or optimum functioning did not receive significant attention for almost another century. Following World War One in the USA, emphasis on wellness and manipulation of the environment began as a means of maintaining discipline in military medical settings and was found to be inadvertently therapeutic. Menninger, in the 1930s, advocated a total treatment setting where the institution would be responsive to the patients' needs rather than the patients being forced to adapt to the institution (Patusky, 1989).

In the UK, Jones developed an entire treatment modality focusing on the social interaction of the milieu as the active therapeutic ingredient to create a therapeutic community (Patusky 1989). Jones (1953, cited by Leach 1978: 142) claims:

> . . . in some but not all psychiatric conditions, there is much to be
> learned from observing clients in a relatively ordinary and famil-
> iar social environment so that their usual ways of relating to
> other people, reactions to stress, etc., can be observed. If at the
> same time clients can be made aware of the effect of their behav-
> ior on other people, and helped to understand some of the moti-
> vation underlying their actions, the situation is potentially
> therapeutic.

In a therapeutic community, staff and patients alike partici-pate in democratic day-to-day decision making on matters con-cerning ward activities and functioning. Although the staff hold ultimate authority, emphasis is on patients' self-governance and increased responsibility for living and learning. All aspects of the patients' lives are seen as presenting opportunities for growth toward wellness. In belonging to a therapeutic community, patients begin to feel themselves to be participants in active and productive group endeavors (Leach, 1978).

Creating and maintaining a therapeutic milieu is not only a responsibility of nurses, but requires the involvement of all personnel, including dietary, cleaning and secretarial staff, as well as the multi-disciplinary team, patients, family members and visitors. The nurse provides group leadership and promotes interaction, communication, and structured socialization in order to foster the patient's sense of personal worth and to increase social competence. This requires an environment in which people feel safe and secure without relying on coercive or directive management (Thelander & Ribble, 1997). The milieu has healing potential because situational conditions can be set up to enable people to build on their strengths and capacities.

Although the milieu is much more than furniture, decorations and physical structures, these things are important. Safety measures, cleanliness, harmonious colors, and comfortable furnishings all positively influence the behaviors of staff and patients. Colors such as pale blues, greens and shades of purple are known to have a soothing effect on people (Leach, 1978). Nurses also attend to objects in the environment that might contribute to the sensory overload or sensory deprivation of patients who might become agitated in noisy, crowded environments, or more isolated and withdrawn in barren and inactive environments.

The role of environment is not to be underestimated. The physical milieu generates and sustains subtle messages and impressions about the value, worth and expectations of people, through what is present and what is absent. For example, the nurses' station that is surrounded by wired glass with only a small window where communication can occur, conveys a message of danger and protection. Nursing from a salutogenic perspective requires the nurse to be mindful of environments that perpetuate hopelessness and inability and alter, if feasible, the physical arrangements to promote expectations of hope and possibility. The following story by Simon Champ illustrates the power of the physical climate in contributing to a sense of self, health and illness.

Simon Champ: consumer story and reflection

The language of flowers

Twenty years ago, as a patient in an overcrowded ward my mind was filled with confusion as delusions frustrated my ability to really comprehend what was happening to me. At some stage my parents visited me in the ward. Later their visit from interstate would seem like a dream.

Still, my parents talk about that visit. There was the shock of seeing their son ill but there was also the bureaucracy and conditions of the hospital. Nothing had prepared them for that experience.

Years later one thing that struck me was that psychiatric hospitals back then never had a gift shop. Nowhere to buy a bunch of flowers, a get well card or a box of chocolates. I try to rationalize the fact by telling myself it would have been uneconomical but I think the lack of flowers spoke of other things.

In medical wards, families and friends so often announce themselves with gifts and flowers but visitors to the psychiatric wards where I was a patient came bewildered and, worse, often in shame. How could my son or daughter come to be in a place such as this they'd ask. For back then, for many families, psychiatric wards did not seem places of healing but the end of the road. A place of last resort and great shame.

Nowadays consumers talk about the right to privacy but back then visitors were often thrust into the confusion of the ward and a visit from family or friends was punctuated by the other patients' interruptions. The only place that afforded some measure of privacy was the benches in the hospital grounds on fine days. There was little provision made for friends' or families' visits.

I think the lack of flowers perhaps had as much to do with the stigma that surrounded psychiatric hospitals as economics. The lack of privacy for entertaining visitors spoke of many other things. It spoke of outmoded facilities and wards that were long past their use-by dates. It also reflected the legacy of a period when psychiatry had decided families, particularly mothers, caused the illness schizophrenia. It was still influenced by a period when families had been removed from the treatment plans.

—*continued*

—continued

In Australia, policies to mainstream psychiatric services, linking psychiatric wards to general hospitals, reflect changing views about psychiatric care. There are complex debates about these reforms that are perhaps symbolized for me by the fact that on the one hand consumers lose the beautiful gardens and grounds that psychiatric hospitals were usually set in but on the other hand there are now gift shops with get well cards and flowers.

With the improvements in services, be it in the hospital setting or within the umbrella of community care, mental health professionals' attitudes to friends and families are changing. The consumer is seen both as an individual in their own right but also, where family relations are still intact, as a family member with possibly many other relationships within the community. Good nursing sees friends and family as potential resources in a consumer's recovery where the relationships are meaningful and healthy. Even to be hospitalized should not rupture or damage the nature of relations with family or friends. To this end, a nurse needs to help create comfortable spaces for the continuity of friendships and family relations. Part of that may mean supporting others who are significant for the consumers in coming to terms with any change in the dynamics of relationships because of the effects of illness or the needs of a consumer's recovery.

Culture, healing and salutogenesis

Mental health is not the same for everyone. The mental health nurse needs to be cognizant of the lenses of culture, social class and age that shape values, beliefs, perceptions, and practices that guide responses to illness. What may be considered aberrant for one group of people may be an unremarkable aspect of human behavior for another group. For example, hearing voices from spirits is not seen as deviant in societies that believe in the presence of supernatural interventions in the affairs of people (Herberg, 1995). There is no way that a nurse can be versed in the cultural, social or spiritual aspects of hundreds of different ethnic groups that make up contemporary multicultural societies. Even the deepest knowledge of a specific culture may not help a nurse to understand a specific member of that culture, as some people modify, suppress or reject some of the mainstream beliefs and values of their heritage. Given that nurses work with diverse people, developing cultural awareness through personal interest, respect and sensitive questioning is the best approach to developing realistic cultural safety.

In general, non-westernized and indigenous populations tend to view the person holistically, as a cultural and spiritual being living in balance and harmony with land and nature. Natural patterns and rhythms of light and dark, seasons, migration patterns of animals, and so on, have dictated how life developed and is lived (Stuhlmiller, 1998). Traditional concepts of health and healing have also emerged from spiritual and natural beliefs and include prayer, remedies from nature, and ritualistic practices. Different cultures from around the world have developed ceremonies to treat emotional illness, stress and states of 'dispirit-edness.' There are rituals that surround death (e.g., wakes) that are designed to facilitate the expression of grief and there are rites of passage that mark the transition to adulthood.

There are rituals in some indigenous societies that prepare men for battle and their return from it (Silver & Wilson, 1988). As an example, Native Americans use the ceremonial and purification ritual of the sweat lodge to reintegrate warriors into their communities following military service. The sweat lodge is a dome-shaped tent of heavy canvas with a shallow pit in the middle that holds rocks that have been heated in a fire. Water is ladled onto the rocks to intensify the humidity. The extreme heat of the sweat lodge, combined with sensory deprivation, singing and restricted mobility, brings about altered states that contribute to an improved mental state. In addition, the cathartic process, guided by the wisdom of a respected elder within a supportive community, gives the warriors a meaningful place within the cultural context to be honored for their sacrifices and, at the same time, diminish their sense of isolation and withdrawal. The sweat lodge holds physical, symbolic and metaphysical significance that provides holistic integration of mind, body and spirit (Stuhlmiller, 1994).

Health and healing, in this example, is viewed as a positive process that is more than an absence of signs and symptoms of disease. It involves broader environmental, sociocultural and behavioral determinants and is not restricted to biologic or somatic wellness. In the holistic paradigm, illness is inevitable and perfect health is not the goal. Instead, the aim is for the best possible adaptation to the environment and caring for one's body (Herberg, 1995). This view is consistent with Antonovsky's (1987) fundamental premise that stressors are omnipresent and not necessarily bad. Also, the consequences of the stressors may at times be salutary, contingent on the character of the stressor and the successful resolution of the tension.

Antonovsky (1979) argues that the sense of coherence is universal. He admits that while cultural patterns vary widely (e.g., group solidarity for one culture may be based on individual strength, whereas in another culture, group strength may be based on obedience and passivity), all cultures promote practices that allow members to make sense of the world or develop a sense of coherence for that group. Comprehensibility is a facet of all cultures. Cultural patterns of social organization provide a continuous series of experiences that build up the GRRs that are crucial to a strong sense of coherence, and these GRRs enable people to see their lives as meaningful (ibid.).

The salutogenic orientation is congruent with the humanistic tradition (see chapter 3). Based on the work of Maslow (1968, 1987), Rogers (1951, 1961), and others, humanists view people in a holistic manner—that is, greater than the sum of their parts. Humanism is a European philosophy that focuses on and values the individual person's abilities, potential and achievements. It subscribes to a positive and optimistic view of humanity. From a humanist perspective, the individual person is understood to be characterized by growth, learning, changing and gaining insights relevant to reaching their own potential (Murray, 1991).

Maslow, like Antonovsky, studied healthy people; and they both recognize that people need to feel a sense of meaning and belonging, that life has a degree of order and predictability, and that the basic resources or needs for living will continue to be available. They believe that people with a high sense of coherence (Antonovsky) or those aiming for self-actualization (Maslow) persevere and overcome obstacles as they work towards developing their potential.

The culturally sensitive and salutogenic approach to facilitating mental health is based on the humanistic principles of respect, acceptance, genuineness and empathy in all interactions. The emphasis is on promoting possibility, understanding and caring, rather than focusing on deficits, diagnosis, or giving advice. With a goal of self-empowerment, people are viewed holistically as being able to develop creatively and responsibly through self-understanding. This approach considers that each person possesses both abilities and potential, wisdom and capability. The nurse aims to develop a therapeutic relationship in ways that enable the person's strengths and capabilities to be uncovered and built on.

Respect is the theme that is common to ways of nursing that are congruent with salutogenesis, humanism and indigenous approaches to health and being. Salutogenesis is a departure from pathogenesis in that it 'salutes' or respects the health and ability of all people. Indigenous cultures are founded on respect for the power of nature and the person's place in it. Humanism locates and respects the power within the person to play a part in their own destiny. These are the basic premises of this chapter.

Saluting health is an overall approach to care that is particularly relevant to mental health nursing, where some of the issues that underpin distress and suffering have to do with the person's experiences of disrespect and lack of understanding. To be present, respectfully enter the life of another person, seek understanding, and helpfully guide the person toward wellness are the imperatives of mental health nursing.

Discussion questions

The final section of this chapter makes the claim that salutogenesis and the concept of the sense of coherence is culture-free or consistent with all cultural beliefs as well as the basic tenets of humanism. What do you think?

Discuss the following questions with a group of nurses.

■ What cultural beliefs about health, illness and mental health do you know about?

—*continued*

—continued

- What ceremonies, rituals and cultural practices have you heard about and how are they aimed at healing members of that culture?
- Identify the elements of the ceremony, ritual or practice that contribute to healing.
- Compare and contrast those elements to the sense of coherence, and concepts of comprehensibility, manageability and meaning.
- In what ways do cultural healing practices align with concepts of humanism?
- Discuss how salutogenic mental health nursing differs from other models of nursing that you have been exposed to.

References

American Heritage Dictionary Second College Edition, 1982. Houghton Mifflin Company, Boston.

Antonovsky, A. 1979, *Health, stress and coping.* Jossey-Bass, San Francisco.

Antonovsky, A. 1987, *Unraveling the mystery of health: How people manage stress and stay well.* Jossey-Bass, San Francisco.

Antonovsky, A. 1993, The sense of coherence as a determinant of health. In: A. Beattie, M. Gott, L. Jones & M. Sidell (eds), *Health and well-being: A reader.* Macmillian, London.

Champ S. 1998, A most precious thread. *The Australian and New Zealand Journal of Mental Health Nursing,* 7: 54–9.

Cowley, S. 1999, Resources revisited. Salutogenesis from a lay perspective. *Journal of Advanced Nursing,* 29(4): 994–1004.

England, M. & Artinian, B. 1996, Salutogenic psychosocial nursing practice. *Journal of Holistic Nursing,* 14(3): 174–95.

Frankl, V. 1961, Logotherapy and the challenge of suffering. *Review of Existential Psychology and Psychiatry,* 1: 3–7.

Frankl, V. 1963, *Man's search for meaning. An introduction to logotherapy.* Pocket Books, New York.

Herberg, P. 1995, Theoretical foundations of transcultural nursing. In: Andrews, M. & Boyle, J. (eds), *Transcultural concepts in nursing care.* Lippincott, Philadelphia (pp. 3–47).

Horsfall, J. 1997, Psychiatric nursing. Epistemological contradictions. *Advances in Nursing Science,* 20(1): 56–65.

Johnson, B. 1997, *Adaptation and growth. Psychiatric–mental health nursing,* 4th edn. Lippincott, Philadelphia.

Jones, M. 1953, *The therapeutic community.* Basic Books, New York.

Kobasa, S. 1979, Stressful life events, personality, and health. An inquiry into hardiness. *Journal of Personality and Social Psychology*, 37: 1–11.

Kobasa, S. 1982, Commitment and coping in stress resistance among lawyers. *Journal of Personality and Social Psychology*, 37: 1–11.

Kobasa, S., Maddi, S., Puccetti, M. & Zola, M. 1985, Effectiveness of hardiness, exercise and social support as resources against illness. *Journal of Psychosomatic Research*, 29: 525–33.

Lazarus, R. 1991, *Emotion and adaptation*. Oxford University Press, New York.

Leach, A. 1978, Environmental management. In: J. Haber, A. Leach, S. Schudy & B. Sideleau (eds), *Comprehensive psychiatric nursing*. McGraw-Hill, New York.

Maslow, A. 1968, *Toward a psychology of being*, rev. edn. Van Nostrand Reinhold, New York.

Maslow, A. 1987, *Motivation and personality*, 3rd edn. Harper & Row, New York.

Murray R. 1991, Theoretical foundations for understanding the developing person. In: R. Murray & M. Huelskoetter (eds), *Psychiatric/mental health nursing. Giving emotional care*, 3rd edn. Appleton & Lange, Conn (pp. 15–72).

Onega, L. 1991, A theoretical framework for psychiatric nursing practice. *Journal of Advanced Nursing*, 16: 68–73.

Patusky, K. 1989, Milieu therapy. In: L. Birckhead (ed.), *Psychiatric mental health nursing. Therapeutic use of self*. J. B. Lippincott, Philadelphia (pp. 251–75).

Peplau, H. 1952, *Interpersonal relations in nursing*. G. P. Putnam's Sons, New York.

Peplau, H. 1990, Interpersonal relations model. Principles and general applications. In: W. Reynolds & D. Cormack (eds), *Psychiatric and mental health nursing. Theory and practice*. Chapman & Hall, London (pp. 87–133).

Rogers, C. 1951, *Client-centered therapy. Its current practice, implications, and theory*. Houghton Mifflin, Boston.

Rogers, C. 1961, *On becoming a person*. Houghton Mifflin, Boston.

Rotter, J. 1966, Generalized expectancies for internal versus external locus of control of reinforcement. *Psychological Monographs*, 80: 1–28.

Seeman, M. & Evans, J. 1962, Alienation and learning in a hospital setting. *American Sociological Review*, 27: 772–83.

Silver, S. & Wilson, J. 1988, Native American healing and purification rituals for war stress. In: J. Wilson, Z. Harel & B. Kahana (eds), *Human adaptation to extreme stress. From the Holocaust to Vietnam*. Plenum Press, New York (pp. 337–54).

Stuhlmiller, C.1994, Action-based therapy. In: M. Williams & J. Sommer (eds), *Handbook of post-traumatic therapy*. Greenwood Press, Connecticut.

Stuhlmiller, C. 1998, Understanding seasonal affective disorder and experiences in Northern Norway. *Image. Journal of Nursing Scholarship*, 30(2): 151–6.

Sullivan, G. 1989, Evaluating Antonovsky's salutogenic model for its adaptability to nursing. *Journal of Advanced Nursing*, 14: 336–42.

Sullivan, G. 1993, Toward clarification of convergent concepts. Sense of coherence, will to meaning, locus of control, learned helplessness, and hardiness. *Journal of Advanced Nursing*, 18: 1772–8.

Tedeschi, R. & Calhoun L. 1995, *Trauma and transformation. Growing in the aftermath of suffering.* Sage, Thousand Oaks, Calif.

Thelander, B. & Ribble, D. 1997, Assaultive patients. In: A. Burgess (ed.), *Psychiatric nursing. Promoting mental health.* Appleton & Lange, Conn (pp. 587–605).

Winkelstein, W. 1972, Epidemiological considerations underlying the allocation of health and disease care resources. *International Journal of Epidemiology,* 1: 69–74.

6
Interpersonal nursing for mental health

Key concepts
in this
chapter:

■ health and well-being
■ human change, growth or transition
in illness ■ interpersonal nursing
■ meaning ■ nurse–patient relationships
■ nursing theories

Introduction

According to Meleis (1991), the concepts central to the discipline of nursing are interaction, client, environment, transition, problem-solving, nursing therapeutics and health. Meleis (1991: 101) proposes that:

> The nurse interacts (interaction) with a human being in a health illness situation (nursing client) who is in an integral part of his socio-cultural context (environment) and who is in some sort of transition or is anticipating a transition (transition); the nurse–patient interactions are organized around some purpose (nursing process, problem solving, or holistic assessment), and the nurse uses some actions (nursing therapeutics) to enhance, bring about, or facilitate health (health).

This inclusive definition of nursing highlights the interaction of at least two people and the actions of a nurse for the purpose of achieving change in the direction of positive health or well-being for the patient or client.

As straightforward as this might appear, what is therapeutic in relation to supporting the bio-psycho-social-spiritual and existential aspects of a person with a mental illness, is highly individualized. These aspects of care rely on person-to-person or 'interpersonal' relating in order to more fully understand the distress and determine specific health possibilities and goals.

125

The exchange between the nurse and the person remains one of the most fascinating, challenging and ultimately rewarding aspects of nursing practice. This chapter will explore nurse-person interactions and interpersonal nursing as described by key nurse theorists.

Interpersonal nursing and nursing therapeutics

Meleis (1991: 112) defines nursing therapeutics as the actions aimed to assist people in meeting their needs for health and health care, to enhance adaptation capability, to develop self-care abilities, and to maintain or promote health and well-being. This assistance is provided through an active process of interaction between the nurse and the client. The focus of interpersonal nursing is to make this interaction more effective or therapeutic.

Among the nurse theorists most concerned with the characteristics of interpersonal nursing, nurse–patient relationships, and nursing therapeutics are Peplau, King, Orlando, Paterson and Zderad, and Travelbee. Before describing the relevance of these nursing theorists to mental health nursing, a mini-history of nursing theory will help to locate their contributions.

The evolution of nursing theory

Nursing theory is as old as nursing itself. How best to care, comfort, and promote healing have always been quintessential questions for the discipline of nursing. Florence Nightingale is credited as being among the first nurses to articulate nursing therapeutics in statements such as, 'put the patient in the best condition for nature to act upon him' (Nightingale, 1859). The heyday of nursing theory, however, is between 1950 and 1980. Formalized attention to the development and documentation of nursing theories grew out of a need, in the United States in particular, to determine what should be the focus of nursing in educational curricula. The questions posed by nurse educators were: what is nursing, what is its focus, and how is nursing distinct from other disciplines. Do these questions sound familiar?

Meleis (1991) organized the significant people and events that shaped nursing theory development into the stages of:

1. practice
2. education and administration
3. research
4. theory
5. philosophy.

From the late nineteenth century to the early twentieth century, the predominant concern of nurses was practice—to provide comfort and care to people who were ill, distressed and suffering.

The second stage, focusing on education and administration, was activated by Columbia University Teachers College, New York, in the mid-1950s in an effort to develop graduate programs for nurse educators and administrators. Educators had to consider the roles and concepts that differentiated basic from advanced education (i.e., diploma, bachelor's degree and master's degree). Consequently, nurses such as Peplau, Henderson, Hall, Abdellah, King, Wiedenbach and Rogers, all graduates of Columbia in that era, began theorizing about nursing. Because advanced education in nursing was not available at the time, each of these theorists drew ideas from other fields of study that they had been exposed to (Meleis, 1991).

The research stage was an outgrowth of the attention to nursing curriculum development, teaching and learning strategies, and administration. A means for evaluating, critiquing, and communicating these developments was needed. *Nursing Research*, the first journal of nursing research in the world, began publication in 1952. The journal was designed to report scientific investigations in nursing and aimed to legitimize nursing as a scientific endeavor. As a result, at this stage objective criteria characterizing the scientific paradigm began to be applied to nursing work (Meleis, 1991).

In 1965 the American Nurses Association ushered in the fourth phase of theory growth by issuing a position paper stating that the most significant goal of nursing was to further develop theoretical nursing. Nursing theory conferences sprang up and influential writers with backgrounds in philosophy (e.g.,

Dickoff & James, 1968) began to promote theory development. Meta-theorists emerged, defining theory and its components, and discussing ways of critiquing nursing theories. Theory building and testing became one approach for generating scientific knowledge for nursing. In this environment, in 1972, the National League for Nursing demanded that all nursing schools in the United States adopt a nursing theory to guide their curriculum as a requirement for accreditation (Meleis, 1991).

Following an active period of theory generation between the mid-1970s and 1980, nurses became involved in the fifth phase, which consisted of reflection on the conceptual and philosophical aspects of nursing practice and the premises underlying nursing theory and research. Diversity became embraced and valued. The acknowledged complexity of human beings, contextual variables, and holism called for more congruent and subtle research tools (Stevenson & Woods, 1986). The ties to quantitative research methods subsequently loosened to include other approaches that nurses found more amenable to their concerns.

Since the 1980s, qualitative research methods have attracted enthusiasm among nurse researchers. Alternative approaches to knowledge development such as critical theory, feminist theory, and phenomenology (Allen, 1985; Allen et al., 1986; Benner, 1984) have emerged to enable a deeper examination and refinement of nursing concepts and theories. With the ensuing analysis and understanding, nurses have become even more aware of the need to use frameworks that allow for an integrative, holistic and contextual description and understanding of nursing phenomena (Meleis, 1991).

Discussion questions

What exposure to nursing theory have you had? In a nursing tutorial session, discuss the following questions:

- What nursing theories or theorists have you heard about?
- What do you remember about the theory or theorist?
- Discuss the relevance or irrelevance of nursing theory to your work?

Interpersonal and interaction nursing theory and theorists

Peplau (mid-1950s)

The first 'formal' nursing theorist and undisputed grandmother of psychiatric nursing is Hildegard Peplau. As a nursing student in the 1920s, Peplau was exposed to the writings of Nightingale. She was struck by Nightingale's emphasis on bodily processes and the focus on what nurses should or ought to do to for patients. She also found that Nightingale's task-oriented approach to nursing—revolving around rules, duties, activities, and the 'proper conduct' of nurses—ignored the problems or concerns of patients as described by themselves (Peplau, 1992a). Of course, Nightingale was a product of her time—the era of the Industrial Revolution, with the rapid rise of hospitals and the need for cleanliness and safety.

After completing her nurse training, Peplau worked as an operating room supervisor and later headed the infirmary at Bennington College, Vermont, where she received her undergraduate degree in interpersonal psychology in 1943. She obtained her master's degree in psychiatric nursing in 1947 and education doctorate in curriculum development in 1953 from Columbia University. She worked at Bellevue and Chestnut Lodge psychiatric facilities, with prominent psychiatrists such as Frieda Fromm-Reichman and Harry Stack Sullivan. As a member of the Army Nurse Corps during World War Two, she served in a neuropsychiatric hospital in England. She developed and taught in the graduate program of psychiatric nursing at Columbia Teachers College until 1954 when she went to Rutgers University, New Jersey and developed and chaired the graduate psychiatric nursing program until her retirement (Howk et al., 1998).

Peplau has published two books and over 100 papers. She has held a variety of national and international leadership positions and has been the recipient of numerous prestigious achievement awards. Clinically, she is noted for her advocacy for patients, and she is known for having physically stood to block seclusion room doors and demanding that patients be dealt with in more humane ways (personal communication, 1995).

Peplau's theory of interpersonal relations, particularly for mental health nursing, evolved mainly from the interpersonal orientation of H. S. Sullivan, the humanistic perspective of Maslow, and the personality theory of Miller. Sullivan was trained as a classical Freudian analyst, but as he developed his interpersonal theory, he came to rely more on concepts from the social sciences than psychoanalytic theories (Peplau, 1992b). Maslow studied mental illness through a study of mental health—the opposite of analytical theorists. He believed that the person was always in the process of developing potentialities to better or self-actualize (Maslow, 1970). Miller's work focused on the principles of social learning (Howk et al. 1998). Drawing on these works, Peplau aimed to have the nurse move away from a disease orientation to one whereby the psychological meanings of events, feelings and behaviors could be explored and incorporated into nursing interventions.

Peplau's theory is based on psychodynamics or 'being able to understand one's own behavior to help others identify felt difficulties, and to apply the principles of human relations to the problems that arise at all levels of experience' (1952: xi). The emphasis is on getting to know the patient but, more importantly, knowing oneself. Fundamental to psychodynamic nursing are the concepts of interpersonal relations, which are embedded in the various phases of the nurse–patient relationship. Originally, Peplau outlined four phases: orientation, identification, exploitation and resolution (1952). Because each phase overlaps and interlocks, in later writings Peplau combined the identification and exploitation phase into the working phase.

Peplau's phases of the nurse–patient relationship. During the *orientation phase*, an individual has become aware of a health problem and professional assistance is sought. During this phase, the nurse introduces herself or himself and becomes involved in an exchange, exploring the problem from the patient's perspective and determining what can be done given boundaries and roles. During this encounter, the nurse either conveys receptivity and interest, or fails to do so (Peplau, 1997: 164). The initial meeting makes a great deal of difference to the health outcome of the patient and is partially determined by how the nurse feels about helping others. For example, does it make a difference if someone is admitted at the end of a shift when the nurse is tired and wants to go home? In the orientation phase, full participation of the patient in exploring the facts and decisions in their life will help them to locate their illness in a life context.

Movement to the *identification phase* occurs when the patient's impressions of their illness are somewhat clarified and they begin to respond positively to people who seem to offer the help they need. For example, they may take on the attitudes of cheerfulness, optimism and problem solving as they identify with nurses who are themselves optimistic and helpful in assisting in solving problems. The nurse permits exploration of feelings so that the illness experience can be survived and positive aspects of the personality can be strengthened (Peplau, 1952).

The *exploitation phase* is typified by the patient taking full advantage of the help being offered through the relationship. As certain goals are reached, new goals are identified. This phase overlaps with the identification and resolution phase of the nurse–patient relationship. Power shifts from the nurse to the patient as the patient begins to focus on new goals (ibid. 1952).

The *resolution phase* entails the patient and nurse relinquishing ties to each other (ibid. 1952). Nurses help the patient to re-organize himself or herself by reflecting on what has occurred and what is possible for the future. The ability to conduct other interdependent and meaningful relationships of the person's own choosing is explored in this phase.

Peplau's idea of roles in the nurse–patient relationship. Throughout the various stages of the nurse–patient relationship, the nurse takes on different roles as stranger, resource, teacher, leader, surrogate and/or counselor (Peplau, 1952). The first role is that of stranger. Because most often the nurse and patient will not know each other, common courtesy, acceptance, and emotional support is to be extended. In the role of resource person, the nurse helps the patients interpret their illness and plan of treatment, and answers questions. The skill of the nurse is to determine what style and approach to education will be most beneficial—be it factual, experiential or counseling.

The teaching role is the combination of all roles and 'always proceeds from what the patient knows and it develops around his interest in wanting and being able to use additional medical information' (Peplau, 1952: 48). In later writings, Peplau expands on the role of teacher to include instructional teaching or information giving and experiential teaching, using the experience of the learner to develop learning (Howk et al., 1998).

Leadership functions of nurses are directed towards open discussion and participation in shared decision making. This means that patients are treated with dignity, respect and worth as the nurse gathers information about what the patient is experiencing and helps the patient meet the situation at hand. Leadership in nursing requires an understanding of the interpersonal dynamics of the nurse–patient relationship (Peplau, 1952).

Surrogate roles in nursing often occur spontaneously. Being a surrogate means to stand in for another person. The patient may identify with the nurse in a particular way that symbolizes a prior relationship. For example, a nurse may remind the patient of a mother, brother, teacher, friend, enemy or lover, toward whom the patient has a range of feelings. In the surrogate role, the nurse helps the patient become aware of the similarities and differences between the nurse and the person of whom they are reminded.

> Permitting the patient to re-experience feelings in new situations of helplessness, but with professional acceptance and attention that provokes personality development, requires a relationship in which the nurse recognizes and responds in a variety of surrogate roles.
> (Peplau, 1952: 57)

Nurses in the counselor role facilitate conditions that enable patients to reveal their problems to themselves and others so they might be able to re-experience the feelings and view their difficulties in a new way or from a new perspective (Peplau, 1952: 61). Counselling functions in nursing include helping the patient understand the conditions required for health, providing those conditions when possible, identifying threats to health, and using the evolving interpersonal relationship to facilitate learning. Listening and other interpersonal techniques used by the nurse will help the patient understand and notice what is occurring in the current encounter so that the techniques can be integrated with and applied to interpersonal interactions outside the mental health setting. The role of the counselor is central to mental health nursing.

Peplau acknowledges that nurses have other roles as well (e.g., consultant, tutor, safety agent, mediator, administrator, recorder, observer and researcher). However, the roles outlined here are the most relevant to understanding interpersonal relations in nursing.

Reflective questions

Peplau describes the multiple roles of the nurse as stranger, resource person, teacher, leader, surrogate and counselor. Think about your experiences as a nurse and explore the following questions.

■ Can you relate to the roles identified by Peplau? Give examples.
■ Are there any other roles, not identified by Peplau, that you think should be included?
■ How do you think the roles of the nurse may change within the phases of the nurse–patient relationship?

While the ideas espoused by Peplau are central to the authors of this book, her work has been critiqued and criticized. Regardless, Peplau's work has had a far-reaching impact on nurses around the world. In the main, however, we believe that Peplau's basic concepts and practices are sound and consistent with effective mental health nursing that values both patients and nurses as people.

Other nurse theorists—specifically, King, Orlando, Travelbee, and Paterson and Zderad—also consider that interpersonal dynamics are central to nursing. They share similar concepts and assumptions, yet the focus and emphasis of each theorist varies to some extent. Several nursing transactions will be examined using different theoretical perspectives after a brief overview.

King (mid-1960s)

Imogene King graduated from a hospital school of nursing in 1945, obtained her baccalaureate degree in nursing education in 1948, master's degree in nursing in 1957, and doctoral degree in education from Columbia Teachers College in 1961. Much of King's career has been spent as an educator. Her theoretical framework for nursing 'goal attainment' was influenced by the systems theory of von Bertalanffy. King set out to explain the complexity of the organized whole in which nurses are expected to function. Systems theory is best illustrated by present-day views of ecology that acknowledge that all aspects of our environment—land, water, air, plants, butterflies, birds, animals and humans and our creations—have an impact on each other. When applied to people, systems theory acknowledges the interconnectedness of all people in a person's milieu, and all life experiences. Systems theory is most evident in some contemporary forms of family therapy wherein the therapist works with all family members to bring about change in the family system to improve both the patient's well-being and ultimately everybody else's as well.

Because nurses interact with individuals (personal systems), groups and families (interpersonal systems), and communities (social systems), King proposed that a general systems framework could be used to make explicit the focus of nursing care. The components of a systems theory include goals, structure, functions, resources and decision making. If 'the goal of nursing is to help individuals and groups attain, maintain, and restore health' (King 1971: 84), then nurses must understand the dynamic interaction between systems, including the varying goals, values and resources at each level, in order to set goals and agree on the means to attain the goals (King, 1996).

Central to King's theory is the view that communication is an essential process required for effective goal attainment (DeHowitt, 1992). The nurse acts, reacts, interacts and transacts to set mutual goals, plans to provide alternative means to achieve goals, and evaluates to determine if the goal was obtained (Sieloff et al., 1998). The present meaning of the situation and perceptions of goals, needs and values of both nurse and patient will significantly influence the interaction and indeed the outcomes.

Orlando (1960s)

Ida Jean Orlando's theory was prompted by the change in curriculum of the Yale University School of Nursing in the mid-

1950s when psychiatric concepts were integrated into the entire curriculum. Influenced by Peplau, she was concerned that nursing might become dictated to by organizational demands and not patient needs. Like Peplau, she focused on nurse–patient interactions aimed to clarify and resolve problematic situations.

Orlando (1961: 339) proposed that:

> Nursing responses to patients are based upon observations of the patient's verbal or nonverbal behavior and are influenced by perceptions, thoughts, and feelings related to the patients' action that prompt the nurses reaction or vice versa.

Nursing actions include a continuous process of reflection as the nurse aims to explore observed behavior, share perceptions, and validate the meanings with the patient. Exploring, sharing and validating perceptions helps to minimize misinterpretations and enhance understanding of our own and others' actions and reactions (Schmieding, 1987).

Nurses deal with the needs of a patient in an illness situation by engaging in immediate exploration of the patient's perceptions, thoughts and feelings (Orlando, 1961: 65). When nurses supportively explore these personal and interpersonal actions, the patient experiences insight into feelings and behaviors, which may then improve. When the patients' interpersonal needs are met, they feel safe, they are likely to feel a sense of adequacy, and therefore are less inclined to feel helpless or continue to express extreme distress.

Travelbee (1960s)

While undertaking her master's degree at Yale University, Joyce Travelbee was influenced by the theory of Orlando. Travelbee also credits May (1958), a prominent existential theorist, and Frankl (1963), an originator of existential psychotherapy, with influencing her theory. According to Travelbee (1971: 7):

> Nursing is an interpersonal process whereby the professional nurse practitioner assists an individual, family, or community to prevent or cope with the experience of illness and suffering and, if necessary, to find meaning in these experiences.

Each nursing encounter has the potential for exploring meaning and being helpful.

Because nurses work with people who suffer and experience pain, the nurse must aim to understand the patients' suffering. Therefore, nurses should not shy away from being connected with patients. Human relationships help people to cope with suffering (Meleis, 1991). In establishing a human-to-human relationship, the nurse and patient progress through stages that include the original encounter, emerging identities, empathy, and sympathy, and eventually rapport. A person's attitude toward suffering will contribute to how effectively they cope with illness (Travelbee, 1971).

Paterson and Zderad (1970s)

Josephine Paterson (with a background in public health) and Loretta Zderad (in psychiatric nursing) taught graduate students together while they were completing their doctoral studies in the 1960s. Their theory evolved in the 1970s while observing clinicians and teaching a hospital course on humanistic nursing. They were concerned with what goes on between a nurse and a patient and focused on the significance of continuous growth of the nurse through interaction. For Paterson and Zderad, nursing is a lived dialogue that incorporates an intersubjective transaction in which a nurse and patient meet, relate, and are totally present in ways that include intimacy and mutuality (Paterson & Zderad, 1970–1971).

> Nursing brings a person together with a nurse because of the call of that person for help and the response of the nurse. The encounter is influenced by all other human beings in the patients' and nurses' lives and by other things, whether ordinary objects (such as utensils, clothes, furniture) or special objects (such as life-sustaining equipment). The dialogue during these encounters occurs in a time frame as experienced by both partners. When there is synchronicity in timing, the inter-subjective dialogue is enhanced.
> (Meleis, 1991: 349)

Paterson and Zderad's theory was influenced significantly by existentialism and phenomenology. Existentialists (e.g., Frankl, see chapter 5) aim to understand what it means to be fully human and find meaning in existence. Phenomenologists (following Husserl's philosophy) seek the foundations of knowledge in human experience. Paterson and Zderad deem that

Table 6.1 Main concepts of different nurse theorists

Theorist	Definition and goal of nursing therapeutics	Nurse–patient relations and nursing
Peplau	Nursing is a therapeutic, educative, goal-directed, mutual growth-promoting interpersonal process between a nurse and patient, with an aim toward stimulating movement toward health. Psychodynamic nursing is being able to understand one's own behavior to help others identify felt difficulties, and to apply principles of human relations to the problems that arise at all levels of experience.	The nurse–patient relationship is an interpersonal field, which can be examined as a basis for greater self-understanding and learning. It is likely that the nursing process is educative and therapeutic when the nurse and patient can come to know and respect each other as people who are alike, and yet different, and as people who share in the solution of problems.
King	Nursing is a process of human interaction (action, reaction, interaction and transaction) between a nurse and client whereby each perceives the other in the situation and through communication; they set goals, explore means, and agree on the means to achieve goals. Their actions indicate movement toward goal achievement, to maintain, restore and promote health.	Nursing therapeutics involve a process of perception and communication between person and environment and between person and person, represented by verbal and non-verbal behaviors that are goal oriented transactions that involve informing, sharing, setting of mutual goals, and participation in decision about goals and means.
Orlando	Nursing is responsive to individuals who suffer or anticipate a sense of helplessness. The avoiding, relieving, diminishing or curing the individual's sense of helplessness, finding out and meeting the patient's immediate need for help. The goal of nursing is an increased sense of well-being, increase in ability, adequacy in better care of self, and improvement in patient's behavior.	Nursing therapeutics involve the direct function of initiating a process of helping the patients express the specific meaning of their behavior in order to ascertain the reason for their distress, and helping the patient explore the distress in order to ascertain the help he or she requires so that the distress may be relieved; the indirect function is calling for the help of others.
Paterson and Zderad	Nursing is a human discipline involving one human being helping another in an inter-human and inter-subjective transaction that contains all of the human potential and limitations of each unique participant. Humanistic nursing is a goal in itself; that is, to help patients and self to develop human potential and to come toward health and well-being through choice and inter-subjectivity.	Nursing therapeutics involves a dialogue of being and doing, providing nurturing and comfort for improved well-being. Nurse–patient experience is an intersubjective transaction with empathy, involvement and an active presence. To provide nurturing and comfort involves experiencing, reflecting and conceptualizing. Nurses offer alternatives, support responsible choosing, share self, knowledge and experience.

—continued

Table 6.1 *Continued*

Theorist	Definition and goal of nursing therapeutics	Nurse–patient relations and nursing
Travelbee	Nursing is an interpersonal process and service vitally concerned with change and influence of others; an interpersonal process whereby the nurse assists an individual or family to prevent, cope with the experience of illness and suffering; and if necessary, assist the individual or family to find meaning in these experiences, with the ultimate goal being presence of hope.	The nurse–patient relationship is an experience between an individual in need of the services of a nurse and a nurse for the purpose of meeting the needs of the individual. Nursing therapeutics require use of self, disciplined intellectual approach to patient problems, and helping patients find meaning in their experiences.

nurse self-awareness influences patient progress; thus, nurses should aim to experience therapeutic interactions as meaningful for both self and patient. Of the five phases of phenomenological nursology (study of nursing) that they propose (Paterson, 1971), the second phase, the 'nurse knowing of the other intuitively,' may be most relevant to mental health nursing. By seeing the world through the eyes of the patient, the nurse becomes an empathic and therapeutic insider.

Table 6.1, adapted from Meleis (1991), outlines the main concepts of the nurse theorists as a quick reference guide for clinical application.

Keeping a journal

All nurses are theorists. Nurses draw on personal, professional, disciplinary, and scientific concepts and theories to assess and plan the focus and goals of care. Underpinning each nursing action is a personal belief and rationale for the action taken. This exercise is aimed at uncovering and making explicit your own ideas or theories about nursing. The exercise can be carried out by yourself in a journal or with a group of nurses on a big sheet of paper. Following the examples of the nurse theorists discussed in this chapter, generate your own theoretical framework for mental health nursing.

—continued

—*continued*

- *Write down in one sentence your definition of nursing.*
- *Identify several goals of nursing.*
- *Define what the nurse–patient relationship consists of.*
- *Describe in one or two sentences what nursing therapeutics are.*
- *Using your newly generated theoretical framework for mental health nursing, examine the care of a patient that you are currently working with and describe how your care is organized around your theoretical concepts.*

Nursing transactions

Scenario 1

Wendy's situation. Fourteen-year-old Wendy was carried into the local hospital emergency room by her stepfather at 11:30 on a Sunday night, having been found by her younger sister collapsed on the bathroom floor. Unable to stand or sit up unaided, Wendy was semi-responsive, mumbling something unintelligible over and over. She seemed frightened and upset, although extremely lethargic. Vital signs were taken and bloods were drawn for toxicology. The tests revealed that Wendy had high levels of a prescription analgesic in her system and that the peak levels were lethal. A gastric lavage was performed immediately and Wendy was held overnight for observation. Her vital signs had returned to normal in the morning and when questioned about the pills, Wendy responded hesitantly that she had had a really bad headache, the worst ever, and that she thought that these pills (used by her brother following his dental surgery) would stop the pain. She began sobbing and turned her face into the pillow. The rest of the morning, Wendy remained quiet until her stepfather returned to pick her up.

Brad's response. Brad, the nurse who admitted Wendy, took the vital signs and a brief 'on the run' history. The stepfather reported that Wendy had refused dinner, spent the evening in her room blasting music and arguing with a schoolmate on the telephone. Brad's primary concern was to stabilize her vitals and find the cause of Wendy's problem, as she was beginning to lose consciousness. Brad had to work quickly and independently, as all other staff were involved in a multi-vehicle car crash. When Brad went to draw the blood, he noticed that Wendy had several burn scars on her forearm which seemed familiar to him. Yes, nearly a year ago Brad had treated Wendy for burns. At that time, Wendy said that she had been trying to fix her butane curling iron when it had exploded on her. Brad began to put the stories together and thought, 'Self-harm. How could this be; she is so young and pretty? If she is self-harming, it's for attention—besides, attention seekers deserve what they get!' Brad followed the procedure for poisoning, charted his suspicion of an intentional overdose and decided that someone else could deal with it—he would rather attend to the accident victims in the next room who were not responsible for their injuries!

Theoretical examination. From King's perspective, Brad would think about Wendy in the context of having personal, interpersonal and social concerns with varying goals and aspirations. Wendy is a teenager with issues relevant to her age, such as peer acceptance and other adolescent transitions. She is a member of a family which includes her place in the family system and relationships with a sister, brother, stepfather, and possibly others whom Brad does not know about. She is a member of a larger community which includes her schoolmates, one of whom she has been arguing with.

Brad knows very little about the circumstances of her relationships. For example, does her stepfather resent her, is he hurtful to her, or over-protective? Is the schoolmate, with whom she has been arguing, someone who spread an ugly rumor that has led to ridicule and bullying? She has ingested pain-killers, which signals some kind of pain. Whether her pain is experienced physically, psychologically, or both, Brad does not know. The levels ingested are potentially lethal. Is this by intention or accident? She is reported to have skipped dinner. This in itself may or may not be remarkable. She also appears frightened and upset, mumbling something repeatedly and the next day, is sobbing. Brad notices the scars and begins to add up a story. Is it a reasonable conclusion?

Brad's immediate goal is clear: to provide emergency care. However, Wendy has provided many cues of distress that beg for interpersonal nursing. From King's perspective, this requires that Brad check out his perceptions with Wendy and her family, and together set some goals such as adjustment to stressors, for example. This cannot be achieved if Brad fails to explore this situation further. Therapeutic nursing has been halted with Brad's unilateral decision that self-harming 'attention seekers' are not worthy of his care.

Taking the Paterson and Zderad approach, the emphasis shifts to the intersubjective meaning whereby Brad would put himself in Wendy's place and attempt to understand her situation, distress, and need for nurturing, comfort and empathy. After all, the root meaning for nursing is nurturing! Brad would attempt to recall his teenage years and challenges in living. He might recall occasions of pain and what kinds of help or nurturing he might have wanted. An interpersonal dialogue that includes intimacy, mutuality and the potential for growth, despite the limitations of the present emergency situation, has not been realized.

Scenario 2

Karen's situation. Thirty-five-year-old Karen was scheduled to receive outpatient wound debridement on her hand following a fireworks accident on New Year's Eve. Karen just happened to be in the path of some sparklers that had been lit and tossed aside and landed on her. The burns were deep, creating nerve damage; so while the procedure of removing the dead flesh was not too painful, the wound was nonetheless grotesque and the procedure upsetting.

Karen, herself a nurse, had worked a double shift on New Year's Eve and wanted to go home. Her work colleague with whom she shared a ride had promised, 'We'll only stop in for one drink and then leave.' Now she was having to arrange her life around burn treatments, skin grafting and plastic surgery—not the way to start a New Year!

On her first visit, Vicki, the burns nurse, performed a careful but expedient debridement. She was all action and no talk. At the end of the treatment she left the room saying, 'I will be back to do the bandage, just stay here.' Karen waited, thinking that Vicki would return in 5–10 minutes. After 30 minutes had passed, Karen, contemplating her soon to be permanently scarred hand, began thinking about the infection she could pick up in the office while waiting to be bandaged. In fact, she had just heard a report to that effect on *60 Minutes* (television program). She went out to inquire about the delay and exclaimed to the staff, 'Vicki took off and left me; does that mean I should finish up myself?'. Vicki returned immediately to the room with a cold glare in her eyes and said, 'You know, you're not the only one around here. I went to get you a bandage and had to attend to an emergency as I was coming back.'

Vicki's response. Vicki, having worked a seven-day stretch, had 12 more scheduled treatments to complete before she was due to pick up her eight-year-old son and attend a parent–teacher meeting concerning his aggressive behavior. As Vicki assessed each case, she tried to work out how she was going to get everything done in time. She decided to double her efforts and work on two treatments at the same time. She said very little to Karen during the procedure as she didn't want to get involved in any chatty conversations that would distract her or keep her from getting away quickly to attend to the other patient. Furthermore, she already felt nervous and anxious, knowing that Karen was a fellow nurse. As she worked on Karen's injuries, she thought to herself, 'There is something about this woman that I don't like. I feel like she is evaluating my every move.'

When Vicki finished the procedure, she went out to get some larger bandages and told Karen to stay put. On the way to the supply cupboard, she looked into the room of the other person she was treating. She noticed some fresh blood coming from the patient's wound and decided she had better deal with it and that Karen could wait. After what seemed to be a short time, she heard Karen out in the hall assertively announcing that 'Vicki had left her.' Vicki thought to herself, 'I was right, Karen is one of those impatient know-it-alls!'

Theoretical examination. Using Peplau's lens of analysis, Vicki has bypassed the basic steps of interpersonal nursing. She has not introduced herself, outlined the procedure, checked out Karen's perspective, revealed her need to keep on schedule, or agreed upon how they might work together to meet the situational demands. Although Vicki is highly aware of her own prejudices toward Karen, she is not mindful of or is ignoring the impact that this will have on her care of Karen. As fellow nurses, you can be sure that there are some identification dynamics as outlined in the surrogate role. An early pleasantly stated observation such as, 'It's not every day that I work on a nurse,' may have helped to decrease or free the tension.

Vicki and Karen probably share a similar goal, that of expedient wound treatment and healing, but the potential for growth or learning is not present. Acknowledging the concerns of the other does not require much time. If Vicki had simply mentioned that she also had another treatment going on at the same time, it is quite possible that Karen would understand Vicki's lengthy absence and even respond by offering to bandage herself with what was available.

Making meaning out of suffering would be a key concept to focus on when viewing the situation with Travelbee glasses. Both Vicki and Karen, as nurses, are no strangers to suffering. Working on a burns unit, Vicki is challenged every day to make sense out of the suffering that results from damage caused by burns, as well as the pain and discomfort she herself often inflicts by carrying out the procedures. She has learned to put her feelings on a shelf at work, but emotions of grief and inadequacy catch up to her from time to time. In an effort to regain a sense of control, she often gets aggressive in dealing with her son. Coping at work has become a matter of professional efficiency. She has become extremely proficient in her work but perhaps at a cost to herself, the patients, and her family life.

Karen reminds Vicki of a smug 'know it all' which makes her feel inadequate and feelings of aggressiveness begin to surface. She figures the best thing to do is to keep her mouth shut and get this procedure over with. It is no surprise that after attending to the urgent need of the other patient, she has taken an unexpected amount of time returning to Karen. Karen, in response, interprets these signals as 'This nurse is showing me who is boss here, she has even put me at risk of infection!' Karen then decides to assert her authority and announces that she can take care of herself.

Both Peplau and Travelbee would focus on expanding Vicki's self-awareness and insight because it affects her ability to communicate therapeutically and establish relatedness with Karen. As Peplau (1952) underscores, the kind of person that the nurse is makes a substantial difference in what each patient will learn as a recipient of nursing care. Travelbee (1971) also asserts that the nurse's perception of the patient will greatly influence the quality and quantity of nursing care delivered to the ill person.

Scenario 3

Jim's situation. Jim, diagnosed with bipolar illness 12 years ago, is well known to members of the local mental health team. Presently he has been off his medications for six weeks—although he told Molly, the community mental health nurse, that he was still taking them. Two months ago Jim met an interesting woman at a barbecue. Feeling inadequate, dull and boring, Jim decided that the only way he could make himself attractive to her was to get off the pills and reclaim his energy. He always feels more motivated and adventurous in his 'natural state.' Living life in a pharmaceutical straitjacket was getting to him. In addition, if he wanted to get romantically involved with this new woman, he wanted his penis to work. After all, he didn't need that additional embarrassment.

After three successful dates, Jim was feeling no limits to his abilities and started showering his girlfriend with expensive gifts. He decided to surprise her with a trip to Tahiti. When he went to the bank to withdraw $10 000 cash (nearly all of his savings) to pay for the airfare and the five-star hotel he had booked, the teller noticed Jim's over-the-top behavior and informed the bank manager, Pete, who had known Jim for years. Pete stepped in to inquire what was going on and Jim reported his wonderful news and surprise trip to Tahiti. Pete reminded him, 'After this withdrawal, you will be left with only $132.' 'Hey, you only live once,' Jim responded. Jim became angry and belligerent when Pete would not supply the money in cash. He persuaded Jim that it would be safer to pay the travel agent by cheque and to bring in the bill the next day. Jim left the bank in a huff and Pete called the mental health centre.

Molly's response. Molly, the community mental health nurse, was used to getting calls like this about Jim. It seemed that everyone liked and cared about Jim and wanted to protect him from himself during his episodes. Molly had known Jim for five years and on several different occasions had stepped in to bail him out of a tight spot. The last time had been to retrieve a refund for a deposit Jim had placed on a Ferrari sports car. Molly liked Jim when he was stable and felt more like a sister to him than a mental health nurse. After talking to Pete, she knew she had to act fast to avoid further trouble at the bank the next day. She decided to re-schedule her afternoon appointments and go over to see Jim.

When she arrived, Jim was drinking champagne and entertaining his girlfriend with stories of conquest. In fact, it appeared that several bottles of champagne had been consumed and that Jim was feeling euphoric. Molly became quite angry—she hated this side of Jim. When he stopped taking his medication, he became an arrogant show-off, God's gift to women; the kind of guy that Molly detested. She preferred Jim to be the agreeable, compliant person who basically did what she told him to do. Molly, now realizing she was going to have to step in once again, went over to the sink and poured the rest of the champagne out, announcing at the same time, 'The party's over!', When Jim's girlfriend asked, 'Who are you?', Molly replied, 'I'm Jim's psych. nurse.'

Theoretical examination. Jim's sense of adequacy springs to mind when thinking about Orlando's concerns. Molly, knowing Jim for five years, has certainly acquired some sense of his behavioral patterns. Although she wants to prevent a worsening of Jim's health crisis as well as financial disaster, she needs to consider ways of accomplishing both, and at the same time maintaining Jim's dignity without creating additional distress. Stepping in, tipping out the champagne, and announcing herself to be Jim's psychiatric nurse in front of someone she does not know would undermine Orlando's nursing principles. In what ways could she convey respect regarding Jim's need to feel adequate in front of his new girlfriend and set up a situation with Jim where they can privately explore the limits and reasonableness of his actual and potential behaviors?

Using the King model, Jim and Molly would examine the goals that Jim is trying to achieve. Isn't it understandable that Jim is excited about his new intimate relationship and wants to buy gifts and have a holiday? Exploring Jim's feelings about being in a drug straitjacket might enable Molly and Jim to find new ways to understand his behavior and organize some medication changes. This is the responsibility of the nurse in interpersonal nursing. Realistic goals can only be set when the nurse and patient thoroughly understand each other's perspective and the blocks to achieving those goals.

The above scenarios have not been exhaustively examined and you may be able to think of a number of different ways to approach each situation and apply the concepts of the nurse theorists. These theorists do, however, provide us with a nursing focus to consider and build upon.

Discussion questions

Group work in nursing enables multiple perspectives and approaches to care to be considered. In a nursing tutorial session or with another group of nursing colleagues, examine in further detail the three scenarios presented in this chapter. Each scenario has already been examined from two different theoretical perspectives. Using the nurse theorist's quick reference guide to clinical application (Table 6.1) apply the three remaining theoretical perspectives to each scenario and discuss:

■ the strengths and limitations that each differing perspective brings to the specific nursing care approach
■ how nursing theory helps to clarify, organize and articulate care
■ what other interpersonal interactions might have been used to lead to more therapeutic outcomes.

Apply your own nursing theory generated in the previous exercise (keeping a journal) to each scenario.

Interpersonal nursing for you, me and us

The theorists examined in this chapter describe the inter-personal nurse–patient relationship (Peplau, Travelbee), inter-action (King, Orlando) and dialogue (Paterson & Zderad) as central to nursing. They emphasize the importance of knowing yourself and knowing the patient. Because nursing is an experience that occurs between two or more people, each person is reciprocally affected. The nurse, however, is respon-sible for being aware of the potential and actual impact that his or her communications and actions are likely to have on patients.

The nurse must also recognize the complexity of the people being nursed and learn about the perceptions (Orlando, Paterson & Zderad), meanings (Travelbee), goals (King) and expectations (Peplau) that shape the person's experience. Inter-action is the tool by which nurses gather this information, assess needs and consider resources. The therapeutic use of self enables the nurse and patient to work together toward growth and understanding (Peplau), goal attainment (King), meeting needs (Orlando), improving well-being (Paterson & Zderad) and finding meaning (Travelbee).

These theorists have drawn on humanism, existentialism, phenomenology, symbolic interactionism, and interpersonal and human developmental theories to inform their ideas about nursing practice. Embedded in these theories are the nursing domain concepts of interaction, client, environment, transition, problem-solving, nursing therapeutics and health. As the nursing client is in continuous interaction with his or her envi-ronment, the nurse monitors, regulates, maintains and changes the environment (Meleis, 1991). The nurse uses an interpersonal process to therapeutically effect the person's transition toward health.

The health–illness transition is an experience that creates possibilities for understanding and growth for both the patient and the nurse—it is a mutual process. Valuing the patient's back-ground and perceptions as well as the nurse's intuitions and self-understandings, form the bedrock of therapeutic relations as the nurse acknowledges the uniqueness and individuality of each person and situation. The nurse uses his or her senses to perceive and validate existential health–illness transitions of others and interacts in ways to promote health goals and self-development (Meleis, 1991).

All of the interactionist theorists agree that nursing involves the potential for human growth. Nursing fellow humans is an important and significant endeavor. The nurse, who is maturing through life experience, interacts with a person who is undergoing a changing life situation within a health care system that is in flux. The interpersonal nursing theorists highlight the intrinsic value of creating human connections in the midst of change. Interpersonal nursing for you, me and us affirms that in this process of being together, meanings about the dignity of people and the worth of life are explored, shared and enhanced.

Reflective exercise

The nurse theorists examined in this chapter all emphasize the importance of the nurse–patient relationship, dialogue or interaction. Effective interpersonal nursing is about understanding and clarifying communication that occurs within this exchange. One of the best forms of feedback that the nurse can get is directly from the person he or she has cared for. Following your next nursing interaction:

■ Ask the person you have nursed to describe what they have learned or gained from the encounter.
■ Share what you have learned with them in return.

References

Allen, D. 1985, Nursing research and social control. Alternative models of science that emphasize understanding and emancipation. *Image: Journal of Nursing Scholarship*, XVII(2): 58–64.

Allen, D., Benner, P. & Diekelman, N. 1986, Three paradigms for nursing research: Methodological implications. In: P. Chinn (ed.), *Nursing research methodology. Issues and implementation*. Aspen Systems, Rockville, Md.

Benner, P. 1984, *From novice to expert. Excellence and power in clinical nursing practice*. Addison-Wesley, Menlo Park, Calif.

Commonwealth Department of Health and Aged Care 1999, *Learning together. Education and training partnerships in mental health*. AGPS, Canberra. (Publication no. 2570)

DeHowitt, M. 1992, King's conceptual model and individual psychotherapy. *Perspectives in Psychiatric Care*, 28(4): 11–14.

Dickoff, J. & James, P. 1968, A theory of theories. A position paper. *Nursing Research*, 17(3): 197–203.

Frankl, V. 1963, *Man's search for meaning. An introduction to logotherapy*. Beacon Press, Boston.

Howk, C., Brophy, G., Carey, E., Noll, J., Rasmussen, L., Searcy, B. & Stark, N. 1998, Hildegard Peplau, Psychodynamic Nursing. In: A. Tomey & M. Alligood (eds), *Nursing theorists and their work*, 4th edn. Mosby, St. Louis, MO (pp. 203–18).

King, I. 1971, *Toward a theory for nursing*. John Wiley & Sons, New York.

King, I. 1992, King's theory of goal attainment. *Nursing Science Quarterly*, 5(1): 19–26.

King, I. 1995, A systems framework for nursing. In: M. Frey & C. Sieloff (eds), *Advancing King's systems framework and theory of nursing*. Sage, Calif.

King, I. 1996, The theory of goal attainment in research and practice. *Nursing Science Quarterly*, 9(2): 61–6.

King, I. 1997, King's theory of goal attainment in practice. *Nursing Science Quarterly*, 10(4): 180–85.

Maslow, A. 1970, *Motivation and personality*, 2nd edn. Harper and Row, New York.

May, R. 1958, Contributions of existential psychotherapy. In: R. May, E. Angel & H. Ellenberger (eds), *Existence. A new dimension in psychiatry and psychology*. Basic Books, New York.

Meleis, A. 1991, *Theoretical nursing. Development and progress*, 2nd edn. Lippincott, Philadelphia.

Murray, I. 1997, How can clients and carers become allies? *Nursing Times*, 93(27): 40–1.

Nightingale, F. 1859, *Notes on nursing. What it is, and what it is not*. Harrison & Sons, London.

Orlando, I. 1961, *The dynamic nurse–patient relationship*. G. P. Putnam's Sons, New York.

Orlando, I. 1990, *The dynamic nurse–patient relationship. Function, process and principles*. National League for Nursing, New York.

Paterson, J. 1971, From a philosophy of clinical nursing to a method of nursology. *Nursing Research*, 20(2): 143–6.

Paterson, J. & Zderad, L. 1970–1971, All together: Through complementary synthesis are the worlds of many. *Image. Journal of Nursing Scholarship*, 4(3): 13–16.

Peplau, H. 1952, *Interpersonal relations in nursing*. G. P. Putnam's Sons, New York.

Peplau, H. 1992a, Notes on Nightingale. In: D. Carroll (ed.), *Notes on nursing. What it is and what it is not*, commemorative edn. J. B. Lippincott, Philadelphia (pp. 48–57).

Peplau, H. 1992b, Interpersonal relations. A theoretical framework for application in nursing practice. *Nursing Science Quarterly*, 5(1): 13–18.

Peplau, H. 1997, Peplau's theory of interpersonal relations. *Nursing Science Quarterly*, 19(4): 162–7.

Schmieding, N. 1987, Problematic situations in nursing. Analysis of Orlando's theory based on Dewey's theory of inquiry. *Journal of Advanced Nursing*, 12: 431–440.

Sieloff, C., Ackermann, M., Brink, S., Clanton, J., Jones, C., Tomey, A., Moody, S., Perlich, G., Price, D. & Prusinski, B. 1998, Systems framework and theory of goal attainment. In: A. Tomey & M. Alligood (eds), *Nursing theorists and their work*, 4th edn. Mosby, St. Louis, Mo (pp. 300–13).

Stevenson, J. & Woods, N. 1986, Nursing science and contemporary science. Emerging paradigms. In: G. E. Sorenson (ed.), *Setting the agenda for the year 2000. Knowledge development in nursing*. (Publication No. G-a170, 3M, 5/86.) American Nurses Association, Kansas City, Mo.

Travelbee, J. 1971, *Interpersonal aspects of nursing*. F. A. Davis, Philadelphia.

7

Conundrums of care: paradoxes in interpersonal relationships*

Key concepts in this chapter: ■ advocacy ■ boundaries ■ caring
■ closeness ■ interpersonal relationships
■ partnerships with consumers
■ safety nets ■ self-disclosure ■ touch

Introduction

Consider the following situations:

1. A person you have been nursing reveals that they have developed a sexual attraction toward you and that they fantasize about being with you romantically.
2. A person you have been working with tells you that her mother has suddenly died and asks you to attend the funeral and be available for emotional support.
3. You are assigned a new patient and find out that the person is your best friend's stepfather.
4. A person you have been nursing has asked for your phone number and would like to ask you out for dinner after being discharged from hospital. You are fond of the person and would like to pursue a friendship and possibly more.
5. You wake up suddenly in the middle of the night from an upsetting nightmare about a traumatic incident that a patient has confided to you.
6. A person you are nursing tells you that you remind them of a former lover who was very kind, considerate, trustworthy, and whom they felt very safe with.

* The author wishes to thank Jen Bichel for her contribution to this chapter.

7. A person you have been nursing informs you that they have stopped taking their medication to see what will happen.
8. A nurse tells you confidentially that he is having sex with a patient after hours in a rarely used room in the hospital.
9. The mother of a young girl you have been nursing asks if you would work privately during your time off, to assist her when she is discharged home.

These are just a few of the kinds of scenarios that a mental health nurse may encounter. For many nurses, the specific context and circumstances will dictate clear solutions. For other nurses, however, some of these situations can create controversy, conflict or emotional turmoil. Notice that the patient's medical diagnosis has been omitted so that you might consider what difference, if any, it would make in your response.

The boundaries between professional and personal conduct in mental health nursing are not as clear as we might like to think. Professional care in nursing is highly personal and unique to the person of the nurse; therefore, striking the right balance between personal involvement and professional duty is an ongoing challenge. Because nursing involves close person-to-person contact, the very nature of caring sets up some of the kinds of paradoxes and dilemmas that will be explored in this chapter. Several methods to help monitor therapeutic involvement (or safety nets) will be described.

The nature of nursing

Caring

Caring is a core concept in nursing and many nurses consider that this is what distinguishes nursing from other professions. Caring is about protecting, enhancing, and ensuring that patient respect and dignity are maintained. It conveys to the person that they are important, special, worthy, and that their concerns matter. To communicate caring within the therapeutic relationship, the nurse conveys compassion and tenderness and aims to help the person create meaning out of their situation (Brady, 1997). This is accomplished by the nurse in a uniquely personal way that includes varying forms of communication that are reciprocal but asymmetrical—meaning the exchange is two-way, but the focus is on helping the patient.

There is no specific formula for providing professional and caring nursing; however, both the nurse and the person will recognize when appropriate care has been given and received. The patient will experience the nurse as committed, involved and honest. The nurse will have a sense of satisfaction knowing that they have made a positive difference in the experience of the other. Both people in the relationship have the capacity to develop and be enriched from the caring transaction. The caring nurse in essence chooses 'being with' rather than 'doing to' the person being nursed.

Can nursing occur without caring? Brykczynska (1997) claims that without caring, nursing practice is without soul, incomplete and insincere. From this perspective, nursing delivered in the absence of caring is nothing more than a set of tasks that lack potential for bringing about holistic health. However, feelings such as kindness and tenderness cannot be forced, but are likely to emerge from a concerned involvement with and for the person being nursed and their family and/or support network.

Because caring comes from a personal commitment, it is not without its risks. Involvement with another person, at any level, creates the potential for harm and intensifies feelings of vulnerability. Caring creates a meaning in personal involvement with other people and projects; and events matter and provide direction and motivation for people (Benner & Wrubel, 1989). It is because these processes are important that people may become stressed when their involvement and concerns are threatened, blocked or ignored. Caring in nursing therefore creates an exchange that has the potential to offer both rich rewards and challenges.

Caring in nursing creates conditions of trust that enable the patient to use the help offered and feel cared for. That is why 'nursing can never be reduced to mere technique because humour, anger, tough love, administering medications, and even patient teaching have different effects in a caring context than in a non-caring one' (Benner & Wrubel, 1989: 4).

Closeness

Nurses have close physical and emotional contact with patients. Nursing sometimes requires entering the personal space of the body to perform invasive treatments or clean up blood, sputum, vomit, feces, urine, pus and other discharges that can be disgusting and embarrassing for the person being nursed. In what other profession are the genitalia, for example, made public to an uninvited stranger? At the same time, ensuring safety, comfort and support requires intimate and sometimes sustained contact that includes access to the emotional life of others. Consequently, 'doing things for people that they would normally do for themselves in private if they were able, involves crossing social boundaries and breaking taboos' (Lawler, 1991: 30). This closeness places nurses in challenging and difficult positions.

Peplau has long acknowledged professional closeness as a special kind of involvement with a patient, client or family group. She describes professional closeness as follows:

> In it, the professional person employs nonverbal gestures, such as occur in physical closeness, and empathetic linkages, such as are associated with interpersonal empathy. However its focus is exclusively on the interests, concerns, and needs of the patient. The nurse is aware of her own needs, but sees herself as separate from the patient and detaches her self-interest from the patient situation so that she may act as an stimulus to, and as a agent for, favorable change in the patient. (Peplau, 1969: 345)

Although the nurse's close contact with patients is widely understood to have therapeutic potential, historically this has not always been the case (Savage, 1990). At one time, the allocation of nursing work was based on seniority. As seniority increased, the nurse moved away from the 'dirty work' or basic care to more technical tasks requiring less intimacy (Lawler, 1991). This approach was perceived as advantageous in protecting the nurse from anxiety by reducing the contact and involvement that he or she had with patients (Menzies, 1970). Distancing was encouraged as a form of self-protection. Furthermore, as nursing became a vocation fit for upper-class women, emotional distance from patients was a means to desexualise relationships that involved close bodily proximity (May 1991).

With the advent of primary nursing a couple of decades ago, the importance of continuity of care as delivered by one nurse was thought to allow the development of a 'close' relationship that would have greater therapeutic impact. Not only would it ensure continuity of care, but also foster emotional understanding and commitment on the part of the nurse. According to Lee (1993: 28), primary nursing began 'as an attempt to recapture the personal nature and responsibility of a one-to-one nurse–patient relationship.' It provided the impetus for the nurse and the person being nursed to approach each other as equal partners, and acknowledged that establishing a sense of closeness was not only important, but was actually beneficial in terms of patient outcomes (Lee, 1993).

In a detailed study of intimacy in nursing, Savage (1995) found it to be a form of rapport that encourages openness. Nurses used strategies such as touch, humor, and body posture to promote and manage their closeness to patients. The self-disclosure that closeness prompted was seen to be central to the therapeutic process. Self-disclosure was seen to be reciprocal; however, for nurses, self-disclosure need not occur verbally—it can be expressed through the body (ibid.: 4).

Debates about the therapeutic value and consequences of closeness and distance in nursing continue. As nurses are invariably involved with the pain, distress and suffering, as well as joy, success and recovery of others, they are inevitably in circumstances conducive to closeness. Ultimately the level of involvement depends to some degree on the nurse's own level of comfort with interpersonal relations. Nursing is one profession in which satisfaction, happiness and success are dependent to a great extent on the skills a nurse has developed in promoting good interpersonal relations (Burton, 1977).

Menzies (1970) supports the view that nurses find the effort required to keep distant from patients more stressful than the demands of nursing itself. Her research indicated that the stress inherent in nursing was compounded by the organizational structure and ethos that persistently worked against the development of a social relationship between the nurse and patient. This is supported by Lyons (1997) in a study of occupational therapist students in a mental health setting, which found that they experienced professional detachment as distressing; and they perceived that organizational values directed them to practice the art of deception, and to be something they are not.

Types of interpersonal relationships

While it is impossible to draw a sharp distinction between the anticipated outcomes of the nurse–patient relationship and the way in which these goals are accomplished, certain ways of being and relating tend to communicate care and lead to therapeutic outcomes. The next section examines the issues and challenges specific to relating in mental health nursing.

Most textbooks of nursing outline distinctions between social, intimate and therapeutic relationships. Social interactions are defined as the everyday kinds of exchanges that occur between people in the course of living. They include casual chitchat about the weather, common interests and activities, giving and receiving advice, lending or borrowing things, and helping one another out. Social communication includes equal self-disclosure, spontaneity, and equal opportunity for personal needs to be met. Intimate relationships are most often considered to be one-to-one love relationships where there is a mutual exchange of affection that includes sex (Shives, 1998; Keltner et al., 1991).

Therapeutic interactions have a goal of enabling the patient to express their thoughts, feelings and concerns about what is going on in relation to their health and illness, with the nurse providing assistance and support in problem solving. Therapeutic communication relies on patient self-disclosure, with the professional close enough to be involved but impartial enough to be helpful. Along with showing concern, compassion and interest, the nurse maintains a perspective on the situation that the person they are nursing may lack.

These definitions may seem clear and obvious. In practice, however, the features specific to each type of relationship are not mutually exclusive. For example, characteristics of a non-sexual intimate relationship that includes mutual respect and admiration can occur within the context of a therapeutic relationship. A therapeutic relationship may also involve social relating.

Social interactions often form the gateway to establishing therapeutic relationships. Take for example 14-year-old Jim who is admitted to the hospital because of poor self-image and suicidal depression. Sue is assigned to Jim and makes repeated attempts to initiate therapeutic contact by offering time and a listening ear to learn about his life and current situation. Each attempt is met with opposition, with Jim saying, 'I don't feel like talking about it—my life sucks and there's no point in being reminded of it.'

Sue understands from Jim's mother that he used to enjoy playing with a frisbee. Sue just happens to have a frisbee in her car and decides to ask him to play. To her surprise, Jim lights up and says OK. While playing, Jim remarks about Sue's throwing skill and she reveals that she is part of an ultimate frisbee team. Jim has never heard of such a game and wants to know more. This is the first time since Jim's admission that he seems to be taking an interest in anything.

As a nurse Sue understands the therapeutic possibility that this activity is bringing to bear—a connection and opening for getting to know Jim. But in the course of playing, she is becoming aware of a fond feeling for him—as a little brother who needs protection and reassurance that he can make it through this rough patch and discover worthwhile reasons for living. Sue feels compelled to hug Jim at the end of the game but realizes that her own feelings of connection may be overriding his. Instead, she offers a high five. Jim asks if Sue can make plans to play the next day.

This story illustrates several important aspects of relating in mental health nursing. Establishing contact is a necessary first step in getting to know the person and the problems that they are experiencing. When the nurse was met with rejection, she sought an alternative approach through active engagement. Her self-awareness allowed her to acknowledge the feelings of protection and desire to physically embrace Jim. She demonstrated restraint in order to avoid creating a situation that could overwhelm Jim and jeopardize their beginning relationship—after all, this was their first meaningful contact. It is because she cared about Jim and his future, that she searched for a way to connect.

Because nurses have backgrounds and experiences as people, these shape our nursing interpretations and make it questionable whether nurses could be objective or neutral across a range of interpersonal nursing situations. If you are asked to care for a person who inflicted an injury on someone else while intoxicated, and as a child you were beaten by a drunken parent, it will be highly unlikely that your previous experience will not influence your care of the person. In all interactions, your own background, feelings and responses to patients (and their responses) will influence their sense of you as a nurse and your nursing.

Since nurses are involved in the private aspects of a person's life, nursing practice can be considered to be intimate and therefore strict relationship boundaries may not be feasible or even desirable. Furthermore, the idea of maintaining a constant fixed position and establishing 'emotional borders' is to ignore the important therapeutic connections that can be made when roles, relationships, and responses are flexible. That is not to say that no boundaries are preferable. Keeping a sense of professional purpose is essential.

Elements of therapeutic relationships

Empathy, self-disclosure and advocacy are frequently identified elements of the therapeutic relationship. Examination of these concepts and their association with other concepts helps to explain boundaries within nurse–patient relationships.

Empathy involves identifying and understanding another person's situation, feelings and motives (see chapter 2). The language of empathy moves the nurse into the patient's space (Keltner et al., 1991). This is non-invasive if the empathy is correct—if it is the patient's feelings and not the nurse's. Recognition of a patient's feelings allows the nurse to understand the feelings without absorbing them.

Empathy has the potential for the nurse to focus on similarities between himself or herself and the person being nursed, leading to an inaccurate perception of the person's feelings. Therefore it is essential for the nurse to continuously reflect on practice and explore her or his own feelings, reactions to specific patients and levels of interpersonal involvement, and to clarify the purpose of the nurse–patient relationship.

In responding empathically, Havens (1986) explains that using emotion descriptors will convey a feeling of support. For example, the nurse might say, 'If that had happened to me I'd feel scared.' When the nurse empathizes with a patient, he or she temporarily adopts the feelings of that person for the sole purpose of accurately understanding the experience from the person's perspective. Experiencing empathy can reduce the patient's emotional burden.

Patient self-disclosure refers to revealing personal information. The aim in mental health nursing is to create an atmosphere where the patient can feel safe and comfortable enough to talk about their life and problems of living, and examine solutions without fear of rejection. To foster self-disclosure, the nurse uses verbal and nonverbal communication to set the stage. An interested, open, and outgoing stance that includes the use of open-ended questions helps establish the trust required for deeper communication. After all, is it reasonable to expect someone to trust a person whom they do not know?

The standard rule for nurse self-disclosure is to abstain from disclosing personal problems or providing information that may reverse the focus of concern from the patient to the nurse. By-and-large, this principle is sound. However, a skilled nurse may purposely create a distraction for the person by telling a personal story that enables the person to take a break from their problems or look beyond to other possibilities.

Nurse self-disclosing statements may include, for example, 'When I'm angry it's sometimes because I am frustrated and disappointed that something I tried didn't work out' or 'With some people I'm ashamed to admit to making mistakes; and this happens to other people I know.' This type of self-disclosure may help the patient feel more at ease or provide clues to help them unravel their difficulties.

The level and depth of self-disclosure is dependent on both the patient and the nurse and their comfort with themselves and each other. Meaningful connections cultivate mutual interest. A patient may suspect that you live in the local area and ask if your home was affected by the recent storm. To describe the damage that has led to your relocation and disrupted life will likely solicit a response of concern. To share your distress as well as the coping methods that enable you to continue your work can be very instructive to others. In return, their understanding of your situation may help to decrease your anxiety about needing to seem in control and cheerful when you are not feeling that way. Regardless of your situation, the people you nurse must feel assured that you are capable and competent to care for them.

In mental health nursing, there is great concern that self-disclosure may lead to unsafe or untoward consequences. The nurse who gives out her or his address, telephone number, or any number of details without having a therapeutic reason, or recognizing potential ramifications, is acting irresponsibly.

People with mental health problems may be seeking friendship or support beyond the confines of professional settings. It is understandable that a person may wish to continue a relationship that they have found to be meaningful or useful. It is also flattering to know that you are liked and that a connection has been made. However, it is neither reasonable nor often times therapeutic to extend nursing relationships beyond the work environment unless you are employed in a setting where such arrangements are supported.

Patients need to be reminded that it is not unusual to feel a special involvement because they have opened themselves up. The nurse has also made himself or herself available to the patient in a way that is unique. It is important for patients to recognize their own ability to trust and open up to another person. Through the therapeutic relationship, the nurse provides an opportunity for the person to realize that they can communicate and connect with others.

Self-disclosure in mental health nursing is a sensitive issue that is best managed by each nurse in their own way and at their own pace. Beginning nurses are urged to err on the side of caution, test out their interactions, and note responses little by little. New graduates are well advised to seek supervision from an experienced mental health nurse who can help examine interpersonal relationships so that blind spots, strengths and insights can be identified and built upon.

Reflective questions

Students and employees alike are required to wear a name badge that identifies them as a member of the health care staff. Patients and their families and friends are also entitled to know who is providing care and what their title, position or qualifications are. In some schools of nursing and health care agencies, students and staff are encouraged or even required to cover up or remove their surnames from the badge when working with mental health patients. Think about the following.

—continued

—continued

■ How do you feel about the issue?
■ What reasons might there be to conceal your surname? Assess the validity of your argument?
■ Why would you conceal your surname in certain patient care areas such as mental health and not in others?
■ What message does concealing your surname convey to students, employees, consumers, and the general public about people with a mental illness?
■ Have you noticed that in the mental health settings, people working in some disciplines conceal their surname while others do not? What sense do you make of this?
■ What therapeutic concerns might the name badge issue represent and how might they be dealt with alternatively?

As a patient advocate, the nurse is obliged to support and act on behalf of the patient's best interest. To determine the 'patient's interest' the nurse becomes engaged in the situation with the patient in order to learn what is right and good for them (Hess, 1996). Morally and ethically, the nurse must advocate for the patient's position—that position being free from force or coercion (see also chapter 2).

A true advocacy position is not possible in nursing practice where compliance to treatment is imposed. Four assumptions of compliance in the nurse–patient relationship are:

1. the patient must cooperate with medical care
2. compliance leads to cure; non-compliance leads to morbidity or mortality
3. the best outcome is a medical cure
4. the nurse knows what is best for the patient (Hess 1996: 21).

Practices based on compliance must be questioned even in settings when people are legally treated against their will. The classic writings of Goffman (1961), Laing (1965) and Szasz (1974) offer critiques of the misuse and abuse of psychiatric power. Their work will not be reviewed here; however, many mental health nurses find their views to be illuminating and worthwhile.

How does a mental health nurse respect the wishes of the client and at the same time adhere to the duty of care to protect the patient from the harmful consequences of their actions? On occasions where the person is comatose or not able to make informed decisions, the nurse and other medical personnel have the responsibility to take charge under a universal principle of beneficence.

When patients are not at immediate risk of harming themselves or violating the rights of others, they are entitled to do and be as they see fit. However, it is important (though often difficult) for nurses to learn to accept that the person's right to choose freely includes the right to choose 'wrongly' (Hess, 1996).

A further complication occurs when the nurse actually agrees with the patient's autonomous decision that goes against medical advice. Caught in the bind between client and employer, it is advised that the nurse acknowledge the dilemma and seek counsel. One option is to examine in further detail, with the person being nursed, the ramifications of varying decisions. While nurses encourage independent decision making, they can also demonstrate ways to examine problems from multiple perspectives in order to make well-informed choices.

The nurse can exert a powerful influence over those they nurse, through persuasion. To act responsibly is to know the patient and to understand as fully as possible the arguments that surround the issue. Institutional rules and professional judgments are usually informed by mainstream utilitarian views and when these views are not appropriate, the nurse can point out their limitations.

Nurse advocacy in many mental health settings has its limits. The aim of this discussion is not to render the nurse impotent, but to prepare the nurse for the reality of practice and highlight some of the more fascinating aspects of mental health care that include ethical and moral predicaments.

Partnerships with consumers

The concept of partnership in mental health is another contemporary practice issue that the mental health nurse should be aware of. Based on national and international agendas to 'empower' consumers and their carers to be equal partners in mental health treatment, partnership is in attempt to enable users of services to take responsibility for decision making and safeguard against exploitative practices by professionals. This would seem like a worthwhile nursing endeavor. However, according to Murray (1997: 40), 'The idea of partnership between service users and professionals contains its own con-tradictions. Partnership implies equality, yet inequality is con-sidered necessary in the current system so that the professional can be of use to the client.' As Hughes remarks, 'Professionals profess. They profess to know better than others the nature of certain matters, and to know better than their clients what ails them or their affairs' (1963: 656). The medical profession's long-standing control of treatment and its paternalistic attitude are highly likely to have contributed to the consumer movement and consumers' desire for empowerment.

Peplau's (1969) theory of interpersonal nursing embodies the notions of partnership, as nursing from this perspective is informed by participation, involvement, and collaboration with the consumer and their support network. This is achieved through the nurse and patient coming to know and respect each other as people who share in working to solve a problem. The nurse uses understanding as the basis for providing effective help and stimulates the patient to develop and use his or her own competencies to understand problems and help him or herself.

The ability to demonstrate unconditional regard, and being genuine and empathetic are essential to promoting partnership (O'Donnel, 1993). Nurses must also demonstrate competence, confidence and assertiveness (Peplau, 1969). Nurses who fail to embrace the principles of interpersonal nursing will most likely resist the ideas of partnership. If empowering others means sharing of knowledge and resources, the nurse's sense of power and control may be threatened. Also, patients may not wish to be involved in their care, or perhaps are too ill. In addition, mental health environments are sometimes intimidating and coerce patients to conform to spoken or unspoken rules, and coerce nurses to 'simply get the work done' (Wade, 1995).

In Australia, fostering a culture that values the opinions of consumers and carers was addressed in a series of workshops under the Second National Mental Health Plan—Education and Training Initiative. Groups of consumers, carers, government officials, practitioners, managers, academics, psychiatrists, mental health nurses, occupational therapists, psychologists and social workers joined to discuss education and training of the mental health workforce. Statements of principle were generated. They are as follows:

■ The relationships between consumers and service providers and carers and service providers should be the primary focus of practice and research in mental health. Consumers and carers are therefore major players in the education, training and development of the mental health workforce.
■ Mental health professionals need to learn about and value the lived experience of consumers and carers.
■ Mental health professionals should recognize and value the healing potential in the relationships between consumers and service providers and carers and service providers.
■ Mental health professionals should recognize and value the ongoing potential for recovery of people within the mental health system. (Commonwealth Department of Health and Aged Care, 1999: 1)

These principles challenge the old paradigm of professional dominance that is entrenched within most systems of education and mental health care. Imagine what it would be like if these statements were incorporated into the educational curricula and practice of all disciplines involved in mental health care? Certainly mental health nurses could take a leadership role in supporting such an agenda, as these principles are consistent with the basic values of nursing.

Simon Champ: consumer story and reflection

The consumer movement and nursing

Mental health consumers come from all walks of life and are not a homogenous group. Diversity is perhaps the strength of the emerging consumer movement. Individual consumers have a whole range of experience of illness and treatment, and their

—*continued*

—*continued*

beliefs about mental health issues cover an enormous spectrum. The various networks and associations that make up what has been called the 'consumer movement' include individuals who may have widely differing philosophies and understandings of the causes of and treatment needs for mental illness. Many consumers challenge the very notions of mental illness that are held in society, particularly those of the 'medical model' that dominate in psychiatry. However, consumers subscribing to a variety of philosophies do unite around certain core beliefs, creating what has become a movement to secure rights and ensure that consumers are treated with respect and dignity by the health care system and within the wider society.

As has happened in some other western countries, consumers have become a vital force in contributing to the changing picture of mental health services in Australia during the 1990s. Consumers have also made significant inroads for change in the wider society. They have challenged the stigma and ignorance so prevalent in society and demanded society respect the human rights of people who have experienced mental illness. The emergence of a consumer movement provides many opportunities for mental health professionals, including nurses, to rethink their attitudes to consumers. It has also created new ways for nurses to engage and work with consumers.

In the treatment and care of consumers there is now a new mandate through several human rights mechanisms to work with consumers in ways that ensure that the dignity and respect of the consumer is upheld along with a full recognition of that consumer's rights.

Rights mechanisms and documents that have determined the rights of consumers include the United Nations 25 Principles for the Protection of Persons with Mental Illness and for the Improvement of Mental Health Care, the Mental Health Statement of Rights and Responsibilities (1991) and the National Standards for Mental Health Services (1996).

Rights for consumers go further than guaranteeing optimum care with dignity and respect, they also suggest that consumers have the right to partake in the design and development of policies and services that affect their lives. Where these aspects of rights are being implemented, the involvement of consumers with services, government and education is significantly
—*continued*

—continued

changing these areas, how they function, their concerns and outcomes.

The emergence of a consumer movement in mental health will increasingly impact on nursing in the future. Here in Australia through national organizations and advisory bodies such as the Mental Health Council of Australia (MHCA), the National Coalition of Community Advisory Groups (NCAG) and the Australian Mental Health Consumer Network, consumers are having real influence in the direction and form of mental health policy and projects at the national level. At a state level too, mental health service provision and policy is informed by the expertise of consumer representatives.

Increasingly, nurses will find themselves working alongside consumer representatives, advocates and consultants on committees and boards of management. Health regions and services are now encouraged to budget for consumer participation and involvement. In some services full- or part-time consumer workers coordinate consumer issues and initiatives, ensuring that consumers' perspectives are included in all aspects of the functioning of that service. This includes everything from influencing budgetary concerns to ensuring consumers' satisfaction with outcomes.

Having consumer workers involved in the day-to-day running of mental health services can often call into question existing procedures and routines that professionals have designed, and services need to be responsive to advice from consumer representatives. Consumers should be involved in the review of mental services and when reforms and change are suggested, consumers should be consulted regarding their views and needs. Many consumer workers have a role as advocates. This often includes supporting other consumers in making a complaint about a service or a professional working for a service.

In some health areas, in hospitals and community services, consumers are becoming involved in peer support in rehabilitation and treatment programs. Their experience and perspectives are being seen to add new dimensions to the rehabilitation and recovery of other consumers in hospital or the community.

—continued

—continued

Often professionals and consumers view situations and needs differently. A good example of this is how, when professionals describe what are the most distressing aspects of living with schizophrenia, they may suggest that these are hallucinations or delusions. However, a consumer experiencing the illness may actually prioritize loneliness, stigma or feelings of hopelessness as the most disabling aspects of living with the condition. Listening to either view perhaps suggests different responses to and treatment of the condition.

The lived experience and perspectives of consumers involved in services is an invaluable resource and provides expertise that now needs to be accepted as informing all professional practice, including that of nurses.

Consumer workers draw on their lived experience and consulting with peers to inform their work. Sometimes consumers in recovery will feel more comfortable sharing experiences and concerns with someone who has had first-hand experience of a mental illness.

Consumer workers, often just by their presence and having been employed by a service, become strong role models for consumers struggling with recovery. To know that others have travelled similar paths and now work as advocates or consumer consultants can provide hope and encouragement.

Many communities now have a range of formal activities and support for consumers that grow out of existing services or are provided by non-government organizations. Consumer workers can often provide an introduction to these activities or groups for consumers who need information and support.

Perhaps because of the levels of stigma still existing in the community and because of the value many consumers see in supporting each other, many consumers develop friendships and become part of informal networks of consumers within the community that provide many benefits. Consumer workers are usually aware of these networks that run independently of the health service supporting them because they attest to the richness that some consumers find in associating with other consumers socially.

As more links evolve that encourage consumers to stay in touch with each other in the wider community, there have been many benefits. Beyond the social aspects of being part of a consumer

—continued

—continued

culture, many consumers come to see that indeed the 'personal is political' through consumer networks. Consumers find other more politically aware consumers who raise consciousness about the nature and politics of the health services they receive and society's treatment of people who have experienced a mental illness or disorder.

In Australia during the 1980s and 1990s, many consumers became politically active, lobbying for change for consumers. Consumers who have taken on the role of activists in the field of mental health have challenged not only the low priority given to mental health issues in society but also highlighted issues of abuse and neglect within the system and lobbied for the implementation of human rights for consumers.

Understanding the concerns of consumer activists can provide nurses with a more critical attitude to their practice. The concerns of activists can provide valuable insights and questions about the social, cultural and political contexts in which nurses practice. Consumer activists may also become strong allies for nurses, supporting their own concerns about ensuring quality services, equity of access and adequate funding.

Boundaries

Limit setting includes defining the rules of expected behavior in the clinical setting. Typical rules include honesty, confidentiality and its exceptions, and acceptable means of emotional or behavioral expression. People with mental health problems often require help in finding ways to express themselves, since their difficulties usually entail some sort of alteration in communication. It is therefore important to realize that responses may be extreme and that some guidelines must be in place to help ensure safety and protect the nurse from possible legal action of professional bodies or employing authorities.

It is the actual therapeutic relationship and the personal interplay that occurs within the relationship that enables the patient to concentrate on their abilities and goals in life. If this were not the case, a person with a mental disorder would not require nursing care. Within this therapeutic relationship, however, it is paramount that the nurse maintains a professional boundary and establishes limits within this boundary.

Professional relationships are fairly structured, finite, fiscally based, and nurse and patient power is unequal. Rather than spontaneously occurring, these relationships require specific training and education, and a period of preparation and adjustment, with the professional assuming the responsibility for establishing and maintaining suitable boundaries for the continued existence of the relationship.

In nursing, boundaries can be defined as:

> The spaces between the nurse's power and the client's vulnerability. The power of the nurse comes from the professional position and the access to private knowledge about the client.
>
> (National Council of State Boards of Nursing 1996, cited in Horsfall et al., 1999: 6)

Consequently, it is the nurse's responsibility to establish and maintain professional boundaries, manage patient vulnerability safely, and guard against the misuse of multiple subtle and obvious power advantages.

Potential boundary violations can be physical, emotional, spiritual, financial or sexual (Horsfall et al., 1999). Boundary transgressions can be overtly and covertly communicated by physical contact, speech, gesture or even voice tone. The nurse should always be mindful of the vulnerable position that the people being nursed often find themselves in, and be consciously aware of their own body language, attire, and the content of their conversations.

Whatever the purpose of the interaction, it is expected that mental health nurses will exercise prudent and ethical judgment within therapeutic relationships and appraise their own behavior with individual clients through reflective processes such as journaling and clinical supervision. A few issues relevant to boundaries are worth exploring briefly; these include gift-giving, touch and presencing.

Gift-giving

Gift-giving in health care institutions has always been problematic in so far as the gift could be interpreted as seeking to exert influence to obtain preferential consideration or treatment.

Similarly, the nurse whose satisfaction lies in getting compliments, favors or gifts from patients will set up interactions that accommodate this need (Peplau, 1969). In either case, therapeutic care may become compromised. Token gestures or small gifts such as flowers and confectionery, often given to staff when the person being nursed has been discharged, are acceptable as they are perceived as an acknowledgment of the care received. Gifts that are not inexpensive, or those that are given during hospitalization or treatment in the community, should be carefully evaluated for their intent and may require the nurse to politely decline and give an explanation.

Touch

Everyone requires body contact to reassure them of their presence in the world. The classic studies by Harlow & Zimmerman (1959) demonstrated that tactile comfort provided by mother monkeys was more important to the infant than food. Bowlby's (1969) studies of mother–child attachment also underscored the important role of physical contact in communicating trust, confidence and security, and its impact on emotional development.

In mental health nursing, tactile communication is commonly transitory and at times reciprocal. Touch, when used judicially, can be very reassuring to patients. From a nursing perspective, touch should be used responsibly and the nurse should reflect upon intent, therapeutic potential and the possibility of misinterpretation (Carter, 1981: 121). Warnings about the misinterpretation of touch as promoting affection or sexual advance seems to be a common concern among mental health professionals. Introductory texts of mental health nursing frequently subscribe to a conservative stance of limited use of touch. Psychiatric patients are portrayed as having 'fragmented or uncertain ego boundaries,' so caution is recommended. People who are fearful or mistrusting also require careful assessment and careful recognition of their personal space.

The rules of touch are determined by mores set by the mental health workplace as well as the nurse's own level of comfort. One author has worked in situations where hugs and kisses on the cheek were ordinary actions in the therapeutic community. Alternatively, there are many mental health settings where hugs and kisses are banned, regardless of the circumstances. The beginning practitioner must develop a situational understanding about when touch is threatening and unacceptable and when it might be comforting and reassuring.

Presencing

Presencing refers to being with someone in a way that acknowledges their experience (Benner & Wrubel, 1989). It is about being here now, with one's interest and attention in the present place and moment and nowhere else. That means we are not wondering when we will get a word in edgewise, trying to remember if we locked a door, thinking about the good impression we are making on the person, or the wisdom we are imparting (French & Harris, 1999).

Consumers frequently describe the presence of the nurse as being helpful. In fact, Pearson (1984) claims that the very essence of advanced nursing is 'being there.' Being present in the here-and-now is a basic requisite for establishing a meaningful connection. It communicates a focused interest, awareness and receptivity that enable the person to feel listened to, understood and cared for. People experiencing mental distress or illness have difficulties in one or a combination of the areas of perceiving, thinking, feeling or behaving. Their extreme or distorted affects or behaviors create barriers to effective communication with others, often leaving them feeling alone and alienated. Therefore, the nurse, through presencing, can demonstrate acceptance of the other person's reality. Being there places the nurse in a unique position to help mitigate the negative side effects of illness: alienation and a feeling of being out of touch with the self and with the social context (Stuhlmiller, 1995).

Safety nets for mental health nursing

The circumstances around which people experience mental distress and suffering can challenge and overwhelm the nurse's sense of self, safety and meaning in the world. Patient stories of abuse, violence, neglect, despair and loneliness are quite common. The effects on the listener are also well known. An empathetic listener may be sucked into the traumatic details, experiencing the client's trauma second hand. This phenomenon, formerly known to contribute to professional burnout, has been more recently studied and defined as vicarious traumatization, secondary traumatization or compassion fatigue (Figley, 1995; Saakvitne & Pearlman, 1996; Stamm, 1995).

For example, as a beginning nurse working with Vietnam Combat Veterans, one of the authors heard many grim stories of death and destruction. After about six months, she woke up one night from a nightmare and started throwing hand grenades out of her bed. Having never been in war or Vietnam, this was a clear signal that she had soaked up the experiences of her clients and needed to take care of herself or get help.

To not be affected by the horror and tragedy of traumatic human events is to shut down normal emotions. This ability can serve as useful protection but it can also lead to callous and nihilistic views about humanity that will not be helpful personally or professionally. This final section explores safety nets that nurses can use to help maintain their own health and wellness.

One of the best forms of self-protection in mental health nursing is self-awareness. Keeping to the forefront personal feelings and reactions that develop in the course of interpersonal relating is an occupational imperative. Because the work of mental health nursing entails an examination of what is called forth in the other person, constant review of feelings and reactions is required. As the nurse assesses his or her reactions, he or she must decide what emotions are acceptable, unacceptable, or of concern. In other words, to care for others, the nurse must first know, and care for, herself or himself.

Journaling is a form of reflective practice that is useful to assess one's own cognitive, psychomotor and attitudinal ability in order to improve practice and increase confidence. Such a process is ultimately self-protective for the nurse in ongoing practice situations. It involves writing about nursing situations and the personal thoughts, feelings, actions, responses and understandings related to those encounters. Garratt (1992) believes that the reflective process enables the nurse to work through the many layers of cloudiness that conceal the actual significance of an experience, thus resulting in enlightenment or deeper understanding. According to Gallop (1997), gaining insight into how one's personal emotional baggage impinges on experiences helps us to know where we end and others begin. In addition to this, an appreciation of the difficulties of the human circumstance and an increased understanding of self places one in a much better position to listen attentively and reflect upon the human condition of others (Gallop, 1997).

A number of techniques have been developed to help prevent vicarious traumatization of the therapist and to facilitate the client's emotional exploration and resolution of mental distress without requiring the person to disclose specific content or details. One such approach, known as trauma incident reduction (TIR), has proven successful in reducing the stress associated with traumatic events (French & Harris, 1999; Gerbode, 1995). Although specialized training is required to conduct TIR, nurses can, and perhaps already do, apply some of the principles such as creating a safe space for the person to work out their own issues. The strength of the method is in its elegant simplicity of empowering the individual to confront their own issues without the interference, interpretation, suggestion, leading questions, and directing of the client to the therapist's world view. TIR should not, however, be attempted by a novice nurse.

Using a method of non-directive facilitation, the therapist can help bring to the person's awareness troubling emotions connected to events. Simply ask the person to picture the situation in their mind as if it was a movie that they were viewing from beginning to end. When they reach the end, have them just describe to you the emotions connected to the movie that they just viewed in their mind. In viewing the movie over and over and providing a summary of only the emotions each time, you will begin to notice a change in the emotional content. The basic nursing skills, including full attention, acknowledgment and presencing, enable this approach to be useful. While space does not permit a full explanation, further reading can be found in Stuhlmiller (1996) and Stuhlmiller and Thorsen (1997).

Barker (1997) has developed a similar emotionally protective technique that he calls *the blue banana*. He developed this method to spare the client from negative judgment or backing away by the nurse who might be uncomfortable with or call to question delusional material that a patient reveals. The patient is instructed to name and discuss their difficulty as 'the blue banana.' The following example from Barker (1997: 247) illustrates how a nurse can helpfully address difficulties without specific knowledge of the problem:

Nurse: So, how are you today?

Person: Not good, it is getting worse. I don't know how much more I can take.

Nurse: I see. Tell me a bit more about what is getting worse.

Person: Well, it's the blue banana, isn't it? It's back!

Nurse: Uh-huh It's back. So it's been away?

Person: Yeah. Well, not long, but I thought that I was on top of that, y'know.

Nurse: Umm. I see. (pause) So when did you first notice this 'blue banana'?

Person: Oh, I dunno...maybe...oh, years ago. It comes and goes, y'know.

Nurse: Yes. So you noticed this 'years ago'. Do you remember when exactly?

Person: Well . . . yeah, when I was at college. I was studying for exams . . . and . . . yeah, that's when it started.

Nurse: Right! So did it affect you then?

Person: Well . . . I couldn't keep my mind on things . . . anything. And . . . I just couldn't shut it up.

Nurse: OK. And now it's back. How does it affect you now?

This method of exploring a person's difficulties does not deny the problem, but forces both the nurse and the patient to focus on the emotional consequences of the Blue Banana in the past and the present. Such a technique avoids the nurse pursuing the minutiae of a person's delusional, hallucinatory or traumatic experience for no good therapeutic reason, given that others have probably trodden this path before. This approach also avoids the temptation for the nurse to project their own emotions, meanings or consequences onto the patient. Similar to TIR, this 'context-free' method of interviewing can be used at times to help protect the nurse from over-exposure to material that may be distressing; and it allows the interviewee to be in charge of their story without revealing things that may be embarrassing.

One method of interpersonal evaluation is to gain direct feedback from the patient. This allows you to evaluate your nursing, learn from the feedback and gain satisfaction from positive outcomes. Such processes are also protective for the nurse. Most people you nurse can describe what has been useful or not useful specific to your nursing care. Nurses are often surprised to learn that some aspect of care that they might have considered insignificant was in fact quite important and meaningful to the person. Direct feedback provides unparalleled information that can be used to understand and improve your effect on others. Do not hesitate to ask questions such as: 'How was this for you?', 'What concerns or questions do you have?' or 'What have you learned?'. It is recommended to end some important nursing encounters with a question that leaves the person reviewing positive or growth-promoting possibilities. Ask the person to summarize what has occurred and offer your impression of the interaction as well. This concluding activity can be revealing, confirming, and useful for planning and organizing care. In addition, the process of validating the experience reinforces the importance of the interpersonal encounter.

Clinical supervision is another feedback mechanism through which interpersonal interactions can be examined, and emotionally problematic issues can be processed and eventually left behind. There are many definitions of clinical supervision. One representative definition is:

> Clinical supervision is a regular, protected time for facilitated, in-depth reflection on clinical practice. It aims to enable the supervisee to achieve, sustain, and creatively develop a high quality of practice though the means of focused support and development. The supervisee reflects on the part she plays as an individual in the complexities of the events and the quality of her practice. This reflection is facilitated by one or more experienced colleagues who have expertise in facilitation and the frequent, ongoing sessions are led by the supervisee's agenda.
>
> (Bond & Holland, 1998: 12)

Clinical supervision is known to improve nursing effectiveness by clarifying, extending or validating one's efforts in the clinical setting. Evaluation studies indicate that increased morale and confidence, decreased absenteeism and workers' compensation claims, and increased retention of staff have been documented (Butterworth & Faugier, 1998). Increased job satisfaction also has implications for improved care and consumer satisfaction.

While there are numerous models of group and one-to-one clinical supervision, a structured program may not be available in every workplace. For that reason, finding an alternative opportunity for reflection may require initiative on the part of the nurse. New graduates may be able to identify an experienced nurse who is willing to examine practice issues with them on a regular basis. Beginning practitioners and veteran nurses can find clinical supervision a valuable way to examine interactions from alternative perspectives as well as an effective way to rejuvenate themselves.

Each profession has a set of standards or code of conduct that outlines the duties and ethics of practice. Two publications available from the Australian and New Zealand College of Mental Health Nursing (ANZCMHN) entitled: *Standards of practice for mental health nursing in Australia* (ANZCMHN, 1995) and *Towards ethical mental health nursing practice* (Horsfall et al., 1999) offer guidelines for safe and ethical mental health care. Mental health nursing standards, codes and policies outline issues regarding accountability, professionalism and self-regulation. Consequently mental health nursing standards can also help the nurse manage boundary issues and determine safe practices for self, colleagues and patients.

A nurse story and reflection

Mutual attraction

I met a wonderfully sexy man one day while swimming in the Veterans Hospital swimming pool. It was the staff swim lunch hour and I noticed myself trying to avoid eye contact as minutes earlier, the first time our eyes met, there seemed to be an overwhelming, instant connection. I felt really drawn to this man and did manage to engage in small talk about the pool temperature and luxury of having the pool nearly to ourselves. He asked how often I swam and he said that he just happened to have meetings at the hospital that corresponded with the swim hour. I saw him during one other lunch swim but avoided contact as I felt a mutual attraction but was too shy to pursue it.

Several weeks later, this same man was admitted to the Vietnam Veterans psychiatric unit that I worked on. I was shocked but not surprised. It turns out that Mark had kept forenoon appointments with an outpatient counselor who had arranged for him to join the staff swim. Mark was randomly

—continued

—continued

assigned to me as his primary nurse which also meant he was to attend my psychotherapy group. At first, I thought it might be interesting and that I could keep professional objectivity. Mark had spent 15 years in prison for a murder he had committed just after discharge from Vietnam. Fresh out of jail, he was exploring a life of freedom. Admittedly, he was attempting to integrate his Vietnam as well as prison experience and in the safety of a therapeutic community and milieu of the Vietnam Vets Program, exploring new and covered-over feelings.

I had a couple of one-to-one meetings with Mark and it became apparent that the initial attraction we shared was still alive. In the second meeting, Mark revealed that he had been thinking about me and had some fantasies about being together romantically but was worried that his thoughts might be sick. 'You see, I have spent so much time in jail, I don't know what is normal or pathological any more. I don't even know how to judge my feelings. Perhaps they are all just sick delusions.' Mark described to me what I thought to be some tender, romantic and caring desires. At the end of his disclosure, I confirmed that I found his fantasies normal and appealing but because of the situation, not possible to carry out with me.

I explained that I was glad he felt comfortable to reveal his feelings and that being in therapy would open up all kinds of dormant feelings that required sorting out. I told him about how beginning to open up in the presence of young female nurses who were accepting and supportive, often stimulated feelings of connection that could be mistaken for love. I gave him the standard explanation of the surrogate role and its significance by suggesting that this meant relating to others in such a way in the future was possible for him.

This was different though. I also felt an attraction in return and admitted it to him. I did not deny my feelings as I knew that I was blushing in his presence anyhow. To deny my feelings would be to deny Mark an opportunity to understand and judge his effect on others. I thought it unfair to reflect back and lie. At the end of the meeting, I told Mark that, given my attraction to him, it would be best that he work with someone else. I was not rejecting him but rather was concerned about my ability to be helpful during such an important time of his recovery. I also told him

—continued

—continued

that I had consulted my colleague Paul, and asked for help about my feelings but did not reveal the details of our conversation. After much discussion, Mark and I agreed to cherish the awakening we both shared and to hold it in a special place—not to be acted on or forgotten.

My safety net during this time was to consult with Paul, a trusted colleague whom I worked with. The day Mark was admitted to the program, I told Paul about the 'lust at first sight' pool encounter. He said, just keep track of those feelings and let him know as things evolved. After telling him that Mark had been assigned to my group, we both agreed to see if the feelings would pass. When they didn't, I told Paul that I needed help. We decided that I must discuss this with Mark and suggest a transfer to another therapist.

This story is reminiscent of numerous situations that occur between nurses and patients. Unfortunately, not all encounters have good outcomes. An inevitable aspect of nursing includes becoming genuinely interested in the people you are caring for. The point at which that interest grows into mutual affection and love can be difficult to detect. However, attending to cues, self-disclosure and seeking trusted counsel will help to identify when involvement is becoming too close, ineffective, blurred or potentially harmful.

Discussion questions

Return to the introduction of this chapter. In a nursing tutorial session, discuss each situation listed with members of the group. In discussing your responses to each situation, consider the following questions.

■ What cues, if any, might you notice that would indicate such a situation was developing?
■ What would you do?
■ Whom would you talk to and/or consult for help about the situation?

—continued

—continued

■ In your response, how can you convey acknowledgment and understanding of the person's feelings and wishes without discounting, minimizing or negating them and, at the same time, make your position clear?
■ What situation generated the most discussion in the group? Why?
■ What situation would you personally find most challenging to deal with?

Summary

Caring is an interpersonal process that obliges the mental health nurse to put the patient first, physically and mentally, and to be receptive and responsive to their needs. People experiencing a mental illness seek the comfort, security and support that caring provides, and want the nurse to make them feel like a valuable and worthwhile individual. Caring allows the person to develop a sense of hope, encouragement and confidence in their ability to make positive change. The potential to be caring is often sustained through nurses caring for themselves and each other—a cooperative sense of teamwork.

The issues identified in this chapter are cause for celebration. If the nature of mental health nursing work was unambiguous or simply a matter of routinized actions, a chapter about conundrums would not be necessary. The fact that nursing involves changing and evolving relationships with others makes it not only a necessity, but an exciting and stimulating endeavor.

References

Australian Health Minister's Advisory Council National Mental Health Working Group 1996, *National standards for mental health services*. AGPS, Canberra.

Australian Health Minister's Conference 1991, *Mental health. Statement of rights and responsibilities. Report of the mental health consumer outcomes task force, adopted by the AHM, March 1991*. AGPS, Canberra.

Australian and New Zealand College of Mental Health Nurses Inc. 1995, *Standards of practice for mental health nursing in Australia*. ANZCMHN Inc., Adelaide.

Barker, P. 1997, *Assessment in psychiatric and mental health nursing. In search of the whole person*. Stanley Thornes, Cheltenham, UK.

Benner, P. & Wrubel, J. 1989, *The primacy of caring. Stress and coping in health and illness*. Addison-Wesley, Menlo Park, Calif.

Bond, M. & Holland, S. 1998, *Skills of clinical supervision for nurses. A practical guide for supervisees, clinical supervisors and managers*. Open University Press, Buckingham, UK.

Bowlby, J. 1969, *Attachment and loss. Attachment, vol. I*. Basic Books, New York.

Brady, P. 1997, The therapeutic relationship. In: B. Johnson (ed.), *Adaptation and growth. Psychiatric–mental health nursing*, 4th edn. Lippincott, Philadelphia.

Brykczynska, G. 1997, *Caring. The compassion and wisdom of nursing*. Arnold, London.

Burton, G. 1977. *Interpersonal relations. A guide book for nurses*. Tavistock, London.

Butterworth T. & Faugier, J. (eds), 1998, *Clinical supervision and mentorship in nursing*, 2nd edn. Chapman and Hall, London.

Carter, F. 1981, *Psychosocial nursing. Theory and practice in hospital and community mental health*. Macmillan Publishing, New York.

Commonwealth Department of Health and Aged Care 1999, *Learning together. Education and training partnerships in mental health*. Publication number 2570. AGPS, Canberra.

Figley, C, 1995, *Compassion fatigue. Coping with secondary traumatic stress disorder in those who treat the traumatized*. Brunner/Mazel, New York.

French, G. & Harris, C. 1999, *Traumatic incident reduction*. CRC Press, Florida.

Gallop, R. 1997, Caring about the client. The role of gender, empathy, and power in the therapeutic process. In: S. Tilley (ed.), *The mental health nurse. Views of practice and education*. Blackwell Press, Oxford (pp. 28–42).

Garratt, S. 1992, Reflective practice as a learning strategy. In: G. Gray & R. Pratt (eds), *Issues in Australian nursing 3*. Churchill Livingstone, Melbourne (pp. 213–28).

Gerbode, F. 1995, *Beyond psychology. An introduction to metapsychology*, 3rd edn. IRM Press, Menlo Park, Calif.

Goffman, E. 1961, *Asylums. Essays on the social situation of mental patients and other inmates*. Anchor Books, New York.

Harlow, H. F. & Zimmerman, R. 1959, Affectional responses in the infant monkey. *Science*, 130: 421–32.

Havens, L. 1986, *Making contact. Uses of language in psychotherapy*. Harvard University Press, Cambridge, Mass.

Hess, J. 1996, The ethics of compliance. A dialectic. *Advances in Nursing Science*, 19(1): 18–27.

Horsfall, J., Cleary, M. & Jordan, R. 1999, *Towards ethical mental health nursing practice* (#3 of the monograph series). The Australian and New Zealand College of Mental Health Nurses, Hobart.

Hughes, E. 1963, Professions. *Daedalus*, Fall: 656.

Keltner, L. Schwecke, L. & Bostrom, C. 1991, *Psychiatric nursing. A psychotherapeutic management approach*. Mosby Year Book, St. Louis, Mo.

Laing, R. 1965, *The divided self. An existential study in sanity and madness*. Penguin Books, Baltimore.

Lawler, J. 1991, *Behind the screens. Nursing, somology, and the problem of the body*. Churchill Livingstone, Melbourne.

Lee, J. 1993, A history of care modalities in nursing. In: K. Kelly & M. Maas, *Managing nursing care. Promise and pitfalls*. Mosby, St. Louis, Mo (pp. 20–38).

Lyons, M. 1997, Understanding professional behavior. Experiences of occupational therapy students in mental health settings. *American Journal of Occupational Therapy*, 51(8): 686–92.

May, C. 1991, Affective neutrality and involvement in nurse–patient relationships. Perceptions of appropriate behavior among nurses in acute medical and surgical wards. *Journal of Advanced Nursing*, 16: 552–8.

Menzies, I. 1970, *The functioning of social systems as a defence against anxiety*. (Reprint of Tavistock pamphlet 3.) Tavistock, London.

Murray, I. 1997, How can clients and carers become allies? *Nursing Times*, 93(27): 40–1.

O'Donnel, M. 1993, How to enable staff to empower patients. *Nursing Standard*, 8(12): 38–9.

Pearson, A. 1984, The essence of advanced nursing is being there. *Nursing Mirror*, Sept. 4: 16.

Peplau, H. 1969, Professional closeness. A special kind of involvement with a patient, client, or family group. *Nursing Forum*, VIII(8): 342–60.

Saakvitne, K. & Pearlman, L. 1996, *Transforming the pain. A workbook on vicarious traumatization*. Norton & Co., New York.

Savage, J. 1990, The theory and practice of the new nursing. *Nursing Times*, 86(1): 42–5.

Savage, J. 1995, *Nursing intimacy. An ethnographic approach to nurse–patient interaction*. Scutari Press, London.

Shives, L. 1998, *Basic concepts of psychiatric nursing*, 4th edn. Lippincott, Philadelphia.

Stamm, B. 1995, *Secondary traumatic stress. Self-care issues for clinicians, researchers, and educators*. Sidran Press, Lutherville, Md.

Stuhlmiller, C. M. 1995, The construction of disorders. Exploring the growth of PTSD and SAD. *Journal of Psychosocial Nursing and Mental Health Service*, 33(1): 20–3.

Stuhlmiller, C. M. 1996, Narrative picturing. Ushering experiential recall. *Nursing Inquiry*, (3): 183–4.

Stuhlmiller, C. M. & Thorsen, R. 1997, Narrative picturing. A new approach to qualitative data collection. *Qualitative Health Research*, 7(1): 140–9.

Szasz, T. 1974, *The myth of mental illness. Foundations of a theory of personal conduct*. Harper & Row, New York.

Wade, S. 1995, Partnership in care. A critical review. *Nursing Standard*, 9(48): 29–32.

Mental Health
Nursing Practice

8

Emotions: anxiety is contagious

Key concepts
in this
chapter:

- anxiety reduction
- being with the consumer
- cognitive reconstruction
- feelings, verbalization
- generalized anxiety disorder (GAD)
- holistic assessment
- interpersonal aspects of anxiety
- nurse management of own anxiety
- post-traumatic stress disorder (PTSD)
- relief behaviors
- substance abuse and dependence
- therapeutic relationships

Introduction

Anxiety is a common human experience. All people feel levels of anxiety greater than their own normal levels from time to time. Nurses will work with consumers whose anxiety levels may be less than their own at a particular point in time and with many patients in general hospitals who are anxious in relation to hospitalization, the suddenness, severity or mysteriousness of their medical diagnosis, surgery or a range of practical and social worries. In the community or in mental health settings, RNs will work with consumers whose anxiety levels range along a continuum. For most consumers, an anxiety disorder will not be a primary reason for consulting the health system. However, in mental health settings, most consumers will experience some distressing anxiety on top of the difficulties associated with other psychiatric diagnoses (Greene, 1997). Nurses in any setting will frequently be working with anxious consumers,

186 Interpersonal nursing for mental health

family members or staff. It is therefore essential to gain an understanding of human anxiety, to assess direct and indirect signs of anxiety, and develop a range of nursing practices to help people lower their anxiety levels.

Prevalence rates of anxiety disorders

According to the recent Australian Bureau of Statistics (ABS) study of a representative sample of 10,600 Australian adults, anxiety disorders constitute the most common psychiatric diagnoses attributed to women across the life span. Women born overseas have a slightly higher rate of anxiety disorders in comparison with Australian-born women; overseas-born men do not have higher rates of anxiety than men born in Australia. The largest group of psychiatric diagnoses made of men in the study related to alcohol and other drug use and/or abuse; the second highest grouping for men was anxiety disorders. Ten per cent of the adult population are deemed to have experienced anxiety symptoms to the extent that they could have received a specific anxiety diagnosis at some stage during the 12 months prior to the interview (ABS 1998). Epidemiological studies in the USA place the rate at 12.6 per cent of the adult population (Harris & Keltner 1997). Anxiety is the most prevalent single psychiatric disorder of the present era.

The percentage breakdown of disorders among the 12 per cent of women deemed eligible for an anxiety diagnosis (ABS 1998) is:

- post-traumatic stress disorder (PTSD) 4.2%
- generalized anxiety disorder 3.7%
- social phobia 3.0%
- panic disorder 2.0%
- agoraphobia 1.5%
- obsessive compulsive disorder 0.4% (definitions appear later in this chapter).

For the seven per cent of men deemed eligible for an anxiety diagnosis, the percentage breakdown is:

- social phobia 2.4%
- generalized anxiety disorder 2.4%
- post-traumatic stress disorder 2.3%

- agoraphobia 0.7%
- panic disorder 0.6%
- obsessive compulsive disorder 0.3% (ABS 1998).

These figures are important because they draw our attention to the unexpectedly high proportion of people—especially women—in our society with residual post-traumatic stress disorder; around the expected level of generalized anxiety disorder among the population; and the unexpectedly high percentage of people who live with a social phobia—especially men.

The national survey data indicate that the ways women express anxiety are more likely to be considered to be a psychiatric disorder. If the use of alcohol can be understood to be at least partly related to its anxiolytic (anti-anxiety) effect, then men's higher levels of substance use may indicate self-medication for relief of anxiety. In the ABS study, 9.4 per cent of men were deemed to use alcohol harmfully or be dependent upon alcohol, as well as three per cent who reported harmful use or dependence on other drugs. Among women, 3.7 per cent were deemed to be harmfully using or dependent upon alcohol and just over one per cent harmfully using or dependent upon other drugs (ABS 1998).

Sex differences in expression of anxiety are also evident in different age cohorts. Men between the ages of 18 and 24 experience the highest level of anxiety (9%) and the highest level of substance abuse (21.5%) across the age spectrum. Women between 45 and 54 years of age experience the highest level of anxiety disorders (16%); but the 18- to 24-year-olds register the highest rate of substance abuse (11%) across the age range (ABS 1998).

Because anxiety is such an uncomfortable human experience, many of us have learned to distract ourselves from the discomfort or to avoid specific anxiety-creating situations. For example, a person who has experienced fear in response to parental disputes, may, as an adult, leave the room when conflict escalates, change the topic or placate the aggressor before the exchange proceeds too far, or lash out physically to decrease the time in which the tension builds up between the antagonists. These mechanisms may work well for some years of their lives; however, they mitigate against learning how to deal with conflict constructively for their own and other people's benefit.

Peplau (in O'Toole & Welt 1989) calls these distracting or avoiding strategies 'relief behaviors'. These are common human responses to the physical and emotional discomfort associated with anxiety.

Relief behaviors

When a person perceives a serious threat to self, relief behaviors occur automatically. In other words, such responses are unconscious and have been drawn upon over long periods of time. Each of us develops characteristic patterns of relief behaviors that provide some inner protection from perceived threats (Smith-Alnimer 1996). These are all helpful to some extent, but if they prevent us from experiencing the anxiety, then we cannot learn to consciously deal with such situations in constructive or healthy ways. Peplau (1989) outlines four primary patterns of relief behaviors: acting out, somatizing, withdrawal, and learning or realistic problem solving.

Acting out is one pattern of relief behavior. Holoday-Worret (1996: 28) defines acting out as 'behavior displaced from one situation to another in response to inner tension . . . ; the individual acts out on impulse instead of feeling, thinking, or discussing the tension-causing situation when it happens'. The real issues or interaction causing the person's inner conflict is not dealt with. Often acting out results in other people's distress. In a non-therapeutic environment, everybody then attends to the negative consequences of the acting out, not the actual internal impetus behind the person's behavior.

Somatizing is the second pattern of relief behavior named by Peplau (1989). When anxiety is unconsciously converted to a troubling bodily sensation, the person is distracted by her or his palpitations, headache or trembling, for example. Somatizing removes the individual's awareness of anxiety or emotional distress and the person worries about specific aspects of their physical health instead of finding the underlying cause of the anxiety and actively dealing with it.

Withdrawal is another pattern of relief behavior. This may include physical removal of self from the threatening situation, a sort of psychic numbing that some very traumatized people experience, or withdrawal into one's self. Extreme patterns of withdrawal include depression, when the person seems to be inaccessible to others, and withdrawal to internal thoughts, ideas and reverie along the schizophrenia continuum.

The characteristics of these three forms of relief behavior are that they are patterned, involuntary and they eventually fail to protect the person from distress. Peplau's (1989) final pattern of relief behavior is drawing on the psychic energy associated with anxiety for useful learning purposes. Thus, the fourth pattern of behavior is the constructive conversion of anxiety into developing strategies that bypass automatic behaviors and offer an opportunity for growth by broadening a person's repertoire of coping responses in emotionally uncomfortable situations.

Charron (1994) discusses people whose experience of high levels of conscious or unconscious anxiety over long periods of time result in inflexible ways of interacting with other people. She describes two common maladaptive patterns of relating that are likely to emerge: over-dependent behaviors or mechanisms to distance self from others.

Common dependent behaviors include:

- submissiveness
- approval seeking
- indecisiveness
- acting helplessly
- excessive advice seeking
- taking up other people's opinions
- deference toward others, especially those in authority.

Common distancing behaviors include:

- limited authentic expression of feelings
- taking uninvited or inappropriate control of other people
- blaming others for problems
- conveying a sense of personal superiority
- manipulating others to achieve own goals
- behaving angrily when authority is even mildly queried
- assuming moral superiority for self and disdain for others.

Discussion questions

Think of members of your family. Do any of them interact with others using either of the two styles above? What are the short-term consequences of using these behaviors? What are the actual or likely long-term consequences of behaving over-dependently or in a controlling manner?

Discuss these issues with a friend or another student. Outline strategies that a person can use to work their way out of dependent behavior patterns.

Concepts relevant to managing ordinary living

Personal practices and lifestyles that allow both the experiencing of anxiety (as opposed to denial or repression) and an achievement of emotional equilibrium are central to maturity and life satisfaction. Healthy living requires a balance between 'being in control' and having sufficient relaxation.

Control over our lives is a common expectation of middle class people in westernized societies. The experience of anxiety, fear or other strong distress can be felt to threaten our belief that individuals lead rational, emotionally controlled lives characterized by choice (Horsfall 1998). In reality, anxiety is intrinsic to the human condition and some level of anxiety is inevitable in social interactions.

A balance between the experience of anxiety and some intra-psychic management of anxiety to render it bearable may be one of the great challenges of living. To experience anxiety at levels which are emotionally disturbing or impede daily activities of socializing, working, eating and sleeping is clearly an imbalance which requires some effort to change. Similarly, to be quite unaware of anxiety by virtue of denial, overwork, social isolation or the use of legal or illicit drugs may feel safe for some period of time, but even if the person involved is unconcerned it is likely that family members, friends, teachers or work colleagues will consider that something is amiss.

To achieve some satisfying and functional balance between anxiety and calmness, we all draw on unconscious and conscious coping mechanisms. Constructive ways of dealing with stress include talking about the problem with others, distraction by concentrating on fun or work activities, crying, expressing strong feelings to a person in a safe place, introspection, humour, changing posture and breathing patterns by vigorous exercise, sleep, meditation, or discerning at least one aspect of the problem and dealing with it. Less constructive responses to stress include physical violence, being verbally abusive, driving a motor vehicle at high speed, social isolation, damaging property, mistreating pets, excessive use of videos, television or computers, workaholism, excessive physical exertion or sexual activity, or using addictive substances (Forchuk 1993).

Substance abuse

The use of alcohol is a socially endorsed activity in our society. Many Australians manage their alcohol use over a lifetime with apparently limited negative health consequences. Presently it is considered that approximately three per cent of Australians use alcohol harmfully, a further 3.5 per cent are dependent upon alcohol and another two per cent use and/or abuse other drugs (including sedatives, stimulants, marijuana and opioids) (ABS 1998: 18).

A substance abusing person is impaired or distressed about work, school or family role obligations; or they take risks that are health endangering or life threatening; or their use of alcohol or other drugs is such that they have broken the law, even if they have not been charged with a crime. Substance dependence includes:

1. tolerance of the drug, and/or
2. withdrawal symptoms if the substance use is stopped or decreased, and/or
3. previous serious but failed attempts by the person to stop using the drug.

Tolerance means that over time a higher dose of the same drug has to be used to achieve the equivalent desired effect. Withdrawal symptoms involve the person experiencing a known syndrome when the substance use has stopped; for example, physical symptoms in response to withdrawal from alcohol include tremors, rapid pulse rate, raised blood pressure, sleep interference and the possibility of seizures or alcohol hallucinosis.

The consequences of alcohol abuse and dependence are social, financial, psychological, physical and practical. Substance abusers diminish their own health and they invariably interfere with the quality of life of those involved with them, including parents, children, siblings, friends and colleagues. The most significant characteristic of substance-dependent people is the denial or minimization of their alcohol-related problems. They usually play down the negative consequences to themselves and to others, and underestimate the amount of alcohol consumed at specific sittings and overall. The greatest challenge to nurses in busy hospitals and community settings is to take a thorough substance use history from the person, covering all drugs (legal, prescribed and illicit), the type of alcohol used (for example, which beer, wine, spirit) and the amounts and frequency of consumption.

Once relationships between mental disorders, physical conditions and substance abuse are explored, complex combinations of problems are revealed. Almost 18 per cent of the population is deemed to have a mental disorder, however, only ten per cent have a single anxiety, mood or substance abuse problem (ABS 1998).

Co-morbidity is the presence of two or more disorders in the same person—these can be physical, psychiatric or substance-related. Dual diagnosis is the simultaneous presence of a psychiatric disorder and a substance abuse disorder, which interact and worsen each other.

According to the national mental health survey, substance abuse disorders (3.6%) are the largest single diagnosis in the mental disorder category, followed by anxiety (2.9%). The most common co-morbidities are an anxiety disorder in combination with a physical condition (2.6%). Given the above definition, the most common dual diagnosis in the Australian community at present is that of anxiety and substance abuse or dependence (0.6%) (ABS 1998: 29).

These ABS data show that about half of the population (49%) experience either physical (31%) or mental disorders (18%), or a combination. Hence nurses will work with people with anxiety disorders alone; those with anxiety and physical conditions; or people with anxiety and substance abuse disorders.

People with low self-esteem who experience internal and/or interpersonal conflict, uncomfortable anxiety and a sense of social alienation are particularly likely to use alcohol to block out the anxiety, discomfort and/or powerlessness (cf, Stuart & Sundeen, 1991). This cycle may appear to the person involved to be beneficial for some months or years. However, the over use of alcohol has the potential to lower their esteem in others' eyes, create further conflict, raise anxiety levels within relationships, reinforce feelings of powerlessness and fears of being out of control and the further use of alcohol to attempt to block out emotional pain and personal realities.

This cycle can include prescribed anxiolytics (anti-anxiety medication). Drugs such as alprazolam (e.g., Xanax®), lorazepam (e.g., Ativan®) or oxazepam (e.g., Serepax) reduce tension and anxiety but, among other unwarranted effects, they are likely to increase chemical tolerance, create physical and psychological dependence and precipitate rebound anxiety if their use is suddenly ceased. Drug dependence superimposed on an anxiety disorder is very undermining for the people concerned (Mason, 1996). The majority of anxiolytics are prescribed for women, consequently anxiety plus an addiction to prescribed medication is more often a woman's problem. Furthermore, there are few services that offer detoxification, structured programs and support through withdrawal along with teaching stress management strategies.

It is the nurse's responsibility to become familiar with anti-anxiety medication effects, to discern the impact on individual consumers and to teach them about the advantages and disadvantages of the medication over the short and medium term. Anxiolytic medication cannot cure anxiety disorders; these drugs should only be used to lower anxiety levels in the short term so that the consumer is able to be engaged in constructive therapies (Greene 1997).

Definitions

Anxiety is experienced 'when a severe unexpected threat to one's feeling of self-esteem or well-being occurs' (Smith-Alnimer,

1996). Peplau (1952) deems anxiety to be the basic human response to a psychic threat. Anxiety is not entirely observable, hence nurses need to solicit and value consumer information about their somatic and emotional experiences (Simpson, 1991). People who are concerned about their level of anxiety may feel apprehension, jitteriness, helplessness, vague discomfort, uncertainty or self-doubt (Greene, 1997).

Generalized anxiety disorder (GAD), as the name indicates, is an anxiety condition characterized by diverse anxiety manifestations, as opposed to focused experiences such as phobias or panic. Men experience GAD at about the same rate as social phobia and these are the two most commonly diagnosed anxiety states in men. GAD is the second most common overt anxiety diagnosis in women (ABS, 1998). Excessive anxiety and worry occurring more days than not during the previous six months is the primary characteristic of GAD. The worry is 'difficult to control' and is accompanied by three or more physical or mental signs such as feeling keyed up, muscle tension, sleep disturbance, fatigue, irritability or concentration difficulties which impede or interfere with activities of daily living (Greene, 1997). For more details about psychiatric diagnostic criteria, the reader should consult the DSM-IV (American Psychiatric Association [APA] 1994).

Anxiety is expressed directly and indirectly across a range of somatic and psychological manifestations, including the following:

- affective: apprehension, fear, terror, a sense of impending doom, dread
- behavioral: motor tension, hyper-vigilance, hostility towards others, hyper-activity, hand wringing, foot tapping, nail biting
- cognitive: thoughts or fears about dying, losing control, or going mad
- physiological: shortness of breath, choking sensation, palpitations, high blood pressure, faintness, trembling, sweating, urinary frequency, dryness of the mouth, decreased appetite, nausea, diarrhea.

Reflective questions

Consider the affective, behavioral and physiological signs of anxiety outlined above. Which ways do you respond to stress?

Because anxiety sensations are uncomfortable, they are commonly recognized as physical signs. In some situations do you experience: a knot in your stomach?; a sudden need to rush to the toilet?; trouble swallowing?; headaches like a band around your head?; rising nausea, or other physical sensations? In what types of situations or interactions do these occur? Do these physical sensations prevent you from doing things that you want to do?

Consider the relief behaviors of acting out, somatizing, social withdrawal and reliance on alcohol, cigarettes or marijuana. Do any of these mechanisms apply to yourself or your friends? Commonly these behaviors are rationalized (i.e., the person uses plausible excuses to apparently justify them). Rationalization examples include: 'That's just the way he is—he's aggressive'; 'She will never come out with us because she has these headaches'; 'We drink alcohol, smoke cigarettes or smoke marijuana because everybody in our crowd does'. Do you or your friends rationalize some unhealthy behaviors? Might you (or they) benefit from doing something to change the behaviors rather than justifying them?

Post-traumatic stress disorder (PTSD) may occur as a consequence of a person experiencing or witnessing a dangerous or threatening event to which they responded with intense fear, helplessness or horror. This event is re-experienced by the person via recurrent and intrusive images, thoughts, perceptions, dreams, or emotional re-enactment. These result in the person resorting to three or more of the following avoidance strategies: attempting to not think, talk about or remember the event; avoiding activities, places or people that arouse the recollections; being unable to recall aspects of the event; feeling detached from others; having a narrower range of emotions than before; experiencing less interest in life; or having a limited sense of future. As well as these characteristics, the traumatized person will display a range of general anxiety symptoms which may include impaired sleeping, concentration difficulties, irritability, outbursts of anger, hyper-vigilance or an exaggerated startle response (Greene, 1997).

Not everybody who survives an earthquake, sporting disaster, aeroplane crash, rape, assault, industrial accident, violence within the family, robbery, being a political refugee, witnessing murder or a fatal motor vehicle accident or military combat will experience PTSD. However, this is the most prevalent anxiety diagnosis in the Australian population at the time of writing (ABS, 1998). PTSD is the most prevalent anxiety diagnosis in women and this may indicate sequelae of the abuse of power in gender relations whereby females experience higher rates of child sexual assault, spouse abuse and rape. Intrusive obstetric interventions during childbirth, especially in association with uncaring behaviors by doctors and midwives, can also precipitate an acute stress reaction which is likely to become PTSD if it remains untreated (Creedy, 1999).

Phobias are extreme fears which result in the person determinedly avoiding specific situations, locations, feared objects or events. The fear is considered to be excessive by themselves and others.

The essential features of a *social phobia* are a profound and enduring fear of social or performance situations that the person perceives to be potentially embarrassing. Even though the person recognizes that the level of fear is inordinate, if she or he does proceed with the anticipated feared event, a panic attack is likely to occur. Avoidance, anxious anticipation or distress associated with the feared situation impede the person's activities of daily living. The most commonly feared social situations are public speaking, eating in a restaurant, giving an artistic performance, writing in front of others, or using public toilets (Robinson, 1996). If the anxiety does not reach panic level, the person will experience responses such as shaking, vomiting, vertigo, thought blocking or the inability to perform. These then result in avoidance of friends and situations in case an ordinary social event leads to the feared scenario (Greene, 1997).

Social phobias are the third most prevalent anxiety disorder in Australia (ABS, 1998). As this anxiety reveals social causes and consequences, it may reflect the interest of westernized societies in the idealized individual who is confident, articulate and conducts herself or himself in cool and appropriate ways in all situations. This is a fantasy that most people cannot fulfill.

Obsessions are recurrent and persistent thoughts or images that the person experiences as intrusive, inappropriate and distressing.

Compulsions are repetitive and ritualized physical or mental acts that a person must perform to prevent a feared (but comparatively unlikely) event or situation, or to reduce distress in relation to obsessions.

Most people with a diagnosable anxiety disorder will be untreated, take anti-anxiety medication prescribed by a general medical practitioner or seek assistance from private or community practitioners. A small proportion of people with severe levels of obsessive compulsive disorder or panic attacks will be admitted to mental health settings for treatment. In mental health settings, nurses will mostly be dealing with anxiety superimposed on other mental illnesses and sometimes arising from admission processes.

Holistic assessment

When psychiatry deems an individual's anxiety to be 'excessive', nurses need to know what is and has been happening in the person's life in the immediate past and during the last year or so to make a comprehensive psychosocial nursing assessment. In some situations the level of anxiety may actually be appropriate; for example, when there is violence within the family, harassment in the workplace, or the realistic fear of—or actual—unemployment or homelessness.

Precipitants

Often there have been events in the weeks or months before hospital admission that have precipitated or exacerbated anxiety symptoms. These may be internal or external. Commonly, anxiety precipitants constitute a threat to the person's physical or emotional integrity (Stuart, 1998a). External events that are likely to cause heightened anxiety can be practical, involve loss, or relate to social norms. Practical matters can be social, financial or legal; losses often involve 'exits' or 'entrances' in the person's life; and social norm disruptions can be positive, such as being promoted or getting married, or negative, such as getting divorced or being unemployed.

However, much disabling stress is long-term and may be made up of frequent problems involving relationships, parenting, money or work difficulties over years or decades (Stuart, 1998b).

Appraisal of stressors or precipitants

People view experiences in diverse ways and imbue them with unique meanings, interpretations and significance. Cognitive appraisals can be negative, positive or mixed. Negative appraisals include the perception of actual harm or loss, or the threat of anticipated harm or loss. Some events can be appraised as challenging and these pose difficulties, but include the potential for learning, mastery and personal growth (Stuart, 1998b).

Coping resources

It is important for nurses to assess a consumer's resources. Stuart (1998b) outlines the following resource categories:

- intrapsychic (e.g., self-esteem, a good values system, positive motivation)
- interpersonal (e.g., intimate support, active positive family ties, social skills)
- social (e.g., a supportive network, community stability, group involvement)
- economic (e.g., money to buy goods and services to buffer life difficulties)
- culture (e.g., a sense of belonging, cultural cohesion, shared rituals)
- health (e.g., energy, being well nourished, good physical health, being fit)
- intelligence (e.g., knowledge, awareness, access to information, creativity).

Effective coping mechanisms

Useful strategies are often action oriented or involve thinking the problem through, or both. Action-oriented strategies include carrying out a task, seeking advice, and tackling the threat assertively by negotiation or confrontation. Cognitive strategies involve searching for meaning, analyzing, evaluating, problem solving, selectively ignoring some things, and sometimes dropping one goal and opting for something more realistic (Stuart, 1998b).

Ineffective coping mechanisms

Less constructive methods of dealing with anxiety ultimately reduce life choices. Unhelpful coping mechanisms are often unconsciously developed in response to fears associated with conflict and may include repression, denial or projection, as well as relief behaviors. Initially, relief behaviors 'protect' the individual from interpersonal conflict and anxiety. Relief behaviors and substance use commonly cut people off from meaningful and satisfying relationships at home, school, university or work. Even if the person does not consider these to be problematic, others will. Such situations may result in increased distance between people, or conflict. The mechanisms that initially provided protection from anxiety eventually lead to other interpersonal problems. In other words, relief behaviors ultimately fail (Peplau, 1989).

While relief behaviors remain intact, the person has a limited capacity to resolve serious personal issues. This is likely to be experienced as frustrating by the person or others involved in these circumstances. The combination of anxiety, a limited interpersonal skills repertoire and frustration can become increasingly socially disabling. These social disabilities often do not stop there, but impede learning, interfere with achieving educational qualifications, reduce work productivity and decrease social acceptability.

Substance use

Since alcohol is the most common anti-anxiety substance used in our society (Thurston, 1997), it is important that a person's drug use is ascertained for comprehensive assessment purposes. Use of alcohol, illicit central nervous system depressants or prescription anxiolytics may mask levels of disabling anxiety in some people.

Keeping a journal

Consider the above six assessment headings: precipitants, the person's appraisal of the stressors, range of resources, patient strengths, evidence of ineffective coping mechanisms, and substance use. When you go on your next clinical placement, write these headings down at the end of the day and reflect upon what you know about a specific patient. If you cannot put information under most of these headings, spend some time with the person on the following days and gather some more data to help you understand some likely reasons for her or his distress.

Beginning nursing strategies

Psychiatric diagnoses highlight differences between the disorders but, from a nursing perspective, anxiety disorders are characterized more by their similarities along a continuum, from mild anxiety to panic levels (Molloy 1996). Thus, nursing goals to be developed with consumers run across the anxiety disorder diagnoses and include acceptance of the present anxiety (not fighting against it), increasing self-awareness, learning self-help techniques to decrease anxiety, and developing problem-solving skills (Greene, 1997).

The basic nursing strategy is to develop a supportive and trusting relationship with the consumer. The nature of anxiety and fear is such that each person will require interpersonal support to assist in reducing the level of anxiety. Using interpersonal and practical means, the nurse needs to ensure and maintain the consumer's safety, and this is often at an emotional level in the first instance, because she or he is scared and afraid. When the consumer is in a state of panic (an extremely high and disturbing level of anxiety), an emotional sense of safety is equally important, but in such a situation anxiolytic medication is likely to be administered promptly as well. However, the use of anti-anxiety medication never exempts the nurse from the primary responsibility of being with the person until initial levels of anxiety have decreased to some extent. Especially during early interactions with the consumer, the nurse needs to be consistent, calm and reliable (Stuart, 1998a).

Self-awareness is an essential ingredient for nurses who work with many consumers who experience high levels of anxiety. Anxiety is not a contagious disease, but it is palpably transmitted from one anxious person to others (Molloy, 1996). The nurse can be a source of anxiety in interpersonal interactions, with anti-therapeutic consequences for consumers (Peplau, 1989). Likewise, anxious consumers can increase the experience of anxiety in unaware or vulnerable nurses.

Because anxiety has invisible but transferable qualities, the nurse's internal sense of calmness and ability to be patient is important. These qualities are highly desirable and learnable, even though they require personal effort. Fortunately, they will benefit the nurse as a person as well as consumers. If you do not feel yourself to be a calm person, it could be worthwhile to question yourself about your responses to a person who is overtly anxious. It is important to aim to be nonjudgmental about anxious others, since you may be responding to your own inability to tolerate anxious feelings (Arthur et al., 1992).

A common human response to other people who radiate anxiety is avoidance. This response is understandable but it is not therapeutic from a nursing or consumer perspective. If at first you are unable to remain in the presence of a highly anxious person, you will need clinical supervision to assist you to deal with these issues over time. As a student or beginning practitioner, you may wish to observe and discuss strategies with a more experienced nurse who constructively manages her or his own anxiety for the benefit of the consumer.

Working with consumers who express their helplessness, fears and hopelessness is challenging for all nurses. The sense of helplessness and inadequacy arising from frustration in both the consumer and the nurse, may resonate with uncomfortable feelings of professional inadequacy, especially in the neophyte nurse (Peplau, 1989). These responses are understandable. The student or new graduate requires professional support via supervision or mentoring to understand the interactivity of these feelings, to deal with them in ways that are helpful and provide the foundation from which to work constructively with future anxious consumers.

Principles for working with people with raised anxiety

Once the therapeutic relationship with the consumer is established and maintained, then a few principles can guide nursing practice for working with a person who experiences and evokes anxiety (Boggs 1999). The principles are clear and simple, but implementation is an ongoing nursing challenge. However, as these principles involve the therapeutic use of self, they are transferable from the hospital, to the community, into consumers' homes and into your own.

The principles include:

- behaving calmly
- remembering that the consumer is vulnerable and the anxiety is frightening
- remaining with the person until the high level of anxiety passes
- listening to the person, to create empathy and gain assessment information
- using simple language and brief directive sentences
- clearly explaining nursing actions and ward procedures
- speaking clearly at a low but audible volume
- responding to practical or physical needs
- assisting the consumer to identify some realistic anxiety reducing actions
- not overloading the person with information
- lowering environmental stimulation levels—including demanding interpersonal interactions
- exploring logical reasons for, or precipitants of, anxiety.

When you have been able to remain calm with a highly anxious consumer, assure them that the crisis will pass, and stay with them physically and emotionally and you experience the fact that these principles work, this provides strong positive feedback to you as a nurse that your actions clearly helped the person concerned. There is nothing like overt success to increase confidence and the courage to support another distressed consumer in similar or different circumstances in the future.

Supportive counseling and educational interventions

Generalized anxiety disorder and mild to moderate anxiety levels

Ongoing inquiry about, and assessment of, the level of consumer anxiety is essential. For the person to be able to learn effectively, anxiety should only be mild to moderate (Forchuk 1995). Support and teaching strategies for people with these levels of anxiety include the following.

- Ascertain the person's strengths and positive coping strategies and resources.
- Assess consumer willingness to learn and be responsible for personal change.
- Validate and normalize physiological responses to anxiety.
- Teach the person to develop an awareness of anxiety build-up sensations.
- Facilitate discussion and a full description of experiences.
- Teach the consumer to recognize and name the sensation as anxiety.
- Encourage the person to connect anxiety responses to specific experiences, events, interactions or emotions.
- Ask the person to write a diary or graph anxiety levels in relation to events.
- Encourage the verbal expression of feelings.
- Teach the person to express self and needs assertively.
- Develop problem-solving approaches that draw on verbal negotiation skills.

Expressing feelings, speaking assertively, and verbally negotiating with other people will require practice. The nurse can role model assertiveness and negotiation, and support the consumer in her or his efforts to speak openly and clearly. Consumers will vary in their ability to take up these new communication and behavioral skills. Some people will be able to teach themselves from self-help books or benefit from information and instruction. Others will find these ways of communicating and interacting very difficult because they challenge a lifetime of habit and socially constructed and validated expectations.

Obsessive compulsive disorder and phobias (and other disorders such as anorexia) may be characterized by the person's conscious and unconscious fight against anxiety and desperately trying to control out-of-control thoughts or feelings. These long-held patterns of behavior—fighting and controlling—may ultimately be part of a negative spiral. Both Mason (1996) and Sangster (1996), writing as survivors of agoraphobia and obsessive compulsive disorder, respectively, say that one key to recovery is to accept the anxiety, let go of the anxiety, or pass through the anxiety without trying to wilfully control it. This can be achieved by working within an established therapeutic relationship and/or via art. Sangster (1996: 152) writes briefly and eloquently about her use of painting, drawing and writing 'in a free-flowing way—not in the probing dissecting way of my obsessions'.

Post-traumatic stress disorder (PTSD)

There are three dimensions of PTSD: re-experiencing the trauma, avoidance or emotional numbing, and physiological arousal symptoms. The physical symptoms are similar to those manifested in association with other anxiety disorders and nurses should manage these in symptom-reducing ways, according to the individual consumer's disposition, abilities and other resources.

For PTSD to emerge in response to an individual's experience of a disaster, it is considered that disasters created by people (such as shootings, rape or torture) are more likely to be traumatic than natural disasters. Furthermore, people who have experienced previous trauma are more likely to eventually succumb to PTSD; and those who were powerless during the unfolding of the events are most vulnerable to a traumatic stress disorder (Robinson 1996).

PTSD may involve loss and grief as well as anxiety. Especially if the trauma has been recent and it is clear that the person has experienced significant losses, then grieving for these losses is an essential aspect of healing and recovery. For example, in bushfires where homes have been burnt, pets have died and irreplaceable personal memorabilia have been destroyed, the nurse can assume that each member of the family has experienced a range of losses beyond the obvious loss of money and accommodation. The nurse can work with individuals or with the whole family and encourage them to verbalize and share their distress, fears or concerns. It is likely that both sadness and anger will be expressed by different family members at different times. This is part of the grieving process and when these experiences and feelings have been listened to, validated and understood by at least one other person, then the family members are able to let go of the extreme distress associated with the losses.

Some traumatized people become more severely impeded than others. Antidepressant medication can be helpful for these people and may reduce re-experiencing aspects of the traumatic event and other intrusive thoughts. Intrusive thoughts and images include nightmares, flashbacks and uncontrollable waves of fear (Robinson 1996). Antidepressant medication may also dampen conscious avoidance behavior (such as not visiting people associated with the disaster, not driving past certain places and not talking about the event) and unconscious avoidance mechanisms (such as emotional numbing, denial or dissociation). Ultimately, the medication is best used to relieve distressing symptoms and to allow the person to process the pain, and gain some personal understanding of the trauma and their responses. One method for treating people who have ongoing intrusive thoughts, or those who re-experience trauma, is that of eye movement desensitization and reconstruction (EMDR) in which short-term hypnosis is used in combination with cognitive re-framing (Shapiro, 1995). This process can enable the person to integrate the traumatic experiences into their past life and reclaim control over their thoughts and life and develop a belief in the future again.

Because more women than men are diagnosed with anxiety disorders, it is important to consider gendered and cultural aspects of women's lives that may impede self-expression, assertiveness, and open expressions of personal needs and desires within intimate relationships. For some people, their agoraphobia (for example) has childhood and teenage antecedents that need to be unravelled, understood and processed emotionally (Mason, 1996). The self-esteem and well-being of women is often deemed to be intertwined with their concern for other people within their circle of intimacy, especially their children and spouse (cf., Miller 1986); sometimes to their own detriment. In families where there is cultural conflict between one generation and another, the mother may hear and appreciate both viewpoints, but not have the power to negotiate with the two parties towards a better mutual understanding.

Other practical activities

Anxiety-reducing actions can include a range of comparatively simple activities that fit with the consumer's personal preferences and lifestyle; for example, taking regular warm baths, listening to calming music, moderate exercise such as walking or swimming, massage, yoga or meditation (McLellan, 1992). Such activities can be used routinely as strategies to prevent anxiety, interrupt escalating anxiety, or to manage raised anxiety levels.

People's self-care activities should include maintaining good levels of nutrition, taking the time to eat three meals a day and perhaps using multi-vitamin supplements. Many people should decrease their caffeine intake by cutting down on coffee, tea or carbonated drinks, since these and other central nervous system stimulants worsen anxiety sensations. Exercise is particularly helpful in that it improves oxygenation and blood circulation and increases the efficiency of the removal of carbon monoxide, lactic acid and other metabolic by-products (Robinson, 1996). Self-help books written by anxiety survivors may help consumers develop their own problem-solving approach by drawing on the experiences of others who successfully dealt with similar difficulties.

Reducing anxiety

Robinson (1996) suggests that nurses can teach specific anxiety-reducing activities including:

- progressive muscle relaxation, which involves tensing specific muscle groups followed by relaxation
- controlled slow deep breathing
- relaxation tapes with appropriate music and/or voice commentary

■ guided imagery to assist the person to create the image of a safe haven in their mind to enhance relaxation.

The psychobiology associated with anxiety and other psychiatric disorders has been researched for decades, but is still not well understood because of the involvement of the whole body, as distinct from a specific bodily system or domain of medical expertise. Psychoneuroimmunology is a comparatively new study of the links between psychosocial stressors, emotions and the immune system and their combined effects on the central nervous system. It is believed that stressors activate the hypothalamic-pituitary-adrenal (HPA) axis which stimulates the release of cortisol and other glucocorticoids. Anderson (1998) considers that exposure to acute stress results in the over-stimulation of the HPA axis, but long-term experience of the same stressor leads to an attenuation of the adrenal cortical stress response.

Practical, physical and cognitive nursing interventions aim to disrupt the physiological disequilibrium, decrease the stimulation of the sympathetic nervous system and assist the person to regain physical and cognitive resources for improved coping. In effect, the strategies used by nurses, other health professionals and consumers following self-help paths are often practical rather than theory based, unless the theory is that of pragmatic holism (see Isaacs, 1999, for example).

Active exercise

It is a good idea for you to develop a strategy for controlled slow breathing to manage anxiety and to be able to confidently teach patients this strategy. You should practice this exercise three times a day. The basic directions are as follows (adapted from Isaacs, 1999).

■ Comfortably lie flat or sit.
■ At first, hold your breath and count to five slowly.
■ On the count of five, breathe out and say or think the word 'relax.'
■ Breathe in and out through your nose.

—continued

—*continued*

- Focus on your breathing.
- Breathe in for three seconds and raise your chest and stomach.
- Imagine that the incoming air is bringing calmness into your body.
- Breathe out for three seconds from the bottom of your lungs.
- Imagine the tired air leaving your lungs.
- Repeat the six-second breathing cycle for at least five minutes.

Social relations

Part of the assessment of someone experiencing overwhelming anxiety is to identify others who care about the person and are able to be supportive. Because the person has a 'close family' or 'many friends', they do not inevitably constitute a helpful support network. In particular, relationships between partners should be explored. Occasionally, partners and parents of young adults unconsciously (or consciously) support the consumer's negative self-perceptions, low self-esteem and under-estimation of their own coping abilities. If this is the case, spouse therapy or family therapy are more likely to assist the client.

Practical aspects of the consumer's life also require investigation. Some people experience heightened levels of anxiety around the anniversary of past painful events. In these situations, it is important for the nurse's assessment to allow the possibility of finding out about such events, which often involve the death of a family member or a traumatic accident. Then the nurse and consumer can explore the feelings evoked by the event and connect past experiences to present manifestations.

People who have experienced significant life changes during the past year may become overwhelmed by anxiety because they are simply trying to do too much work. This awareness has become increasingly pertinent to the lives of women who are employed outside the home, who have one or more children at home and whose partners are either absent, workaholic or away for extended periods of time. Often child care responsibilities, along with shopping, cooking, housework and social demands are onerous, and these household labors are not shared, or at least they are not divided fairly. Sometimes both partners have unrealistic expectations of the roles and responsibilities of the mother and/or wife, sometimes only the woman makes unrealistic demands on herself, in other cases the woman knows that she cannot do more but her partner expects or demands more. In these complex interpersonal circumstances, spouse therapy is appropriate, if the partner is a positively motivated participant. If not, the woman should be worked with in supportive and holistic ways to determine her own directions and limitations.

Peer support, culture-specific groups or group therapy can provide a valuable counterpoint to the individual focus of much contemporary health professional practice. For some consumers, the focus on their thinking and feeling increases their sense of failure against a social background involving other people's acceptance of their interpersonal difficulties. Groups for people with similar problems allow members to share problems and achievements and learn positive strategies from each other (Molloy, 1996). Group participation allows the person to feel that she or he is not alone with these particular difficulties and this therefore diminishes the sense of shame and the commonly expressed fear of going mad. Other members of peer support groups will be supportive when this is needed, and these opportunities to provide and receive support can be positive and rewarding experiences.

Cognitive changes

Anxiety reactions are whole body phenomena and therefore include physical, emotional, cognitive and behavioral aspects of the individual's functioning. Consequently, a holistic approach will target physical, emotional, intellectual and behavioral interventions for constructive change. Anxiety must be mild to moderate, as opposed to severe or panic levels, for the consumer to be able to concentrate on the thinking processes required for cognitive re-learning. The person must be willing, motivated and committed to change before embarking on such activities.

Catastrophic thinking involves making negative generalizations as a result of one specific negative experience. Examples include believing that you will fail a course because you received less than 50 per cent for one assignment; or casting serious doubts upon yourself as a nurse because you forgot to give something to a consumer who had asked for it. Such cognitions are often present among people who experience anxiety disorders, thus one strategy is to teach the person to realistically and logically appraise their thinking processes with an aim of decreasing catastrophizing and undermining thoughts (Cowan & Brunero, 1997). Transactional analysis, rational emotive therapy or cognitive behavioral therapy provide frameworks for these strategies.

Re-framing involves facilitating a change in the consumer's interpretation of a situation, her or his actions, or the consequences thereof (Peplau, 1989). Often consumers who experience anxiety disorders are coping with a range of difficulties in their lives. They may see themselves as non-coping or inadequate because they have sought assistance; this viewpoint can be re-framed as evidence of a problem-solving strategy with positive potential (Stuart, 1998a).

Many people who are overwhelmed at times by anxiety experience a negative commentary inside their heads. This is called automatic thinking. As well as discussing and reappraising these thoughts, the consumer can be asked to develop her or his own simple and meaningful self-calming statements. These can be used as a mantra for anxiety reducing purposes, or to change problem behaviors associated with the negative thoughts.

Cognitive therapists recognize a triad of negative cognitive patterns, automatic negative thoughts and problematic behavioral consequences (Joyce, 1996). The negative cognitive patterns consist of negative views of the world, self and the future. The automatic thoughts usually involve:

- over-generalizations (e.g., failing a test equals failing a course)
- selective abstractions—focusing on one negative point within a mixed bag
- polarized thinking which involves all-or-nothing (black and white) beliefs
- personalization (e.g., blaming self for something outside your control).

The consequent problematic behavioral consequences include avoiding situations, giving up, submitting to others and acting helplessly.

Keeping a journal

Since many people experience automatic thinking, you can use your journal to document and change some of your own negative automatic thoughts. The following headings and columns could be used:

- *describe the events leading up to the unpleasant sensations*
- *name the feelings involved*
- *write down the automatic thought(s) associated with the emotion or situation*
- *estimate the strength (percentage) of your belief in the negative thoughts*
- *after reflection, write some logical thoughts in response to the situation*
- *estimate the strength (percentage) of your belief in the positive thoughts*
- *imagine the possible outcome if you had responded to the positive thoughts.*

Over time, see if you can reduce the percentage of your belief in recurring negative automatic thoughts; increase the strength of your belief in alternative constructive thoughts, and note what positive changes emerge for you from these reflections.

Some consumers will benefit from yoga and meditation to explore new aspects of themselves, or to develop more effective strategies to manage their life circumstances. Meditation is a cognitive process in that it involves concentrating on a positive image, idea or sensation and holding on to it while in a state of relaxation. Proponents draw on meditation practices to increase their sense of calm, gain access to inner strengths, lower blood pressure and reduce levels of the chemical by-products of physical and psychological stress (Varcarolis, 1996). Other consumers may benefit from being aware of the potential therapeutic benefits of deep tissue massage, music therapy, or contemporary forms of self-hypnosis (Isaacs, 1999).

References

American Psychiatric Association 1994, *Diagnostic and statistical manual of mental disorders* (DSM-IV). APA, Washington.

Anderson, S. 1998, The biological basis of mental illness. In: C. Glod (ed.) *Contemporary psychiatric-mental health nursing*. F. A. Davis, Philadelphia.

Arthur, D., Dowling, J. & Sharkey, R. 1992, *Mental health nursing. Strategies for working with the difficult client*. W. B. Saunders, Sydney.

Australian Bureau of Statistics 1998, *Mental health and well-being profile of adults. Australia 1997*. AGPS, Canberra.

Boggs, K. 1999, Bridges and barriers in the therapeutic relationship. In: E. Arnold & K. Boggs (eds), *Interpersonal relationships. Professional communication skills for nurses*. W. B. Saunders, Philadelphia.

Charron, H. 1994, Anxiety disorders. In: E. Varcarolis (ed.), *Foundations of psychiatric mental health nursing*. W. B. Saunders, Philadelphia.

Cowan, D. & Brunero, S. 1997, Group therapy for anxiety disorders using rational emotive behavior therapy. *Australian & New Zealand Journal of Mental Health Nursing*, 6(4): 164–8.

Creedy, D. 1999, Birthing and the development of trauma symptoms. Unpublished PhD thesis, Faculty of Health Sciences, Griffith University, Brisbane.

Forchuk, C. 1993, *Hildegard E. Peplau. Interpersonal nursing theory*. Sage, Newbury Park, Calif.

Forchuk, C. 1995, Hildegard E. Peplau. Interpersonal nursing theory. In: C. MetzerMcQuiston & A. Webb (eds), *Foundations of nursing theory. Contributions of 12 key theorists*. Sage, Thousand Oaks, Calif.

Greene, J. 1997, Anxiety disorders. In: B. Johnson (ed.), *Adaptation and growth. Psychiatric–mental health nursing*, 4th edn. Lippincott, Philadelphia.

Harris, D. & Keltner, N. 1997, Medication management. In: N. Worley (ed.), *Mental health nursing in the community*. Mosby, St Louis, Mo.

Holoday-Worret P. 1996, Student issues regarding client and environment. In: K. Fortinash & P. Holoday-Worret (eds), *Psychiatric–mental health nursing*. Mosby, St Louis, Mo.

Horsfall, J. 1998, Mainstream approaches to mental health and illness. An emphasis on individuals and a de-emphasis of inequalities. *Health*, 2(2): 217–31.

Isaacs, D. 1999, *The stress solution*. Pan Macmillan, Sydney.

Joyce, B. 1996, Cognitive therapy. In: S. Lego (ed.), *Psychiatric nursing. A comprehensive reference*, 2nd edn. Lippincott, Philadelphia.

Mason, P. 1996, Agoraphobia. Letting go. In: J. Read & J. Reynolds (eds), *Speaking our minds. An anthology of personal experiences of mental distress and its consequences*. Macmillan, Houndmills, UK.

McLellan, B. 1992, *Overcoming anxiety*. Allen & Unwin, Sydney.

Miller, J. 1986, *Toward a new psychology of women*. Penguin, New York.

Molloy, M. 1996, Anxiety and related disorders. In: K. Fortinash & P. Holoday-Worret (eds), *Psychiatric–mental health nursing*. Mosby, St Louis, Mo.

O'Toole, A. & Welt, S. (eds) 1989, *Interpersonal theory in nursing practice. Selected works of Hildegarde Peplau*. Springer, New York.

Peplau, H. 1952, *Interpersonal relations in nursing.* G. P. Putnam, New York.

Peplau, H. 1989, In: A. O'Toole & S. Welt (eds), *Interpersonal theory in nursing practice. Selected works of Hildegarde Peplau.* Springer, New York.

Robinson, L. 1996, The journey threatened by stress and anxiety disorders. In: B. Carson & E. Arnold (eds), *Mental health nursing. The nurse patient journey.* W. B. Saunders, Philadelphia.

Sangster, M. 1996, I have found a way out of fear. In: J. Read & J. Reynolds (eds), *Speaking our minds. An anthology of personal experiences of mental distress and its consequences.* Macmillan, Houndmills, UK.

Shapiro, F. 1995, *Eye movement desensitization and reprocessing.* Guilford, New York.

Simpson, H. 1991, *Peplau's model in action.* Macmillan, Houndmills, UK.

Smith-Alnimer, M. 1996, The client who is anxious. In: S. Lego (ed.), *Psychiatric nursing. A comprehensive reference*, 2nd edn. Lippincott, Philadelphia.

Stuart, G. 1998a, Anxiety responses and anxiety disorders. In: G. Stuart & M. Laraia (eds), *Stuart & Sundeen's principles and practices of psychiatric nursing*, 6th edn. Mosby, St Louis, Mo.

Stuart, G. 1998b, The Stuart stress adaptation model of psychiatric nursing. In: G. Stuart & M. Laraia (eds), *Stuart & Sundeen's principles and practices of psychiatric nursing*, 6th edn. Mosby, St Louis, Mo.

Stuart, G. & Sundeen, S. 1991, *Principles and practices of psychiatric nursing*, 4th edn. Mosby, St Louis, Mo.

Thurston, B. 1997, Substance abuse and dependency. In: B. Johnson B (ed.), *Adaptation and growth. Psychiatric–mental health nursing*, 4th edn. Lippincott, Philadelphia.

Varcarolis, E. 1996, Relaxation. In: S. Lego (ed.), *Psychiatric nursing. A comprehensive reference*, 2nd edn. Lippincott, Philadelphia.

9
Emotions: misery is scary

Key concepts
in this
chapter:

- alcohol and depression
- cognitive restructuring
- connecting with the consumer
- depression ■ facilitating hope
- families and depression
- holistic assessment ■ holistic healing
- interpersonal aspects of depression
- life events, depression and prevention
- suicidality
- supporting consumer strengths
- therapeutic use of self

The prevalence of mood disorders

Mood is a prolonged emotional state that influences the personality and impedes activities of daily living. Depression is an ongoing lowered mood. Mania or hypomania are elevations of mood.

The Australian Bureau of Statistics (ABS, 1998) survey reveals that 5.8 per cent of the adult population is eligible for a diagnosis of affective (mood) disorder. This is consistent with a USA prevalence of five per cent (Harris & Keltner, 1997). In western nations, depression rates have increased markedly since 1945, and they rise steeply as countries become more 'developed'. The Australian data consist mostly of people with major depression, or dysthymia which is a more long-term, but often less severe, form of depression. A very small proportion of people who experienced an episode of hypomania or mania during the twelve months before the survey are also included in the data (ABS, 1998). Technically, the latter group will have a bipolar diagnosis (involving both depressive and hypomanic episodes) and constitute between 0.6 and 0.9 per cent of the total population (Stuart, 1998).

Peak prevalence rates of depression reveal age differences between women and men, with women between the ages of 18 and 24 experiencing the highest rates (11%) of any age cohort (ABS, 1998). This means that young women in our society experience more depression than any other group. The highest rate of depression for men (6%) occurs between the ages of 35 and 44 (ABS 1998).

Overall, seven per cent of women are deemed to be depressed and just over four per cent of men (ABS, 1998). According to the Australian data, women are approximately 1.8 times more likely than men to be depressed and 1.7 times more likely than men to experience an anxiety disorder. On the other hand, men are 2.4 times more likely than women to harmfully use or be dependent upon alcohol or other drugs (these include marijuana, sedatives, stimulants and opioids).

Alcohol use and/or abuse

Substance abuse disorder is the most prevalent diagnosis for men until about 45 years of age, and rates of apparent depression are consistently lower across the age continuum. For women, substance abuse disorders are the least likely diagnosis across the age continuum; anxiety is the highest, and depression consistently the second most common psychiatric diagnosis from 18 years of age until death (ABS, 1998).

The use of a socially endorsed mood altering drug such as alcohol may cloud the picture in relation to any psychiatric diagnosis. Reliable research evidence that enables clear distinctions to be made between primary diagnosis, cause, precipitant and consequence of mood disorders is not available. However, many clinicians believe that depression underlies much alcohol and other drug abuse (Yapko, 1999).

According to Zahourek (1996) 30 per cent of people with major depression, 30 per cent with a non-phobic anxiety disorder, 25 per cent with phobic disorders and more than 50 per cent of patients with bipolar (mood) disorder have an addictive disorder superimposed on their psychiatric diagnosis. This information is consistent with the hypothesis that people with psychiatric difficulties tend to self-medicate with available substance(s) to try to gain relief from psychic distress and intrusive symptoms. If this argument is credible, then in the long term one person's substance abuse disorder may be tantamount to another person's depression or anxiety disorder. Ultimately—no matter which came first—all of these conditions will interfere with activities of daily living such as eating, sleeping, working, parenting and interpersonal relationships.

Co-occurrence of mood disorders with other psychiatric difficulties

More than 80 per cent of people with an obsessive-compulsive disorder experience depression. Similarly, many women with anorexia nervosa are considered to be depressed. If obsessive-compulsive disorders and eating disorders arise from unconscious efforts to stave off severe misery, then the underlying depression will need to be worked through and made sense of for healing and recovery to occur. Nearly half of people with post-traumatic stress disorder (PTSD) experience depression (Stuart, 1998). Depression can also be a concomitant of schizophrenia. For assessment purposes, nurses can inquire, via a thorough ongoing history taking, whether depression preceded or emerged as a consequence of another psychiatric condition.

Holistic assessment

Mood states can be considered to fall along a continuum. Because mood levels vary and, like anxiety disorders, are confounded by a range of interpersonal, practical and physical difficulties, a holistic nursing assessment is crucial for the provision of effective nursing care (Horsfall, 1997).

At the outset, the nurse should endeavor to find out *what the person's perception of the difficulties is*. This is the first step in attempting to connect with the person and beginning to develop a therapeutic relationship.

Practical life circumstances should be clarified. Employment, money matters and child care responsibilities are significant factors among people who are depressed. To have insufficient money for food, housing and power can be depressing or even life threatening. In circumstances such as these, the depression must be considered to be appropriate, and the practical and financial difficulties should be considered the first problem to be remedied. Unequal child care responsibilities are related to depression in women, especially among those with few material resources, more than one child under five years of age and who are not employed outside the home (Brown & Harris, 1978; Horsfall, 1994). The demands of child care are often underestimated by those who do not fulfill these complex responsibilities on a full-time basis themselves: such people include diagnosing doctors, nurses and middle class parents with access to casual, short- or long-term child care choices.

Single women raising children without regular reliable family or outside help are highly likely to be overworked. Women with children and a partner still continue to bear unequal responsibilities for child rearing, housework and cooking (Steen, 1991). Consequently, women with children often perform invisible and under-valued work, experience conflicting demands and become fatigued. Women are often primarily responsible for monitoring health-related issues among all family members. This may include advising a spouse about the dangers of eating too much food with a high saturated fat content and consuming excessive alcohol; helping lonely or frail aged parents; assessing their school-aged children's health; and being concerned about teenagers' vulnerabilities and risky behaviors. As well as these serious worries and responsibilities, women are commonly the primary carers for family members with long-term illnesses and/or disabilities, whether they are offspring, siblings, parents or grandparents. Even when some of these relatives are hospitalized or living in long-term care settings, extra demands are still made on the carer.

Nurses should also inquire broadly about the family to ascertain possible *cultural conflicts within the family* or between the family and others, especially in a tightly knit ethnic community. In some migrant families there can be conflict over religious beliefs and adherence to specific practices; or one member may experience spiritual disquiet which is incongruent with the prevailing family lifestyle (e.g., to be a disbelieving or questioning teenager in a fundamentalist Christian, Jewish or Muslim family).

For some recent immigrants, experiences of warfare, torture, political oppression, rape and transnational relocation can increase the vulnerability to depression and anxiety. Cultural difficulties can overlap with immigration stresses, losses, and subsequent social disjunction (Beeber, 1996). Conflicts within first or second generation immigrant families can be acted out between spouses and/or between generations and be experienced differently by females and males. 'Girls in some cultures aren't supposed to stand up for their rights and are very strictly brought up' (Poloskey cited in Pryor, 1998). This can be an issue for nursing students as well as prospective clients in the health sector. As nurses though, we should not assume that it is only migrant families who experience intergenerational cultural differences.

In our predominantly sexist and heterosexist society, sexual identity fears or confusion can be exacerbated by depression, especially among adolescents and young adults who live in families with a rigid view of sex roles and intolerance of gays, lesbians and silence about bisexuality. It is also possible that while living in a close gay or lesbian community, a person may experience some personal or interpersonal problem, the discussion of which is censored within the group and this situation may increase vulnerability to isolation and depression.

As well as assessing stressors, the person needs to be *assessed for resources and positive coping strategies*. For people living with depression, social support is known to be important for well-being or even survival. Ongoing assessment must include finding out if there are people in the depressed person's social network who are practically and emotionally willing and able to provide close support over time. Just asking if the consumer has friends or family will not provide a realistic answer regarding their availability.

The nurse should not assume that a partner, by definition, does assist the person constructively. It will be helpful for the consumer to determine the *realistic supportiveness of family and friends* (Peden, 1993). Some partners are extremely supportive over long periods of time, with very little positive feedback from anyone for their efforts and perseverance. Other partners blame the depressed person for their predicament, consider the person to be 'weak' and tell them that they should just 'pull their socks up' and everything will be all right.

Other personal resources should be assessed over time. It is important to know how the consumer usually manages stress, if they communicate effectively, and whether alcohol or other drugs are used routinely. Depressed people commonly experience cognitive distortions, so it is also useful to ascertain whether negative thinking impedes their problem-solving and decision-making abilities (Yapko, 1999).

Keeping a journal

Write down at least twelve psychosocial nursing assessment questions you could ask a person who seems to be depressed. These questions are not to be oriented towards a medical diagnosis or focus on psychiatric symptoms. The questions should be open-ended and not imply that you have answers that you want to confirm; but show that you want to explore life experiences with the person.

One of the aims of the questions is to relate events in the person's life to the experience of loss. Headings to consider include insufficient money, overwork and stress, conflict within the family, parenting responsibilities, relocation, and identity issues such as sexual orientation, ethnicity and gender expectations.

Suicidality

Major depression is the most common psychiatric diagnosis among suicidal people. Depressed mood, feelings of worthlessness, feelings of guilt, sleep disturbances and decreased ability to concentrate were the prevalent symptoms among recent young suicide attempters (Fry, 1999). However, most suicidal people are technically not simply mentally ill: they are in a state of crisis, at an impasse, or are experiencing intense emotional conflict. Depressed people should be routinely assessed for suicidality.

There are known suicide risk profiles. These include:

■ having a suicide plan
■ having attempted to commit suicide previously
■ experiencing the death of, or separation from, an intimate partner

- social isolation
- being unemployed (Riley & Kneisl, 1996).

High levels of substance abuse—including tobacco, alcohol and marijuana—are also prevalent among people who attempt suicide (Fry, 1999).

Students need to be aware that these factors are generalizations. For example, being recently bereaved does not necessarily indicate that the person is suicidal; and because the person does not reveal a plan, does not mean that she or he is not suicidal. However, any individual person with medium to severe levels of depression should be assessed for suicidality.

If a depressed person is being assessed in the community, care must be taken to ascertain the actual level of suicide risk. There are at least three aspects of the person's situation that should be assessed in these circumstances: the person's level of commitment to end their life, the ability to make rational decisions, and the presence of active close support for the person. When a consumer is resolute about suicide, adamant that there is no hope, has a suicide plan and the means to attempt suicide, then legal steps should be taken to hospitalize the person. If the person is at risk for suicide according to these (and possibly some other) criteria, then the advantages and disadvantages of hospitalization should be mutually explored.

Fry (1999), in her report on 80 young people who attempted suicide, outlines a three-level interactive risk framework. Perpetuating factors include violence within the family, significant relationship losses and poor interpersonal skills. Predisposing factors involve low self-esteem, substance abuse, exposure to suicide and impulsiveness. Precipitating factors include limited or absent social support, unemployment, erosion of hope and the anniversary of a death or loss.

For many young people in the study, episodes of interpersonal conflict within the family, involving cross-cultural and intergenerational differences, immediately preceded the suicide attempt. Often this would not be the first time that the young woman or man felt distressed, trapped and powerless within these family dynamics. The young people who attempted suicide again were more likely to be unemployed, depressed and lacking hope than those who did not attempt suicide again within the following six months.

Most consumers with suicidal thinking and intent reveal clues to their distress, directly or indirectly, through their actions, verbal comments or emotional state (Marcus et al., 1996). These indicators include:

- making, or changing, a will
- giving prized possessions away
- putting personal or financial matters in order
- making statements such as 'life is not worth living'
- imagining other people living without them 'X would be better off if I was dead'
- indirect verbalizing about non-coping 'I just want to go to sleep and stay asleep'
- conveying a profound sense of hopelessness
- withdrawing from friends
- indicating a strong belief in the impossibility of fixing serious problem(s).

In either the hospital or the community, it is crucial that at least one nurse develop a therapeutic relationship with the consumer (Cleary et al., 1999). Many RNs in hospitals and community health centers use no-suicide contracts. Such contracts should be realistic and adhere to a specified time frame. The nurse and consumer should have agreed-upon strategies that the suicidal person can use if the intensity or fear of suicidal feelings or thoughts increases.

Ongoing assessment of a depressed person's suicidal potential is very important. However, once a suicidal person has been hospitalized, an undue focus on stopping suicide at the expense of a therapeutic alliance and emotional support can be counterproductive. Such an approach by the nurse adds to the person's feelings of objectification and powerlessness. The use of 'special observation', for example, can create ethical dilemmas due to the contradictions between the role of the nurse as an advocate on one hand and the social control of the patient by the nurse under medical orders on the other hand (Cleary et al., 1999).

In Fry's (1999) research into young people who attempted suicide, only 15 of the 80 subjects who were followed up by nurses (or referred on) intentionally self-harmed during the ensuing six months. This shows that the nursing approach used was very effective for the majority of these vulnerable clients.

The supportive interventions were carried out during home visits and/or telephone conversations. The main nursing goal was to increase the person's social support base and decrease isolation to prevent another crisis. A therapeutic relationship involving rapport and trust development set the foundations for the work to be done. The nurse helped teach problem-solving skill development so that the young person could draw on these skills in difficult situations in the future and prevent a downward spiral or the precipitation of another crisis.

Human responses to significant life events

Significant life events in the previous year are reported by depressed people at almost three times the rate of other people. Separations and losses feature prominently in their backgrounds. 'Most psychiatric clinicians are convinced that a relationship does exist between stressful life events and depression' (Stuart, 1998: 362). The relationship is not directly causal, otherwise, for example, all people who experienced a death in the family last year would be depressed. Connecting disruptive life events with grief and depression can be therapeutic and allow people to uncover meaning in their misery, and offer a turning point. This is one important therapeutic aspect of crisis intervention (or secondary prevention) with people who have been recently bereaved, which has been shown to lessen depression and the utilization of health services in the future (National Health & Medical Research Council, 1993).

Death among immediate family members—whether they were close or not—is the most obvious cause of disrupted grieving that may lead to depression (Brown, 1996). Children's grieving can be impeded because they have been side-lined due to high levels of distress among key adults who are unable to focus on the child's concerns and questions. Sometimes children feel an inordinate responsibility for the death of a parent or sibling and if this is not noticed and dealt with at the time, it may lay the foundations for depression later in life.

Marriage, or an intimate relationship involving long-term commitment, from a statistical perspective, protects both women and men from depression (Yapko, 1999). This does not mean that any close relationship will do so. The preventative factors are likely to be the presence of a confidante, someone to share ups and downs with, and a person with whom love and affection is reciprocated. On the other hand, a partnership characterized by poor communication, avoidance of conflict, or verbal or physical aggression is predictive of depression, especially in women.

Contrary to mass media claims, initiating a separation from a long-term partner is felt by most people to be a serious change of life circumstance. Often this step is taken in response to extreme interpersonal difficulties, unresolvable differences or profound humiliation experienced by the person seeking the separation or divorce (Brown, 1996). Separation or divorce from a spouse is a loss, even for the partner who initiates the move. Even though people are aware of divorce rates, anybody might believe 'this will not happen to me'; consequently the separation can constitute the loss of an important relationship and at times engender feelings of failure. These processes often take years to complete, and issues surrounding the well-being of children often remain worrying. Even adult progeny and other family members can be blaming or hostile towards one spouse because of their disapproval. Work with family members after divorce or separation can be a primary prevention intervention to decrease the likelihood of unresolved grief and anger, or depression (Scanlon et al., 1997).

Sexual assault and other forms of physical and emotional abuse or neglect have a profoundly undermining effect on children. In the USA, more than half of substantiated cases of child abuse are neglect, a quarter physical abuse, and ten per cent sexual abuse (Wangerin et al., 1998). Abused children often feel unloved, rejected, emotionally bereft and have low self-esteem; they commonly experience relationship difficulties because of high dependency needs and under-developed effective problem-solving skills. Another common consequence that is relevant to depression, is poor self-differentiation, which means being unclear about appropriate closeness and distance in relationships (Yapko, 1999).

Many studies, during the last decade in particular, indicate that abuse may make significant contributions to enhancing a vulnerability to, or precipitating, a mental illness. Childhood sexual and physical abuse is associated with high levels of depression in adulthood (Scanlon et al., 1997). Depressed women are more likely than non-depressed women to perceive their parents as rejecting, to have survived high levels of poorly handled conflict within the family and to have experienced separation anxiety as a child (Stuart, 1998). It is understood that victimization and powerlessness in formative relationships are the significant factors involved. This does not mean that feeling like a victim inevitably persists into adulthood.

Active exercise

Do this exercise alone or divide the work up between a small group of students.

Find out the most recent rates for childhood (1) neglect (2) physical abuse and (3) sexual abuse. Find out the ages at which the highest levels of these types of abuse occur. Find out sex differences regarding the major types of childhood abuse. If you cannot get detailed and reliable information for any of these reportable abuses, what does this say about how we value children and mental health?

Consult a chapter in a mental health or psychology text that explains the social emotional, and intellectual challenges and issues that are addressed during each human developmental stage. What are the likely consequences of neglect and emotional, sexual or physical abuse for children of specific ages?

Childbirth is perhaps over-associated with depression. Rates of depression within a year or so of childbirth are believed to be between 10 and 15 per cent. The energy expended on birthing, tiredness in relation to settling the baby into a feeding and sleeping routine, and the common lack of adequate physical and emotional support and relief from ongoing child care, housework, employment or social responsibilities can easily lay foundations for depression (Thurtle, 1995).

People who are depressed or emotionally distressed after experiencing a recent death, separation, sexual assault or giving birth, should not be given antidepressant medication in the first instance, as the medication is likely to impede the healthy grieving process. Loss and grief are painful, but to some extent they are inevitable aspects of living. Even though the distress is disruptive to self and others, the expression of grief is therapeutic and should be supported.

Against a background of increasingly high rates of unemployment, under-employment and poverty in low-paid employment in Australia in the last two decades, economic underpinning of depression must always be considered. According to the recent Australian Bureau of Statistics (ABS, 1998: 24) survey, men and women in part-time employment have higher rates of depression than the average. Both men and women who are unemployed have more than twice the rate of depression in comparison with those who work full-time; that is, over 10 per cent of unemployed men are depressed and over 13 per cent of unemployed women are depressed (ABS, 1998: 24). Recent job loss has dramatic consequences; but the long-term absence of an employed parent in a family is likely to have other more insidious consequences for the self-esteem, social skills and optimism among both parents and children (Scanlon et al., 1997).

Under economic rationalist governments, people have to change jobs more frequently and relocate their residence, within a city, or between states to do so: this causes social disruptions among all family members. Employed people may have other more subtle work-based experiences of discrimination, harassment or other difficulties that are, for practical purposes, non-resolvable. A study by the Working Women's Centre in Sydney during 1997 reveals that a high proportion of respondents were bullied in the workplace. Bullying included verbal abuse, threats, 'nit-picking' and being 'ganged up on'. More women than men experienced these tactics: they took sick leave, felt that their personal relationships were negatively affected, experienced disrupted sleep, impeded concentration and depression (O'Rourke, 1998).

In summary, some types of human response to serious events early in life, or those that accumulate over many years, may increase the risk of depression in vulnerable people in either the short term or the long term. Depression can be understood as feeling trapped as a consequence of the failure of previous efforts to change the situation for the better (Horsfall, 1994). For some people, this hopelessness results from negative (depressing) perceptual and cognitive interpretations of their life situation. However, other people's lives are depressing on a number of counts. Working class women, in particular, are objectively and realistically trapped because of an absence of employment options, poverty and having to raise children with very limited material resources (Brown, 1996). These financial, political and environmental factors can interact with an individual's distress and precipitate depression and negative or self-critical thoughts. For some people, harsh family conditions or early childhood trauma means that negative thoughts about self begin early in life (Peden, 1998).

Medical co-morbidities

Between 12 and 30 per cent of people with a general medical condition will experience depression. These physical illnesses include myocardial infarction, coronary artery disease, cancer, diabetes, stroke and dementia. Most long-term and debilitating illnesses, especially those that are painful and/or terminal can—not surprisingly—be accompanied by depression.

Prescribed medication can also cause depression. Classes of drugs that may induce depression include antihypertensives, cardiovascular agents, antiparkinsonian drugs, sedatives, oral contraceptives, steroids and antipsychotic (neuroleptic) medication (Resnick & Carson, 1996). Withdrawal from amphetamines or alcohol may also precipitate depression.

Consumer experiences of living with depression

Experiencing a depressive episode, or living with a depressive or bipolar disorder, often involves antecedent distress, the despair of depression itself, negative emotional consequences and fear. The focus of nursing then is to work with the individual's responses to unique past and present life experiences that impinge negatively on their ability to act in their own interest in the world right now (Barker et al., 1997).

Depression also seems to commonly be denied and, partly as a consequence of this, at least a third of people with depression are not medically diagnosed or treated. Resnick and Carson (1996) consider that denial is understandable and may be protective for the person in the early stages of depression and allow them to slowly assimilate thoughts and feelings that would otherwise be overwhelming.

People whose depression recurs, or who experience both hypomanic and depressive episodes, need to acknowledge that it is an ongoing illness. Coming to grips with this reality is extremely difficult. Hoping that each episode will be the last is understandable, but is not necessarily helpful for the person in the long term. On the other hand, to feel helpless in the face of unpredictable moods or to fear relapse is also logical, but this position is not constructive in the long term either. To diminish their sense of powerlessness, consumers often need to teach themselves (and others) about experiences, feelings, demoralizing negative thoughts and types of distress that are warning signals, as they have preceded depression or mood elevation (hypomania) in the past.

Interpersonal aspects of depression

The depressed person who lives and/or works with others is never the only person affected by her or his depression. If anxiety is contagious, then depression is disruptively uncomfortable. RNs in many settings acknowledge avoiding people who are depressed. The interpersonal mechanism at work is that most of us have had negative life experiences involving loss; consequently, being with a person who exudes depression, inertia or misery most likely resonates with our own sadness and results in personal discomfort.

Many depressed people seem to have experienced emotional distance or neglect by key adults during childhood. Parenting adults may have been depressed (Beeber, 1996), alcoholic, workaholic or just not understanding of the emotional and safety needs of children.

Consumers who are prone to depression have often come to believe, within their family of origin, that they are unlovable. They then express harsh emotions such as self-hate and gloom and at times are unable to give or receive affection, or even compliments. This results in interpersonal distancing. Withdrawal, lack of motivation and minimal self-care are self-denying actions evident in depressed people. Rejection of help, denial and irritability reveal an inability to allow others to move in closer to assist and support healing—on top of the self-abnegation and helplessness (Beeber, 1989). Others in the depressed person's proximity feel the withdrawal, distancing and hopelessness, and withdraw, keep their distance and feel frustrated, rejected and helpless (Calarco & Krone, 1991). To be therapeutic, nurses need to break this interpersonal cycle and provide a caring presence.

The reactions of intimates and friends to the person's depression must become part of the holistic nursing assessment. To focus on the individual consumer as if she or he lives a life separated from others denies the reality of our human discomfort in the presence of another depressed person.

If a person has been depressed for years or decades and seeks assistance from a nurse in the community, then as the consumer's well-being improves, the partner's response to the improvements needs to be discussed. At times a spouse selects a depressed partner for their own unconscious need to feel superior to a person whose self-esteem is low, who is not demanding and who is deferential in social interactions (Horsfall, 1997). In other situations, the partner may become unwittingly and distressingly caught up in the dynamics of distancing and powerlessness; and if he or she does not receive support and assistance, the quality of the relationship is likely to deteriorate.

Indicators of depression

There are six domains of living that can be affected by a person's experience of depression. For assessment purposes, nurses need to become familiar with the most common indicators of depression, which include the following.

- Depressed mood*, most of the day, nearly every day for more than two weeks. The nurse may recognize a person's lowered mood by their sadness, gloomy demeanor, crying or other expression of misery.
- Behavioral changes, which can include social or emotional withdrawal, decreased effectiveness at work, school or home, and decreased spontaneity or creativity.
- Cognitive changes. These may be evident in the person's negative appraisal of events or occurrences, repetitive negative thoughts, difficulty concentrating*, self-deprecating statements, thoughts of death or suicidal ideation*.
- Feelings associated with depression. The person may express inappropriate guilt*, unworthiness, hopelessness and have limited experience of pleasure*.
- Communication changes. These can be observed in slowed speech, little initiation of conversation, self-absorption and brief verbalization.

■ Bodily concomitants of depression include insomnia*, fatigue*, diminished appetite and subsequent weight loss*, and at times psychomotor retardation*.

The symptoms marked with an asterisk (*) are listed in the DSM-IV psychiatric diagnostic criteria (APA, 1994). It is clear that depression affects the whole person, even though the designated medical diagnostic symptoms focus particularly on indirect physical manifestations of depression, namely, the last group.

In summary, depression negatively affects interpersonal interactions, cognition, behavior and physiology. All of these domains need to be assessed and addressed by nurses according to the consumer's unique difficulties.

Nursing: therapeutic use of self

As with anxiety, the nurse is obliged to reflect on her or his own life experiences to prepare to work with people who are depressed. The therapeutic use of self means that the way the nurse has dealt with significant life events is pertinent to supporting others in diverse health care settings to manage similar transitions. Nurses who have openly shared and worked through grief are better prepared to work with consumers experiencing the range of feelings associated with the pain of grief and loss. On the other hand, 'the more that pain is denied, the deeper it tends to go inside our bodies and souls' (Carson, 1999: 171).

Reflective questions

These questions (adapted from Carson, 1999) may help you clarify your feelings and views about loss.

■ What major losses have you experienced?
■ How did you feel at the time and afterwards?
■ What helped you to deal with those feelings?
■ How might those processes help you work with others experiencing loss?

—continued

—continued

Working with people who have attempted suicide is challenging for many nurses. Have you known someone who committed or attempted suicide? If so:

■ How did you feel when you first found out about the person's suicide attempt?
■ Did any of your behaviors change?
■ How did you to try to understand the suicide attempt?
■ Do you or any of your friends or family still feel guilty or stigmatized?
■ How might any residual feelings affect your ability to nurse a person who has attempted suicide?

The first responsibility of the nurse working with a person who is depressed is to develop a caring connection with him or her. This relationship increases trust and creates a sense of being cared for and reached out to (Beech & Norman, 1995). Establishing a relationship reduces the person's fears, isolation and anxiety, so that they become more amenable to other therapeutic nursing interventions. Because of withdrawal and negativism (Kupper, 1997), the depressed person is probably not immediately accessible to the nurse, so *frequent contact, patience and gentle perseverance* are required. The nurse's expectations about the rate and extent of change and improvement have to be tempered with an awareness of the reality of the slow recovery made by many depressed people.

Acceptance of the person as she or he is, is crucial (Jambunathan, 1996), since the consumer has such a negative view of himself or herself at the time. The person who is depressed needs to be valued for their intrinsic human worth (Beeber, 1996). They are often only aware of what they are not able to do, and in depression it is the 'nots' and 'can'ts' that the consumer is focused on. Acceptance and connection can facilitate the uncovering of meaning in the depressed person's life.

The most important action of a nurse is her or his *capacity to be with the other* anguished person. Jambunathan (1996), in a case study of a person known as Ginny, uses Ginny's words to convey to nurses how they may help a depressed person. After describing her feelings of being overwhelmed and out of control, Ginny observes that others were confused and frightened by her behaviors, but that it is imperative that the nurse is there emotionally for and with the person and aims to be understanding.

When remembering her most scary times, Ginny considered that it was most helpful for the nurse to *listen* while she tried to speak. In these situations it is essential for the nurse to know that his or her own speaking is not necessary, but her or his ability to tolerate painful silence is. With consumers who are depressed, or withdrawn for other reasons, the act of sitting with the person, developing some sort of human connection over time and expecting that the person will eventually be able to speak, provides a silent but hopeful link.

Because helplessness is a common facet of the experience of depression, it is essential that nurses maintain a balance in relation to helpfulness. The nurse needs to be supportive and sometimes guide or assist the person, but not take over. On the other hand, the consumer is likely to benefit from the nurse's acknowledgment of the person's perceptions of helplessness (Kupper, 1997) without reinforcing it. It is therefore a challenge for the nurse to not agree with the person's negative views of self and ability, or negative descriptions or inferences about nursing and therapy, but to express hope in non-exaggerated ways which are personalized and provide an invisible lifeline.

Discussion questions

During a mental health clinical placement there is only one depressed in-patient. How might you feel spending your first ten minutes alone with Chris? Chris is 20 years old, of the same sex as yourself, depressed, has a blank facial expression, sits in the same seat for hours at a time and will only answer a word or two when spoken to. Discuss these questions with a small peer group.

■ What would you do with yourself during that ten minutes?
■ What feelings about yourself as a person and as a nurse might arise?

—continued

—continued

- How would you manage those feelings inside your own head?
- What would you aim to achieve in that time?
- How would you appropriately convey your intentions to Chris?

Varcarolis (1994: 432) considers that 'one way a depressed person avoids recognition of painful feelings is by withdrawing. Withdrawal is a defense against perceived hurts and feelings of rejection.' The nurse may feel rejected by Chris and withdraw. The nurse's expression of frustration or withdrawal may in turn reinforce Chris's feelings of unworthiness. This is a non-therapeutic cycle.

How might you learn to distinguish between your own feelings of rejection and helplessness and those that you pick up from a depressed person? One important step towards improving your ability to be empathic is to separate feelings that come from within you from those that originate from the consumer.

The nurse has to juggle emotional closeness and distance from the consumer, to manage their own and the consumer's dependency. On the other hand, the nurse must not invest hope in the consumer for the sake of her or his own need to see herself or himself as a good, caring and effective nurse. The nurse also has to guard against distancing and avoidance because of the consumer's unhappy disposition, feelings and utterances.

Peplau (1989) calls this a 'caring neutrality' that requires nurses to develop a level of congruence between what they say to and how they act towards consumers. Such personal development cannot be prescribed by educators, employers or consumers, but has to come from the nurse. *Nurse self-awareness and authenticity* benefit the nurse in her or his personal life as well as at work.

Beeber (1989) expects the nurse to be a caring, consistent and reliable person in relation to the depressed person. She considers that the nurse becomes a consumer's 'significant other' to facilitate constructive change and growth. Within the therapeutic relationship 'an empathic linkage' is developed. *Empathy* involves focusing on the person who is depressed—not their symptoms—and developing an open and authentic connection with her or him. Working with other people's painful feelings is dependent upon the nurse's ability to interact empathically.

In the mental health setting in particular, the nurse symbolizes healthy communication and personal competence. The nurse does not necessarily set out to be a role model, but from the consumer's perspective she or he may become one. It can be useful for the nurse to recognize this and be careful about appropriate expression of views, listening and respectful disagreement with others.

At a more subtle level, the nurse's own behavior and language can assist depressed people to *verbally express their feelings*, negotiate with others and solve problems (Kupper, 1997). Even though people who are depressed exude sadness, often they have been unable to convert their feelings of grief or anger into words. When this is the case, nurses can provide invaluable support and interpersonal opportunities for the depressed person to verbalize their pain.

Overall, the aim of the therapeutic use of self is to support the person's strengths and capabilities. By working as a facilitator and resource person the nurse will be able to help the person explore meaning in relation to depression, deal with some of her or his life difficulties, and become more self-aware over time. Resnick and Carson (1996: 782) consider consumer *empowerment* to be a social process that involves the enhancement of 'people's ability to meet their own needs, solve their own problems, and mobilize necessary resources to take control of their lives'. Being with the consumer and role modeling effective communication, assertiveness and problem solving can encourage growth in people who have been depressed and allow them to become more in charge of some aspects of their life.

Hope is a key ingredient for a positive outcome for people overcome by depression (Horsfall, 1997). Authentic, realistic and ongoing gentle reassurance can also be internalized by the depressed person, even if she or he does not respond at the time (Jambunathan, 1996).

Simon Champ: consumer story and reflection

Blu-Tack

If I was asked what has helped me living with schizophrenia and depression I would have to say that medication has helped. However, there have been many other things that have helped, one of the most important being Blu-Tack.

While medication has changed my biochemistry, Blu-Tack, that reusable plastic putty for sticking things to walls, has been essential to my spirit. It has anchored my hopes, dreams, sources of inspiration, artwork and goals to the walls where I have lived.

Different people have very different paths in their journey with a mental illness and use different techniques for recovery; but for me visuals have always been important and above my bed or desk, my walls have usually been host to images that have helped guide me to a better life.

The images may be photographs of my friends and family, reminding me of my connections with others. They might be of nature, helping to ground me and bring beauty into greyer times I have experienced. They might be of art, where echoes within my own spirit have been found, encouraging my own creativity. Sometimes there are faces of inspiring people or an image of a historic moment that give my own life and work courage and hope. At times it has been a written affirmation or a reminder of a personal goal that Blu-Tack held in front of me.

Part of the advantage of Blu-Tack is that it does not leave marks and it does not damage images. It is ideal for the therapy I have developed for myself because I frequently change, add to or re-arrange the relationships between the images on my walls as my own life develops and I find new inspiration, ideas, or my goals are modified. I find the display of images on my walls gives external visual form to the dynamics of my life within.

My working with imagery would not work for everyone, but dealing with a mental illness you need some process to stimulate the spirit and nourish one's path into the future. For some, the inspiration for the path into a better future might come from listening to the lyrics of a favorite song or lines from a poem or book. It could be the words of a spiritual leader or the memory of a football coach's wisdom. Whatever gives a source of hope,

—*continued*

—continued

inspiration or guidance needs to be highlighted and kept before you on the path to that future.

For many people experiencing a mental illness, one of the hardest aspects of depression or the effects of psychosis is the loss of a vision of the possible, or a clear picture of a fulfilling future. After treatments begin to take effect, one of the most common roles a nurse is called upon to take up is that of motivation expert.

In an extreme depression, a consumer may be in need of encouragement to go from one hour to the next, or it may be that a nurse is helping someone to find the inner strength needed to pursue long-term goals involved in living independently. The degree of challenge for the consumer may change from individual to individual, but each must be encouraged to find within themselves a mechanism for giving hope and motivation for life's journey. Some may have had one that has been stalled by illness and the nurse just needs to re-awaken or re-start a belief system, but for other individuals the experience of living with a mental illness may require a whole new approach to finding motivation and inspiration for life.

There are now a great variety of techniques available to develop motivation and help one choose a vision for one's future. However, they may need modification for illnesses like certain of the schizophrenias or forms of depression where loss of motivation is actually part of the illness. Nurses should be familiar with as many of these techniques as possible and the ways they can be modified for consumers' needs.

As in so much of the work of a nurse, one's role in ensuring a consumer has a degree of motivation to pursue their optimum future must be that of a facilitator, giving the consumer the means to create motivation in their own life or find the avenues for ongoing support for their goals in the times when there will be no nurses to help.

For the time a consumer is in a nurse's care, a nurse needs to understand how motivation has worked for this person before and help strengthen that process. It might be trying to help find a tape player to play a tape of New Age affirmations, providing the address of a peer support group or it might be finding that Blu-Tack. Whatever the process, restoring the mechanisms of motivation for the individual consumer is as essential to their future as compliance to any medication regimen they might require.

Nursing principles and actions

Because the whole of the person's practical, physical and emotional life is disrupted by depression, it is incumbent on nurses to consider all of these aspects of living when considering the needs of depressed people. After reviewing outcomes from different types of therapies used with depressed people, Yapko (1999) concluded that those with the best (and almost equal) success rates are interpersonal, cognitive and behavioral approaches. Such comparative evaluations support the view that the nurse should develop a repertoire of approaches to cater to each individual's difficulties. This evidence also indicates that nurses should teach consumers to improve interpersonal communication skills, challenge examples of inappropriate negative thinking and encourage action and initiative.

The first nursing principle is to support the consumer's autonomy as much as possible. If the person is very depressed, activities of daily living will feel unduly demanding; in these circumstances the nurse may need to divide activities into step-by-step 'do-able' tasks. It is important to patiently persevere with the person's slow actions in relation to bed making or preparation for a shower, rather than submitting to frustration and taking over the person's tasks and making them feel even more inadequate. In these situations, the nurse may have to be directive; that is, tell the person clearly and succinctly what has to be done.

To aid healing, nurses should encourage holistic health enhancing practices. Depressed people often require common-sense help with sleep management. This may include decreasing the use of stimulants such as caffeine, and sedatives such as alcohol, as they interfere with sleep patterns. Daytime naps are often counterproductive and therefore should be discouraged; and the consumer needs to limit emotional, intellectual or physical stimulation in the time immediately before retiring to bed. Soothing baths or warm drinks may relax the person and improve their sleep quality. Some consumers make use of nutritional supplements that are considered to enhance sleep; these include calcium, magnesium, some of the B vitamins and tryptophan (Gallenstein, 1996).

The depressed person may benefit from self-nurturing and pleasurable activities, such as communing with nature, aesthetic or spiritual pursuits (Beeber, 1996). These could include walking, going to art classes, or taking up yoga.

Because of their feelings of low self-worth and lack of energy, people who have been depressed for months are probably poorly nourished and under-hydrated. In hospital, the nurse must encourage the consumer to eat small servings of nutritious food and maintain their water intake regularly throughout the day. Junk food may exacerbate feelings of depression and should be avoided, especially if the person has a very small appetite.

Exercise can intervene effectively to break the experience of lack of energy. The nurse can encourage the consumer (and perhaps participate in) rigorous daily exercise, even if it is only for five minutes at a time initially. Nurses can explain that physical exertion relieves stress and tension (Kupper, 1997); and many depressed people experience tension and anxiety as well as mood alteration. Exercise can offer the consumer something specific to focus on that is demanding but achievable, and creates a distraction from distressing ruminations.

Other important nursing strategies are to provide the consumer with information about depression and treatment and to encourage people to draw on or broaden their social support networks. At times, consumers need to tell an empathic listener about certain aspects of their life story, particularly if they have some sense that it is significant. It can be healing to help the person connect particular experiences with loss or grief to allow the person to make some sense of the chaos and despair in their life.

Nurse-facilitated group therapy can be helpful for depressed people. Instead of working with consumers in a one-to-one situation to express their feelings, connect events with feelings and improve assertive communication, these can be accomplished by people supporting each other in a group situation. Group therapy particularly allows participants to recognize that they are not alone and gain a sense of self-worth by helping others as well as themselves. Peden (1998) has been working with depressed women over a number of years and has incorporated positive self-talk (affirmations) and simple strategies to stop thinking negative thoughts (thought stopping) into group work. Her research has shown that that the participants' mood level has improved significantly, along with a significant decrease in negative thinking.

Some depressed people have internalized their anger, which has been suppressed for a long time, due to fears (or lack of internal and external permission) associated with expressing powerful feelings. The nurse needs to allow the person to express hostile feelings in a safe environment. Like anxious people, those who feel depressed are often unable to recognize, express or name feelings. The nurse can support the person to do this. Naming can be an empowering activity in that the consumer can name her or his own feelings as those experienced by all people, not as unique and dangerous.

According to Yapko (1999), it is important for the recovery of people who are depressed to be as active as they can, to learn new interpersonal skills and to question and change some of their negative interpretations of experiences. These include improving or developing the following:

- assertive and direct communication
- critical thinking to distinguish between facts and inferences
- realistic views about what can be controlled and what cannot
- an acceptance and tolerance of ambiguity
- a change in personal attributions to stop the person concluding that *everything* is bad, that negative situations will last *forever* or that it is invariably *their fault* that something went wrong
- a recognition that past victimization does not determine the future
- an ability to compartmentalize overwhelming misery or anger and not allow it to flow over in their interactions with others all the time
- the ability to differentiate self from others, especially a partner or child
- self-responsibility that stops blaming others and allows some interpersonal risk taking.

This repertoire of skills increases the person's ability to make informed choices, solve problems effectively, and actively take charge of their life. Many depressed people will need professional support to learn and maintain these life skills. However, others may benefit from reading self-help books based on rational emotive therapy (for example) that teach how to recognize and change illogical thinking (or negative attributions).

The relevance of challenging and changing habitual negative thinking styles (*cognitive restructuring*) is becoming increasingly central to therapeutic work with people who are depressed. Lam and Cheng (1998) point out that people who use self-defeating thinking can often produce what superficially seems to be evidence to support their negative views of self, events or others. It is therefore crucial that RNs who work in mental health settings come to recognize clients' automatic thoughts, selective use of 'evidence' and the use of all-inclusive (global) terms such as 'I'm useless,' 'I can't do it' or 'I'm no good.'

One key to dealing with these negative automatic thoughts is to interrupt global claims and supportively encourage the person to define what is meant by 'useless' and ask—by guided discovery—what exact (concrete) evidence there is for being 'unable' to carry out a specific action in specific circumstances. Lam and Cheng (1998) outline a three-pronged approach within the therapeutic relationship that involves asking the consumer to define frequently used negative global terms, coming up with other possible interpretations of events, and teaching the person to distinguish between fact and belief (or inference). 'Homework' is a traditional component of cognitive and behavioral therapies and Lam and Cheng (1998) indicate that it is important for the client to gather actual evidence from others to help reinforce their efforts to dispute their habitual negative thoughts and interpretations.

It is important to *offer feedback to consumers about their progress* (Yoder & Rode, 1990). To do this, mood level and symptoms should be clearly recorded in the nursing notes. Often people who are depressed cannot see their own improvement, which emerges slowly. If nurses can say exactly what the person can do now that they could not do some days before, that is more convincing to a person with a pessimistic disposition than vague claims about 'improving'. It is helpful to periodically review the person's achievements to reinforce the gains and provide evidence of personal effectiveness and competence.

Antidepressant medication

Most depressed people who are hospitalized or medically treated in the community are prescribed antidepressant medication. Antidepressants can be life saving for people with severe depression. This medication usually increases sleeping ability, appetite and energy levels, decreases feelings of hope-lessness and lifts the person's mood.

Antidepressant medication does not offer a cure for depres-sion. Ideally, the medication is used to lift severe depression, so that other therapeutic and social changes and supports can be worked out with the consumer. 'Depression sufferers who only take medication, and who do not receive psychotherapy, have a significantly higher rate of relapse' (Yapko, 1999: 212).

It is the nurse's responsibility to provide appropriate infor-mation about the drugs and their actions (positive and nega-tive). It commonly takes up to three weeks for the therapeutic effects of tricyclic antidepressants (e.g., amitriptyline) to be felt; in the meantime, the unwanted effects often create discomfort.

In a UK study of 255 mental health service users who took antidepressants, 47 per cent said that the unwanted effects were either severe or very severe (Rogers et al., 1993). The negative effects of psychotropic medication are called side-effects: from a consumer perspective all consequences of taking the antide-pressant medication are merely effects. These side-effects are varied: some are a nuisance and others dangerous. Tricyclic antidepressants are the most common category of antidepres-sants prescribed during the last 35 years. Their side-effects include:

- dry mouth
- constipation
- blurred vision
- weight gain
- sedation
- orthostatic hypotension
- changes in sexual functioning
- gastric irritation
- tachycardia
- urinary retention
- diaphoresis.

That is, the drugs may have anticholinergic, metabolic, neu-rological and/or cardiovascular consequences (Rawlins et al., 1993). The first six of these unwanted effects are also experi-enced by people who take monoamineoxidase inhibitors (MAOI) (e.g., phenelzine sulphate). This second category of antidepressants should not be the first prescribing option; they require detailed dietary advice from nurses and others and can be dangerous if the restrictions are not adhered to.

Unwanted effects are probably a major reason for consumers not taking prescribed medication. Anticholinergic effects (dry mouth, constipation, blurred vision, urinary retention and diaphoresis) are commonly experienced before the more therapeutic effects of raised mood, sleep improvement (Rogers et al., 1993) and increased energy levels. As the nurse, you need to find out how the consumer feels about taking the medication, what her or his fears are about the medication and what effects of the medication they consider worrying or unacceptable.

The third major category of antidepressant medication is the serotonin re-uptake inhibitors (SSRI) (e.g., fluoxetine). These drugs are similar in effectiveness to the tricyclics, but with fewer troubling side-effects such as weight gain, urinary retention, blurred vision or heart dysrhythmias. Despite the claim to specificity, SSRIs produce unwanted effects which can include nausea, headache, sexual dysfunction, anxiety, weight loss, akithisia, insomnia, tremors, rash or diarrhea. Antidepressant medication can provide chemical support and symptom relief to most depressed people, but not to everybody (Yapko, 1999). Independent researchers have expressed concerns about possible suicidal consequences of the unanticipated distressing experiences of agitation, akithisia and anxiety among about five per cent of users of fluoxetine (e.g., Prozac®) (Boseley, 1999).

Families and depression

Even though genetics is popularly endorsed as an aetiology of mood disorders, depression is not caused by heredity alone. A group of researchers, including geneticists and psychiatrists (Kendler et al., 1992), concluded from their large scale study of twins that the heritability of moderate to severe depression is modest and similar to that for peptic ulcers and coronary artery disease. The team found that the more stringent the definition of depression (in line with medical diagnostic criteria), the lower the rate of apparent genetic heritability.

Claims for the genetic transmission of depression are less supportable than similar claims regarding schizophrenia or bipolar disorder; however, these conditions do not arise from genetic factors alone either. According to Stuart (1998: 355), 'there is wide agreement that heredity and environment play an important role in severe mood disorder'. She points out that if one parent has a depressive disorder, a child has between a 10 and 13 per cent chance of developing depression. For bipolar disorder the chances are raised to 25 per cent for the child with one parent with the disorder. In monozygotic twins the concordance rate for bipolar disorder is considered to be between 40 and 70 per cent (Stuart 1998). If bipolar disorder were merely a genetic inheritance, then the concordance rate would be 100 per cent for monozygotic twins.

Coyne and Fechner-Bates (1992) summarize research findings on depression in the family context. Families with a depressed member have poor communication and problem-solving skills and reveal high levels of tension. Members of the family often make hostile comments about the depressed person's personality and character traits, rather than about the depression per se.

Among those who are married, up to 70 per cent of depressed people describe their marriage as poor before the onset of depression. The marital relationship is characterized by difficulties with intimacy, impulsivity and destructive ways of dealing with conflict. Yapko (1999) considers that about 50 per cent of married depressed people have prior serious marital difficulties; and about 50 per cent of couples seeking marital counselling have one depressed spouse. Depression following a severe life event is more likely when an intimate relationship with the married partner is absent. Brown et al. (cited in Coyne & Fechner-Bates, 1992) also found that depressed women's complaints about their spouses should not be dismissed as part of depression symptomatology, as many were found to actually be very unreliable as partners and providers.

According to Coyne and Fechner-Bates (1992), depressed women are more likely than other women to be married to men with personal and family histories of depression, substance abuse and personality disorders. The diagnosable problems of both spouses pre-date their marriage and the pair have similar adverse childhood experiences and adolescent difficulties. Couples therapy, which involves the skills-learning and problem-solving techniques used with individuals, is likely to be a more effective preventative and treatment approach for many depressed married people.

A significant part of everybody's environment is the family of origin. If family and marital interactions are implicated in the genesis and/or maintenance of depression, then family therapy is an appropriate treatment option. A genogram can be used as an initial family assessment tool to gather detailed information about all family members—living and dead—across three generations.

Family therapy differs from other forms of therapeutic approach in that:

- there is not a focus on one ill, deviant or problem person
- nobody is explicitly or implicitly blamed for the family difficulties
- all children and parents can contribute to positive changes
- different perspectives on problems or issues are offered
- children can feel safe enough to voice their fears
- each family member can see and hear each other's concerns
- communication styles and patterns can be seen in action
- power dynamics are not so easily hidden
- actual conflicts can be expressed and managed with all actors involved
- dynamics of closeness and distance can be observed and explored
- dynamics of parental over-responsibility and under-responsibility and the consequences of these can be explored
- dynamics of exclusion or labeling and scape-goating can be seen, challenged and changed.

For most RNs, couples therapy and/or family therapy require extra education, training and supervision. Because of the power and longevity of family dynamics, family therapy often involves co-therapists, for peer support and to draw on differing viewpoints, strategies and roles. It is important for students and new RNs to be aware that one family member may be depressed, but if that person is living with others then they may be suffering too, or interfering with changes that the depressed person needs to make for recovery.

References

American Psychiatric Association 1994, *Diagnostic and statistical manual of mental disorders* (DSM-IV). APA, Washington.

Australian Bureau of Statistics 1998, *Mental health and well-being profile of adults*. Australia 1997. AGPS, Canberra.

Barker, P., Reynolds, B. & Stevenson, C. 1997, The human science basis of psychiatric nursing. Theory and practice. *Journal of Advanced Nursing*, 25: 660–7.

Beeber, L. 1989, Enacting corrective interpersonal experiences with the depressed client: An intervention model. *Archives of Psychiatric Nursing*, III(4): 211–17.

Beeber, L. 1996, The client who is depressed. In: S. Lego (ed.), *Psychiatric nursing. A comprehensive reference*, 2nd edn. Lippincott, Philadelphia.

Beech, P. & Norman, I. 1995, Patients' perceptions of the quality of psychiatric nursing care. Findings from a small-scale descriptive study. *Journal of Clinical Nursing*, 4: 117–23.

Boseley, S. 1999, Too good to be true? *The Sydney Morning Herald Good Weekend* 18/12/99: 31–41.

Brown, G. 1996, Life events, loss and depressive disorders. In: T. Heller, J. Reynolds, R. Gomm, R. Mustan & S. Pattison (eds), *Mental health matters*. Macmillan, Houndmills, UK.

Brown, G. & Harris, T. 1978, *Social origins of depression. A study of psychiatric disorder in women*. Tavistock, London.

Calarco, M. & Krone, K. 1991, An integrated nursing model of depressive behavior in adults. *Nursing Clinics of America*, 26(3): 573–84.

Carson, V. 1999, The grief experience: life's losses and endings. In: E. Arnold & K. Boggs (eds), *Interpersonal relationships. Professional communication skills for nurses*, 3rd edn. W. B. Saunders, Philadelphia.

Cleary, M., Jordan, R., Horsfall, J., Mazoudier, P. & Delaney, J. 1999, Suicidal patients and special observation. *Journal of Psychiatric and Mental Health Nursing*, 6(6): 461–7.

Coyne, J. & Fechner-Bates, S. 1992, Depression, the family and family therapy. *Australia & New Zealand Journal of Family Therapy*, 13(4): 203–8.

Fry, A. 1999, *Blacktown youth suicide prevention project. Final report*. University of Western Sydney Nepean, Sydney.

Gallenstein, A. 1996, Nutrition and nutritional supplements. In: S. Lego (ed.), *Psychiatric nursing. A comprehensive reference*, 2nd edn. Lippincott, Philadelphia.

Harris, D. & Keltner, N. 1997, Medication management. In: N. Worley (ed.), *Mental health nursing in the community*. Mosby, St Louis, Mo.

Horsfall, J. 1994, *Social constructions in women's mental health*. University of New England Press, Armidale, NSW.

Horsfall, J. 1997, Women's depression. Nursing theory and practice. *Contemporary Nurse*, 6(3/4): 129–34.

Jambunathan, J. 1996, Depression. Dealing with the darkness. *Perspectives in Psychiatric Care*, 32(1): 26–9.

Kendler, K., Neale, M., Kessler, R., Heath, A. & Eaves, L. 1992, A population based twin study of major depression in women. *Archives of General Psychiatry*, 49: 257–66.

Kupper, N. 1997, Depressive and bipolar disorders. In: B. Johnson (ed.), *Adaptation and growth. Psychiatric–mental health nursing*, 4th edn. Lippincott, Philadelphia.

Lam, D. & Cheng, L. 1998, Cognitive behavior therapy approach to disputing automatic thoughts. A two-stage model. *Journal of Advanced Nursing*, 27: 1143–50.

Marcus, P., Lloyd, E. & Rey, A. 1996, The journey scarred by suicide. In: V. Carson & E. Arnold (eds), *Mental health nursing. The nurse–patient journey.* W. B. Saunders, Philadelphia.

National Health & Medical Research Council 1993, *Scope for prevention in mental health.* Commonwealth of Australia, Canberra.

O'Rourke, J. 1998, Bullies scare away workers. *Sun-Herald,* 1/3/98:21.

Peden, A. 1993, Recovering in depressed women. Research with Peplau's theory. *Nursing Science Quarterly,* 6(3): 140–6.

Peden, A. 1998, The evolution of an intervention—the use of Peplau's process of practice-based theory development. *Journal of Psychiatric and Mental Health Nursing,* 5: 173–8.

Pryor, C. 1998, When dad is the word. *The Australian,* 7/11/98: 32.

Peplau, H. 1989, In: A. O'Toole & S. Welt (eds), *Interpersonal theory in nursing practice. Selected works of Hildegard Peplau.* Springer, New York.

Rawlins, R., Williams, S. & Beck, C. 1993, *Mental health-psychiatric nursing. A holistic life cycle approach.* Mosby, St Louis, Mo.

Resnick, W. & Carson, V. 1996, The journey colored by mood disorders. In: V. Carson & E. Arnold (eds), *Mental health nursing. The nurse–patient journey.* W. B. Saunders, Philadelphia.

Riley, E. & Kneisl, C. 1996, Suicide and self-destructive behavior. In: H. Wilson & C. Kneisl (eds), *Psychiatric nursing,* 5th edn. Addison-Wesley, Menlo Park, Calif.

Rogers, A., Pilgrim, D. & Lacey, R. 1993, *Experiencing psychiatry. Users' views of services.* Macmillan, London.

Scanlon, K., Williams, M. & Raphael, B. 1997, *Mental health promotion in NSW. Conceptual framework for developing initiatives.* NSW Health Department, Sydney.

Steen, M. 1991, Historical perspectives on women and mental illness and prevention of depression in women, using a feminist framework. *Issues in Mental Health Nursing,* 12(4): 359–74.

Stuart, G. 1998, Emotional responses and mood disorders. In: G. Stuart & M. Laraia (eds), *Stuart & Sundeen's principles and practices of psychiatric nursing,* 4th edn. Mosby, St Louis, Mo.

Thurtle, V. 1995, Post-natal depression. The relevance of sociological approaches. *Journal of Advanced Nursing,* 22: 416–24.

Varcarolis, E. 1994, Alterations in mood. Grief and depression. In: E. Varcarolis (ed.) *Foundations of psychiatric mental health nursing.* W. B. Saunders, Philadelphia.

Wangerin, G., Glod, C. & Phillips, N. 1998, Victims of abuse. In: C. Glod (ed.), *Contemporary psychiatric–mental health nursing.* F. A. Davis, Philadelphia.

Yapko, M. 1999, *Hand-me-down blues. How to stop depression from spreading in families.* Golden Books, New York.

Yoder, S. & Rode, M. 1990, How are you doing? Patient evaluations of nursing actions. *Journal of Psychosocial Nursing,* 10: 26–30.

Zahourek, R. 1996, The client with dual diagnosis. In: S. Lego (ed.), *Psychiatric nursing. A comprehensive reference,* 2nd edn. Lippincott, Philadelphia.

10

Complex upsetting behaviors: fear and aggression

Key concepts
in this
chapter:

■ anger ■ consumer fear
■ cues indicating aggression
■ de-escalating aggression
■ limit setting ■ low self-esteem
■ nurse fear ■ primary and secondary
■ prevention of violence ■ safety
■ self-control ■ therapeutic milieu
■ violence and society

Introduction

In this chapter, the general focus is violence directed externally towards other people and/or objects in the environment (i.e., not suicide, attempted suicide or physical self-harm). The primary setting we are addressing is a psychiatric in-patient unit. However, the relationships drawn between anger, aggression and violence, and the nursing strategies to prevent escalation and deal with these, are also relevant to everyday life and to nursing people in the community.

Anger is an ordinary human emotion

As with anxiety and depression, anger is an ordinary human experience. Anger in our society is viewed as a negative emotion along with hate, loathing, disgust, envy or disdain. The emotions of love, acceptance, peace, joy, euphoria and grace are contrasted as positive emotions. Emotions just are. They are not inherently good or bad. It is our behaviors and actions, which may be in response to strong emotions, that can become problematic for ourselves and/or others.

Unfortunately, the negative connotations attached to anger are clouded with behavioral outcomes of anger that are not inevitable. Definitions to disentangle these for practical and theoretical purposes can improve clarity in discussion. Stuart and Sundeen (1991) offer brief definitions similar to the following.

* *Anger* is a feeling that is an expression of the anxiety aroused by a real or perceived threat to one's possessions, rights, significant others, security or values.
* *Aggression* is an orientation to act that encompasses both constructive and destructive activities.
* *Violence* is the exertion of force or destruction so as to injure or hurt.

Consequently, anger does not have to lead to aggression, even though it is often assumed that it must. Aggression is also an ordinary component of human life that does not have to result in violence against self or others.

Burnard (1997) considers that the four most common emotions 'bottled up' by people in our society are anger, fear, grief and embarrassment. It is likely that these are connected. When a person has an angry style of interaction they may be suppressing fear, grief or embarrassment. Grief and other emotions are likely to predominate in the interactive styles of those who suppress anger.

Reflective questions

How do you behave when you feel: (1) embarrassment; (2) fear; (3) sadness; (4) anger? If you are not aware of experiencing one or more of these feelings, you might teach yourself to observe your bodily sensations, thoughts and actions in situations that are tense and obviously difficult for others. Ask yourself the following.

* Does your body take up strong emotions that emerge as tension or pain?

—continued

—continued

* Do you have high expectations of yourself and believe that expressions of embarrassment, fear, sadness or anger are unacceptable?
* If you never express anger, could it be masked by other feelings or behaviors?
* If you are often angry, could anger be covering over more sensitive feelings?

Anger is energy

Anger is a form of energy. As energy, anger will seek and find expression, whether it is direct or indirect. Because of our fears associated with violence, anger is often seen to be an outward seeking expression. Anger can be expressed outwardly in words or physical action and in bodily signs associated with an aroused sympathetic nervous system. Anger can also emerge via less recognizable behaviors such as controlling, demanding, being resentful, complaining or organizing to ostracize, undermine or scapegoat. Because these interactive styles are underpinned by anger, anger is a common response to people who whine, demand or control others. At one level, we express their anger for them. This is not therapeutic or helpful; but these interactions can be seen in everyday life.

The more overt forms of anger are *expressions* that communicate specific negative feelings to others. If nurses learn to recognize our own anger and express it openly without resorting to negative forms of aggression, then violence and disturbing indirect expressions will be less common (Peplau 1989). To do this constructively requires interacting with an understanding and assertive friend or partner who can manage the intensity of the expression and realize that the anger arises from within the speaker and is not an attack on the listener. Such practice and principles can stand mental health nurses in good stead for dealing with people behaving angrily in psychiatric settings.

As a routine communication method, the overt angry style, like its indirect counterparts, is ultimately problematic for self and others. Angry interactions are also often a *defense against vulnerability.* Anger directed outward has the short-term advantage, from the actor's perspective, of externalizing distress or fear. For some people in our society, it feels safer to behave aggressively towards others than to allow others to recognize an internal vulnerability.

Externalizing expressions of anger also unconsciously serves to provoke another person to anger, thereby displacing the anger from oneself to others. In this instance, anger is both externalized and distanced. It takes considerable practice and insight into self and others to recognize this interactive style within families, the ordinary workplace, or the psychiatric unit.

Relationship loss and/or low self-esteem

The anger emanating from people who have an ongoing angry style of interaction with others arises broadly from one of two sources. Firstly, people who exude anger over a long time frame have commonly experienced significant relationship loss in childhood or teenage years. (On the other hand, a person whose partner has recently died may unconsciously displace anger onto someone safe and outside the family, such as a nurse, minister or neighbor. If the recipient of the angry expression recognizes that this is unusual behavior for the person concerned, this is an acute angry response to loss. Usually there are tears, distress and grief behind the distancing facade of anger.)

Secondly, and perhaps in connection with loss in childhood, the person who expresses anger in an ongoing way invariably feels inferior or inadequate as a person (Horsfall, 1991). One apparently effective way of camouflaging inferiority and feelings of failure in our society, is to cover them over with anger and to therefore keep other people at a distance, so that they will not guess at the underlying sensitivity and fear. Pre-emptive hostility becomes a mechanism to protect the insecure person from feared rejection (Bailey & Bailey, 1997). One way to recognize this compensatory style is to listen for the put-downs of others, self-aggrandizement and general signs of superficial bravado. These behaviors indicate feelings of insecurity and they aim to act as self-messages to the contrary (Horsfall, 1998). Since these mechanisms serve a self-protective purpose it is likely to be dangerous to blatantly confront such bravado in the presence of others because the person's armor is being pierced in public.

As with anxiety and depression, the expression of anger is strongly gendered in our society. Anger turned inward via hypertension, over-eating, headaches, anxiety, depression or self-mutilation, is the more stereotypical indirect expression of anger by girls and women (McLellan, 1992). Anger turned outward in destructive aggression, sexual violence towards intimates, rape, or physical violence against strangers or property is more common among boys and men. Neither are pro-social or healthy forms of self-expression. But male violence is the most dangerous for friends, family and society in general; and ultimately for the man himself (Horsfall, 1998).

Self anger management

Anger is an ordinary human emotion, but it is often viewed negatively in our society. Nurses need to become aware of their own anger (Peplau, 1989) and manage it reasonably well before they can work constructively with others who are overtly or covertly angry. Angry consumers can be found in every health delivery setting, so nurses will not be able to avoid them. They are in accident and emergency, intensive care, long-term care, among family members, visited by domiciliary nurses, they drop into community health centers and can be found in detoxification units and in psychiatric settings.

To express one's own anger constructively requires valuing oneself as a person, developing assertiveness skills and converting the energy of anger into words to get one's message across without harming self or others. Such challenges are believed to be more difficult for female nurses, given the social proscription of women's expression of anger and expectations of comparative female passivity (McLellan, 1992). However, male nurses are likely to find these demands on self equally challenging, as patterns of aggression and passivity are more common in both sexes than are those of assertiveness.

As well as recommending the venting of anger in a safe environment, Morrison (1997: 357) makes the following suggestions:

* change focus by self-distraction
* use the energy of anger constructively (e.g., by exercising)
* when you are calm, tell the person you are angry with how you feel and what is on your mind
* apologize if you behaved badly
* forgive the person with whom you are angry, if that is reasonable
* relax
* laugh—even at yourself.

Consumer fear

According to Bowie (1996), when theories about the causes of violence are studied for common themes, five motives frequently emerge; these are fear, frustration, manipulation, intimidation, and pain or altered states of consciousness. For hospitalized people, fear is a common experience.

Many consumers of mental health services have good reasons to be afraid. For those who are experiencing their first psychotic episode, the thoughts, feelings and delusions disrupt the usual comparatively predictable sense of reality. People who have been brought to a psychiatric setting against their will or escorted by the police are highly likely to be fearful about what sort of patients will be there and concerned about how the staff will treat them. They are also likely to feel threatened, fearful or angry (Melbourne Consumer Consultants Group [MCCG], 1997).

People who are comparatively newly arrived to the country, or those who speak English as a second language (ESL) may be very afraid because of the unknown environment, lack of information and language difficulties. For political refugees or those from war-torn nations, involuntary admission to a psychiatric setting is likely to be especially frightening. People who are not recent immigrants but have a minority ethnic identification are also likely to have experienced racism and ethnocentrism; hence their distress at being handled by professionals from another culture may increase (Ivey et al., 1993). Serious misunderstandings can occur when a newly admitted ESL person is agitated, yelling or striking out. Perhaps under these circumstances an interpreter would be most useful from the perspective of violence prevention.

Those people who experience frequent panic attacks or are finally being hospitalized because of interminable obsessive-compulsive rituals, are anxious, feel shame and think that psychiatric hospitalization is a sign of personal failure. Likewise, young anorexic women experience other people's fear, their own desperation and alienation and resent hospitalization and the associated social control. Depressed people may be despairing, afraid of going mad and be ruminating about death. People with a borderline personality disorder may fear their emptiness, isolation from human kind and be afraid of, and for, themselves.

To most consumers, being hospitalized in a psychiatric setting means at least fear of the unknown. Even if they have been admitted to that hospital before, the staff may be different, or the atmosphere and protocols may have changed. Fear of violence is prevalent. Most are afraid of other patients with a psychiatric diagnosis, as they continue to be portrayed by both the serious (Williams & Taylor, 1995) and entertainment media as being potentially dangerous. Some will be afraid of the staff, having heard tales of factual or fictional nurse violence in particular; some may have experienced violence at the hands of staff during an earlier admission to the same or a different hospital. Given these circumstances, it should come as no surprise to find that most violent incidents occur during the first week of a person's psychiatric hospitalization, when levels of apprehension and fear of others are at their highest (Rickelman, 1997). Delaney et al.'s (1999) study of 60 aggressive incidents in an acute psychiatric setting in Sydney found that 53 per cent of the incidents occurred within the first five days of admission.

Being admitted to a psychiatric unit will raise issues for the consumer about stigma, personal adequacy and autonomy. Some consumers may be admitted with high expectations of support, assistance and care; if these are not forthcoming they may feel disappointed and disheartened. Others may consider involuntary admission to be especially disempowering and stigmatizing, leading to questions about the reality of their human rights and democratic freedom and raising realistic fears about being controlled by others.

Active exercise

Form a group of three. Recall your last clinical placement. Think of a patient whose behavior you found to be unusual (e.g., they may have been unduly quiet, very demanding, anxious, tearful, argumentative, questioning your expertise). Aim to view such behaviors as complex and not to be taken at face value (e.g., the unduly quiet person had a lot to be concerned about, but was afraid to voice their concerns). Given what you know of the person's social situation, age, English language skills, financial circumstances and diagnosis, did they have any reason to be afraid? If you cannot answer these questions adequately to satisfy yourself or contribute to the discussion, carry out this exercise next time you are on a clinical placement.

Nurse fear and non-therapeutic responses

When a junior nurse or nursing student notices a consumer's behavioral change, senses an increase in tension and becomes intuitively aware of the possibility of violence, *fear* is the first and most universal response. Over time the neophyte nurse will gain experience, knowledge and skills to the extent that recognition of impending violence does not literally lead to flight or fight. The impulse to get away from fear or conflict is understandable, but this results in *avoiding the patient* being a common nursing strategy (Boggs,1999). This is not constructive for the consumer or the nurse in the long term. Bailey and Bailey (1997: 268) consider that 'one of the most serious staff errors is to ignore or to accept disruptive behavior from a patient who is . . . upsetting to other patients.'

The second ordinary response is to behave aggressively towards the person who is showing signs of impending violence, such as increased motor activity. Here professionals are *reacting to interpersonal aggression with interpersonal aggression*, which casts serious aspersions on the nurse's capacity to work constructively with any consumer. Types of behaviors that escalate interpersonal aggression include the use of personal insults, being rude about the person's family or friends, swearing, being argumentative, issuing verbal threats, sneering, or displaying hostile body language. Even in non-health settings, to meet incipient aggression with heightened aggression escalates the tension and threat, and offers less chance of managing the situation constructively, with dignity and words (Turnbull et al., 1990).

Another non-therapeutic nurse response to a consumer who behaves aggressively is to *reject the person*. This is more active than running away or avoiding the person, it involves conveying verbally and/or non-verbally disapproval, blame, or some sort of personal moral superiority in comparison to the consumer. These actions send a message to the consumer of their worthlessness, and therefore increase aggression in someone whose anger is rising and self-control decreasing.

Wishing to punish or humiliate the consumer is another common enough response that is not helpful. In this interpersonal dynamic, the nurse responds to the defiance, highhandedness and/or threatening stance of the consumer and feels the need to meet apparent 'strength' with 'strength'. Neither of these positions are actually strong. The consumer is threatening others, indicating that he or she feels internal and/or external threats. To simply react to consumers at their level of emotional intensity is unthinking, unprofessional and cannot pave the way towards a more constructive resolution.

Some staff who feel fear in response to incipient aggression or an actual violent event, may *respond in an appeasing or placatory way to the person*, in a non-assertive attempt to avoid further violence. Such accommodation aims to 'smooth things over' by coming to a premature compromise or by offering false reassurance (Boggs, 1999). This sends a message of professional powerlessness to the aggressor. For some consumers this will feel like a 'win,' the sort that they have come to experience in their lives outside psychiatric settings. It is a superficial win, in that the person ends up having only power-over-others relationships with everybody, including friends, partner and/or children. This is a classical aggression, submission, aggression dynamic in which neither party is able to use assertive adult communication.

Identification with, or approval of, the violence is another nonconstructive response. This often has a 'macho' underpinning, whereby some sort of male violence may be overtly or covertly approved of by some staff and/or patients. Such collusion may indicate mateship, but it reveals the therapeutic impotence of the nursing staff, as well as a lack of professional ethical practices. One of the most negative outcomes of such dynamics is that patients may compete to become the 'worst,' most destructive patients creating the most havoc, requiring the highest number of nurses to intervene. According to nursing, social work and psychiatrist research informants, this type of collusive environment has recently existed in some psychiatric settings regarding acceptance of, or active support for, the sexual assault of female patients (Davidson 1997).

Safety

Safety is a holistic term in that it includes emotional, cultural, sexual and physical aspects of feeling and being safe. Safety is an interpersonal term in that it ultimately means safety for consumers and safety for nurses.

Keeping a journal

Emotional, social and sexual safety is an issue in the private lives of nurses. Contemporary nursing ideals emphasize caring, tolerance, compassion, altruism, understanding, patience and helping others. If the nurse is over-committed to these behaviors and qualities in personal relationships, then self-denying qualities may not be entirely beneficial for self, or others may take advantage of them. In your journal, explore whether within your friendship and family relationships you are:

- *too kindly to people under difficult circumstances*
- *tolerant of opinions that are hurtful or bigoted*
- *accepting of behaviors that are dangerous or offensive*
- *putting the needs of others before your own*
- *supporting people who should have their actions questioned*

—continued

—continued

■ *helping others but not being offered support in return.*

Carson (1996) considers that heterosexual female nursing students and gay male students may benefit from considering the following profile that indicates the potential for a man to be violent towards a partner:

❋ *he comes on strongly and very quickly regarding sex, love or commitment*
❋ *he is jealous of friends, family, other men, or past lovers*
❋ *he is self-centered, although this may not be clear from his protestations of love*
❋ *when things go wrong he blames others, excluding you at first*
❋ *he does not treat others well, but this may be hidden if you only see him alone*
❋ *some of the things he says scare or threaten you*
❋ *he has strongly held, black and white views about the roles of men and women.*

After reviewing published research in Australia, Canada, the UK and the USA, Bowie (1996) points out that a range of health care, welfare and teaching professionals are statistically at risk of assault in the workplace at the hands of patients, clients or students. This may come as a surprise to undergraduate students, as this information is not widely publicized. Even though nurses in community, general, psychiatric and rural settings (Fisher, 1998) have experienced serious violence in the workplace, it is important that no nurse considers that violence against herself or himself is acceptable. It is also important that employers are not allowed to continue to shirk their responsibilities in these matters.

Violence against patients in health delivery and accommodation settings is not well documented. There is no doubt that consumers of mental health services in Australia have at times, until recently, had their human rights violated in extreme ways, such as by being physically or sexually assaulted while in hospital or being treated by professionals within psychiatric services (Human Rights & Equal Opportunity Commission, 1993, Davidson, 1997). These assaults are unacceptable, immoral and criminal offenses that breach nursing ethics, duty of care and ordinary human decency (Horsfall et al., 1999). A small proportion of nurse perpetrators have been de-registered as a consequence of sexual and physical assault (Health Care Complaints Commission, 1998). The emotional, mental, financial and practical legacy of sexual assaults by nurses (who are by definition in a position of authority and power in relation to mental health consumers who are by definition vulnerable) is tragic (Davidson, 1997). Nurses must do more work collectively and individually to ensure that such violations cease and that perpetrators are prevented from working in health, disability or welfare agencies.

Health departments and hospitals are developing increasingly clear guidelines in relation to ensuring sexual, physical and cultural safety within mental health settings. Nurses must adhere to these policies, protocols and guidelines and implement them in good faith. One basic strategy that is helpful for increasing the sexual safety of women in psychiatric units is the creation of one-sex wards, as women consumers are likely to be at greater risk of assault from predatory men patients than they are from psychiatrists and mental health nurses (Davidson, 1997). As is the case within the family, sexual and physical violence is underpinned or accompanied by emotional violence. Hence, the foundations for a safe mental health environment for nurses and consumers begins with emotional safety that builds upon mutual respect.

Nurse self-control in potentially out-of-control situations

It inevitably becomes the professional responsibility of an RN working in mental health settings (in fact an area of clinical competence) to develop a sensitivity to signs of hostility within a person, an awareness of cues for escalating tension between people, observation skills and preventative strategies. Poster (1996), drawing on a series of studies over seven or more years, considers that high patient acuity, shortages of experienced RNs and limited access to psychiatric beds in the USA, Canada and the UK creates an increased likelihood that any professional in mental health services is a possible candidate for assault. Mental health nurse clinical competence in this domain ultimately means learning to broach the fears, inadequacy or helplessness that underpin consumer violence, and assisting the consumer to fulfill his or her needs in the community by using some more constructive mode of communication with others.

Bowie (1996) considers that the most significant preparation for working constructively with consumers who behave aggressively or violently is self-awareness. This self-awareness leads to nurse self-control, which is essential for prompt effective prevention or intervention. In a potentially violent situation, self-control is a vital prerequisite to action. Self-control is quite different to control of others and to behaving aggressively; it is a finely tuned assertive stance. Any external evidence of the nurse wavering physically, emotionally, socially or cognitively will be recognized by a hyper-vigilant person whose fear, frustration or intent to intimidate is escalating towards violence.

Reflective questions

What type of interactions are most likely to provoke anger in you? If none comes to mind immediately, consider the following:

■ being criticized in front of others.
■ recognizing that another person has made false assumptions about you.
■ being pressured to work faster.
■ having your professional opinion or client assessment discounted.
■ being treated in a sexist way.
■ having your feelings or views ignored.
■ knowing that a person has told lies about you.
■ having inappropriate levels of responsibility demanded of you.

Develop strategies to (1) manage your anger in each relevant situation and (2) inform the other person about your concerns regarding their treatment of you.

The following are strategies for self-control and therapeutic efficacy that nurses can use to prevent violence in an interactive situation in which the potential for violence is recognized (Bowie, 1996).

- Adopt a non-threatening body posture and approach.
- Breathe slowly to maintain alertness and enhance a non-threatened stance.
- Watch the person for small signs of escalation or relenting.
- Listen carefully to what the person is saying.
- Draw on one or two response principles (e.g., do not be antagonistic).
- If the person does or says something that is threatening, count to ten to prevent reacting unthinkingly in words or action.
- Speak after quickly considering one or more possible steps ahead.
- Use few short, clear words and speak at a moderate pace and in a way that will engage the consumer (e.g., by responding to a concern that he or she has expressed directly or indirectly).
- Behave congruently in relation to the person's culture, sex and age regarding eye contact, type of physical touch (if any), humor, or topics of conversation.

Violence and society

Contemporary society tacitly or actively supports many forms of violence at international, national, government, employment, family and interpersonal levels (Horsfall, 1998). News media are permeated with violence, often of the most extreme kinds, such as wars, and in the USA often in the form of mass murders at the hands of one or two individual gunmen, bombers, or even children.

Society at large also appears to support the use and over-use of alcohol. Furthermore, governments, lawyers and media representatives continue to condone both substance use and male violence, and use the former to excuse the latter (Horsfall, 1991). As a consequence of this, young men (in particular) in our society are likely to use alcohol (and some other drugs) in anticipation of justifying a range of antisocial behaviors. The fact that 21.5 per cent of young men between the ages of 18 and 24 abuse alcohol or are dependent upon it (ABS, 1998), is serious cause for concern for nurses and consumers in mental health settings. If the young man has a psychotic disorder as well, it is likely that he will continue to use alcohol and other substances in a desperate attempt to diminish his distress. People who are admitted to psychiatric settings under the influence of alcohol are the most difficult to work with, especially if they do not consider their alcohol use to be a problem that they should do something about.

Consumers speak of violence of various kinds being perpetrated against them by nurses and other personnel when they have been hospitalized. At times they acknowledge that their own behavior at the time was very disturbed. On the other hand, if health policy implicitly and explicitly guarantees consumers a safe and violence-free environment in hospital, it clearly has to be nurses who will provide this. Consumers have frequently experienced violence at the hands of other people outside the hospital; however, they should be able to expect that nurses will not abuse their basic rights and, furthermore, that nurses will offer some understanding and assistance to reclaim their dignity, even during the early hours of a disturbed and disruptive involuntary admission.

Glenister (1997) goes further and declares that some UK mental health nurses are not only violent, but that nurses collectively deny this and use policy phrases such as 'patient-centered care' and 'consumer collaboration' to mask the actual state of affairs. He goes on to say that this violence is not only perpetrated by, and formally ignored by nurses, but it is supported and/or ignored by nursing and non-nursing management. Since consumers do inform nurses and other health professionals about physical and sexual assaults by staff or patients, then it is not only nurses who are abetting these crimes, but senior hospital personnel. Hence, the institution is involved in perpetrating and maintaining violence and neglecting to protect consumers' human rights. At another level, if consumers bring their concerns to public notice via the media or formal inquiries that do not result in charging offenders and stopping the crimes, then society is also supporting institutionalized violence and injustice.

'Violence appears to be an integral aspect of psychiatric services, which must be acknowledged, at some level, by both victim and perpetrator' (Glenister, 1997: 45). Given Poster's (1996) studies and consumer evidence (MCCG 1997), it is clear that today's nurse perpetrator could be tomorrow's victim; and today's consumer perpetrator may be tomorrow's victim. However, as professionals, nurses cannot just accept or normalize workplace violence against consumers or against themselves. Constructive, organized and active whole unit nurse-based approaches to prevention and intervention are necessary.

Health care settings are engaged in some levels of social control and/or coercion on a daily basis and these are contiguous with, but do not inevitably lead to, violence. Such locations include public hospitals, private hospitals, psychiatric units in general hospitals, psychiatric hospitals and community mental health centers (Perkins & Repper, 1998), as well as the offices of general practitioners and psychiatrists in private practice. If a professional in a position of authority in any of these settings makes a referral of a consumer to another agency because they have mismanaged the person and increased the likelihood of violence, then the whole system is complicit in provoking or exacerbating violence. Private hospitals, for example, are not violence-free zones if they do not ensure that admission refusal (or referral) is carried out in ways that are as supportive and calming as possible for the consumer. Psychologists and psychiatrists are not violence free if they ignore consumer requests and concerns and send them back to a nursing unit in a ruffled and frustrated state.

Nurses in public psychiatric hospitals with 'secure' facilities are at the end of a continuum of possible consumer neglect, aggravation or mismanagement by others prior to admission. Violence in acute mental health settings is unacceptable. RNs must be provided with adequate resources and medical and administrative support to ensure an emotionally, culturally, physically and sexually safe work environment for all staff and consumers.

Therapeutic milieu and primary prevention

The ideas and practices associated with a 'therapeutic community' and 'therapeutic milieu' originated with Jones, Bion and others in the early 1950s. Now these practices may be forgotten or derided because they are so old. However, some RNs continue to believe that increases in violence in in-patient psychiatric settings are related to milieu deterioration that results in restricting client autonomy and nurses behaving more reactively than preventively. A less than therapeutic ward environment can arise indirectly from government mental health financial priorities and pragmatic administrative acceptance of under-funding, sometimes achieved by decreasing the number of clinical nursing staff. These factors decrease the sexual safety of women (Davidson, 1997) and physical safety of nurses and consumers (Lanza et al., 1994).

Functional components of the therapeutic milieu include beliefs and practices that affirm the centrality of the nurse–patient relationship to treatment. This is a simple but radical premise, as it not only values the consumer, but respects nurses and nursing practice. Once the therapeutic relationship is established, nurse–consumer collaboration validates consumer experience, feelings and concerns. This means, at one level, that the consumer is the source of therapy, rather than the more common premise that therapy begins with what the professionals know and intend to do. To assist in this process, the basic nursing orientation is to support and enhance consumer self-esteem by acceptance of him or her (Herbert & Queen, 1998), albeit as a troubled person.

Structures that provide external support for the therapeutic relationship and a more therapeutic milieu include management and administrative endorsement, adequate staffing, and a variety of programs to offer consumers activities, diversions and choices. Regular meetings between staff are needed to clarify approaches, keep information channels clear, provide peer support and re-negotiate nursing care plans. As well as these, active daily meetings between as many consumers as possible and as many staff as possible can be convened to ensure that consumer voices are heard together as well as singly, and that staff of all disciplines listen, respond and report back.

The environment within which people are hospitalized, or from which they are seeking assistance (e.g., a community health center, outpatient facility or emergency department), plays a role in either reducing violence or escalating violence by increasing frustration. After a consumer's admission to hospital, there are a range of responsibilities that RNs have in relation to providing a comparatively safe and calm ward milieu (Maude, 1998). These include:

- ongoing building of collegiality and trust between staff
- working cooperatively with consumers
- recognizing cues to imminent aggression
- engaging with the consumer as soon as possible to defuse the situation
- aiming to prevent consumers from behaving in ways they will feel bad about later
- reflection on own nursing practice
- values clarification and self-exploration in relation to issues around violence
- validating nursing achievements in managing threatening people and situations
- reviewing seclusion practices, protocols and consumer outcomes.

Primary prevention: picking up the cues

One significant consumer stressor that increases the likelihood of aggression is his or her scary thoughts and perceptions. Nurses in psychiatric settings will inevitably be working with people who have the potential to become aggressive because of their fear in relation to terrifying thoughts, threatening delusions or command hallucinations. Another common precursor is the process of hospitalization. RNs will also be working with consumers who were not violent two hours before admission, but because of some combination of family, neighbor, medical, crisis team, or police behaviors, their hospitalization is the culmination of multiple threats, indignities, shame, loss or rough treatment.

The *universal application of nurse-based violence preventative strategies* may well be the best form of violence prevention in psychiatric settings. This means that every newly admitted patient is considered to be mentally ill, distressed and in need of nursing assessment and attention. One advantage of the universal approach is that it avoids consumer stereotyping, provocative labeling and relying on biased hearsay.

With prevention as the foremost principle, nursing actions begin with some kind of *professional–personal connection* with each consumer (Herbert & Queen, 1998). Ignoring a client, or offering platitudes, is a major antecedent to violence in psychiatric settings (Rickelman, 1997). Developing rapport, a therapeutic relationship and getting to know the person are essential for individual nursing care and to decrease consumer fear, misunderstandings and confusion.

Another important nursing action is to *knowingly and carefully observe each patient*, to develop a familiarity with their verbal style, gait, body movement, voice level, facial expression range, and their ways of interacting with others in the vicinity. If nurses do not gather this sort of baseline knowledge of the consumer, then subtle cue-revealing changes may not be noticed. Behavioral changes indicating increased alienation, agitation, fear, frustration, tension or distress are then formally invisible and more easily ignored.

A second significant antecedent to aggression or violence is distress or anger in response to frustrating interactions with other patients or staff. Sometimes these interactions are purposeful and well-intentioned; for example, they may be related to nurses trying to give the consumer prescribed medication. Or the tension building may be the over-exposure of a fearful person, with a fragile sense of personal control, to too many people and too much movement, noise and visual stimuli for too long.

In making interpersonal connections with consumers and observing behaviors, nurses should take account of sexual safety issues. Women consumers who behave in sexually disinhibited ways should be particularly protected from sexual assault from sexually opportunistic men in the environment (Davidson, 1997). Men consumers who behave in sexually harassing or aggressive ways towards female staff or patients should have this behavior strongly disapproved of by nursing and psychiatric staff. There must be a hospital and unit commitment to the duty of care towards female patients; and while these male consumers are sexually or physically volatile, they should be treated in areas away from other vulnerable consumers.

Some authors highlight a patient profile indicating violence potential. These factors are: being male, especially between the ages of 26 and 35; substance use or abuse; having a diagnosis of schizophrenia; and not wishing to take psychotropic medication (Rickelman, 1997). If the nurses' expectations of violence are associated with certain types of people, then some nursing biases may be picked up by the consumer. Negative stereotyping of consumers on the grounds of general appearance, clothing style, sex, age, ethnicity, suburb of residence, type of accommodation, and so on, is not likely to be helpful to either party.

Thus, primary prevention of violence begins with the nurses' expectations even before the person's arrival at the hospital or psychiatric unit. Assessment of the potential for violence begins during the consumer's admission and is an ongoing process, especially in acute care or admission wards.

Secondary prevention: responding constructively to the cues

By developing a therapeutic connection with each newly admitted consumer and drawing on interactive and observation skills, the nurse is well prepared to recognize changes that could indicate distress and the potential for aggression. When consumers raise their voice, increase motor activity, glare at others, are physically agitated, sexually harassing others, appear to become increasingly tense, attack furniture, intentionally spill drinks, verbally threaten others, interfere with other consumer's activities, clench fists, or display other behavior changes, these are indicators for nursing action.

Keeping a journal

Recall an incident during which you were intimidated. If you cannot recollect such an experience, make a note in your journal to consider this again in a week or two, as most people in our society have been intimidated at some time within their family, in the schoolyard, in the classroom, or elsewhere.

Make feeling, thinking and behavior column headings. Write down what you can remember, in as much detail as possible, under these headings. Was the ending satisfactory for you? Do you think that your behavior was
—continued

—continued

*influenced by either your feelings or your thoughts?
Analyze the situation to come up with different thinking
responses to personal intimidation to support a more constructive outcome.*

*Have you experienced similar feelings and thoughts to
those above during tense exchanges between consumers,
between nurses and consumers, or between nurses and
doctors while you have been on clinical placement?
Reflect on whether there are connections between
past intimidation with an unsatisfactory outcome and
difficulties that you have in conflictual situations now.
Discuss this with a friend and see if you can come up
with some different strategies that you can practice.*

Prevention of escalation of aggressive behaviors involves making contact with the person, finding the source of the person's distress and assisting with problem solving or alternative actions (Rickelman, 1997). The nurse should walk calmly, but not abruptly or speedily, in the direction of the consumer and plan a few brief questions about his or her well-being and/or comments about what you have noticed. From the consumer's visual perspective you will be seen to be heading in his or her direction (not in a straight line), your manner is unruffled and you appear to be in control of what you are doing and have a purposeful intention. This move is not inherently threatening to either the nurse or the consumer if a professional relationship has been established beforehand.

Use an even-toned voice which is neither unduly loud or inappropriately soft. Say that you would like to talk with the consumer and ask if he or she would like to do so in a quieter part of the room, or elsewhere (Turnbull et al., 1990). If the consumer is willing and able to relocate at this stage, a significant gain has been made because the aggression of one person can feed into that of others. By leaving the main part of the ward, the possibility that other patients may annoy or irritate the person has been diminished. Furthermore, some consumers will 'play up to' or try to impress or intimidate an audience (Bailey & Bailey, 1997). However, the nurse has to consider her or his own level of confidence and safety before moving the person away from others.

Ask the consumer an open question about what is happening to him or her. When the person is silent, give them plenty of time to formulate their thoughts and answer; butting in or changing the topic rapidly will not help. If, after a minute or so, the consumer appears unable to answer, another approach is to say clearly that you have noticed one or two things about the person's behavior that seemed a bit different and you are concerned for their well-being or safety. Your aim is to support the consumer in thinking about and giving voice to their troubles or fears, rather than acting-out violently. When the person appears to be hallucinating, comment on what you have seen and offer medication or other relevant support.

Acknowledge the significance of the consumer's distress if he or she expresses it. Say that converting anger or other strong emotions into words (getting it off their chest) helps to reduce tension. Supportively continue the conversation, as the longer it can be pursued, the more effectively the person is engaged with you and distracted from hallucinations, fear or distress. If the person calms down enough, and reveals his or her concerns, discuss alternative safer ways of dealing with the problem (Ramos, 1996). Ask the person about viable options. It is important that you do not make suggestions first. Asking the consumer to problem-solve affirms their potential for autonomy, control and rationality (Rickelman, 1997). Each of these things is implicitly questioned when a person is admitted to a psychiatric hospital, and this can be experienced as threatening from the consumer's perspective.

It is helpful to use some language that is similar to that used by the person as well as your own. For example, if the consumer is not clear about feelings and uses broad terms such as 'getting madder' or being 'uptight,' incorporate those into the discussion and, as you proceed, name a specific emotion like anger and notice whether that term is comprehensible or appropriate. If the specific word to describe a feeling is rejected or causes agitation, continue to draw on some key words from the consumer's vocabulary. However, the overall aim is for you to explain that distress under the circumstances is understandable, normal and acceptable, but some ways of dealing with it will be better than others for him or her in the longer term. The intention is to maintain the person's dignity, sense of safety and to support personal responsibility (Horsfall, 1998).

De-escalating aggression as secondary prevention

Turnbull et al. (1990) outline a range of verbal and non-verbal nursing skills for de-escalating potential violence. These include the following.

- Take charge of the situation calmly and confidently.
- Keep an open, non-threatening body posture.
- Maintain acceptable eye contact.
- Use the person's name.
- Instruct other consumers to keep their distance.
- Keep a safe distance from the person, but be close enough to engage well verbally.
- Do not corner the aggressor, or yourself, or cut off your access to a door.
- If the person is 'together' enough to choose, offer a choice between two named locations, here or elsewhere, where you can talk with them.
- Ask the person what is happening to him or her.
- Use collaborative terms such as 'we could' or 'what can we do?'
- Offer further simple choices, which might include staying in a room, remaining with the nurse, doing something quiet with another client or taking *prn* medication.
- When you give instructions, make sure that they are clear and achievable.

Make it clear to the person that you are aiming to work with them as an ally and that your intention is to help. Remember that the person may calm down after these interventions, but realize that he or she is in a compromised position and this may lead to concerns about personal dignity and face saving. When possible, create a conclusion that is professionally acceptable but does not leave the person feeling humiliated or socially bruised.

There are also actions and words that should be avoided in such tense situations. Bowie (1996) discusses some of these.

Do not interact with the person in a condescending way. There is nothing more likely to antagonize a frightened and hostile person than being treated like a child. Similarly do not pre-empt the person's actions, guess their motivation or convey the impression that you are a mind reader. It is best to focus on the present and deal with what the person has said and make a matter-of-fact observation about what has occurred. Being judgmental is also likely to escalate aggression.

The words you use should be straightforward. Avoid terms such as 'never,' 'always,' 'must' and 'should' as these are absolute terms which convey an all-or-nothing picture. Other extreme words, exaggeration and over-the-top styles of expression are also unhelpful or potentially antagonistic. Do not make promises. Do not offer emotional or social bribes. Do not offer post-crisis guarantees that are beyond your authority to enact (Bowie, 1996). Such approaches may seem to save the situation in the short term, but you and the consumer are going to have to continue a relationship against a background of unprofessional, unethical behavior and a breach of trust.

If the one-to-one de-escalation strategies do not work sufficiently well, tell the person simply and clearly that you think he or she needs assistance, state the hospital protocol and say that you will send for more nurses. Sometimes it is possible to try the verbal de-escalation strategies again once a number of nurses arrive at the scene. Numbers can indicate strength and safety for all (Maude, 1998). Avoid the group nursing presence being interpreted as a threat by explaining before, during and after their arrival what your intentions are (i.e., to help the person calm down a bit and regain some control).

Limit-setting is 'a process through which someone in authority determines temporary and artificial ego boundaries for another person' (Rickelman, 1997: 616). Hospital rules and protocols should be explained to all consumers on admission. If the consumer is unable to concentrate at that time, then the information should be provided and explained later, when they are able to absorb, discuss and clarify the information. If this is done routinely, then no nurse is left in the dangerous position of inappropriately trying to explain hospital rules and regulations to someone who is having difficulty controlling his or her aggression.

Against a background of continuous assessment, and at least one nurse in the milieu who has a therapeutic connection with the consumer, it may become evident that limit-setting is required. This may occur before de-escalation (if the person is newly admitted and known to have been violent before), in conjunction with a specific de-escalation intervention, or afterwards. Limit-setting is applied to behaviors that explicitly or implicitly break the rules regarding acceptable behavior in that particular setting.

Along the continuum of motives for aggression, from fear through frustration to intimidation, the ratio of support to limit-setting changes (Bowie, 1996: 101–3). If, from the consumer's history, known usual behavior and concerns, you assess that the aggression is fear based, strong interpersonal support is the best violence prevention. If the person's behaviors appear to arise from frustration and he or she has displayed impulsive behavior, then a combination of fear-reducing support and clear limit-setting will be effective. If the consumer's behavior is intimidating, as evidenced by a threatening stance, escalating verbal threats or making unreasonable demands, then clear, firm and repeated limit-setting is most appropriate. In this case, do not reveal uncertainty, do not reveal any signs of fear, and do not threaten the person.

When working with a consumer to set limits on their behavior to prevent self-harm or aggression towards others, the following strategies can be used. Respect the consumer as a person; describe the unacceptable behavior, say what is expected, and discuss alternatives. Clearly state the behavioral limits (Bailey & Bailey, 1997). Explain that they are for everybody's benefit. The consequences of not behaving within the limits should be stated and adhered to as a matter of routine in psychiatric units, so that all consumers are treated equally and all nurses behave equally responsibly. Sometimes a behavioral contract can be made with the consumer; this may include agreed upon strategies that the consumer will use if they consider that their feelings, hallucinations or behaviors are getting out of control.

Because nursing students and RNs new to mental health settings are especially concerned both about consumer violence and 'saying the wrong thing', the following is a brief list of 'do nots' for the neophyte nurse. In a situation in which you feel tension and the possibility of aggression escalating:

- do not ask the consumer why they did or did not do something
- do not touch an angry person
- do not argue, or say 'yes but'
- do not ignore violent behavior
- do not offer an agitated consumer a choice if there is not a choice
- do not threaten anyone who is behaving threateningly.

Managing a violent incident

Contemporary psychiatric settings have formal policies and procedures to follow when a violent event takes place (Maude, 1998). All nurses should be trained in the protocols and understand the philosophy that underpins them (Turnbull et al., 1990). Intervening constructively in a violent incident involves trying to balance adherence to least restrictive principles but maintaining safety and security for everybody. Since consumers have stated that their treatment in psychiatric settings has included violations of their human rights (Human Rights and Equal Opportunity Commission [HR&EOC], 1993), it is important to consider and use the least restrictive option at all times, including during psychiatric emergencies. Strategies may include using sufficient numbers of nurses to immobilize the consumer, having one RN in charge, removing the person from the open ward area, giving prescribed *prn* medication, or using a seclusion room under medical orders and following the associated rules (Ramos, 1996).

Seclusion is defined as 'the supervised confinement of a patient alone in a room which may be locked' (Savage & Salib, 1999). The use of seclusion is not supported by some RNs; however, others view the use of seclusion as falling at the most restrictive end of a therapeutic continuum. Because the end of the continuum has been reached does not mean that constructive nursing principles are ignored, or that because a violent incident is over, that it is finished. The perceived likely benefits of spending time in seclusion should be outlined by the nurse.

During the seclusion process, the consumer should be told what is happening and why, what the next steps are, and when a nurse will be back to talk with them (Rickelman, 1997). In a recent study of 230 seclusion events, Savage and Salib (1999) found that the main stated reasons for the seclusion of patients were violence towards staff; disruptive behavior; and violence towards other patients, with nearly half of the seclusions being for more than one reason. Younger patients and those with a personality disorder diagnosis were secluded most frequently. The average length of seclusion time was less than one and a half hours and no medication was given in 42 per cent of instances (Savage & Salib, 1999).

After seclusion, the consumer will need to be debriefed and their re-entry into the main ward area should be gradual (Ramos, 1996). It can be helpful to explain again what happened before the seclusion, why the actions were taken and how they can be prevented in the future. If there has been an actual violent incident, then the staff will also need debriefing. Nursing staff may require formal and/or informal debriefing. Informal discussion among supportive nursing peers takes time but serves to integrate the experience into the past. After a violent incident, other consumers in the unit should also be given support, information, and the opportunity for debriefing and asking questions.

References

Australian Bureau of Statistics 1998, *Mental health and well-being profile of adults. Australia 1997*. AGPS, Canberra.

Bailey, D. S. & Bailey, D. R. 1997, *Therapeutic approaches in mental health/ psychiatric nursing*, 4th edn. Davis, Philadelphia.

Boggs, K. 1999, Resolving conflict between nurse and client. In: E. Arnold & K. Boggs (eds), *Interpersonal relations. Professional communication skills for nurses*, 3rd edn. W. B. Saunders, Philadelphia.

Bowie, V. 1996, *A guide for the human services. Coping with violence*. Whiting & Birch, London.

Burnard, P. 1997, *Know yourself! Self-awareness activities for nurses and other health professionals*. Whurr Publications, London.

Carson, V. 1996, The nourney marked by violence. In: V. Carson & E. Arnold (eds), *Mental health nursing. The nurse–patient journey*. W. B. Saunders, Philadelphia.

Davidson, J. 1997, *Every boundary broken. Sexual abuse of women patients in psychiatric institutions*. Women and Mental Health Inc., Sydney.

Delaney, J., Cleary, M., Jordan, R. & Horsfall J. 1999, *An exploratory investigation into the nursing management of aggression in acute psychiatric settings*. Central Sydney Area Mental Health Service, Sydney.

Fisher, J. 1998, Violence against nurses. In: J. Horsfall (ed.), *Violence and nursing*. Royal College of Nursing Australia, Canberra.

Glenister, D. 1997, Coercion, control and mental health nursing. In: S. Tilley (ed.), *The mental health nurse. Views of practice and education*. Blackwell, Oxford.

Health Care Complaints Commission 1998, *Annual report 1997/1998*. HCCC, Sydney.

Herbert, J. & Queen, V. 1998, Hospital-based psychiatric nursing care. In: G. Stuart & M. Laraia (eds), *Stuart & Sundeen's principles and practice of psychiatric nursing*, 6th edn. Mosby, St Louis, Mo.

Horsfall, J. 1991, *The presence of the past. Male violence in the family*. Allen & Unwin, Sydney.

Horsfall, J. 1998, Male violence. In: J. Horsfall (ed.), *Violence and nursing*. Royal College of Nursing Australia, Canberra.

Horsfall, J., Cleary, M. & Jordan, R. 1999, *Towards ethical mental health nursing practice*. Australian College of Mental Health Nurses Inc., Hobart.

Human Rights & Equal Opportunity Commission 1993, *Human rights and mental illness*. AGPS, Canberra.

Ivey, A., Ivey, M. & Simek-Morgan, L. 1993, *Counseling and psychotherapy. A multicultural perspective*, 3rd edn. Allyn & Bacon, Boston.

Lanza, M., Kayne, H., Hicks, C. & Milner, J. 1994, Environmental characteristics related to patient assaults. *Issues in Mental Health Nursing*, 15: 319–35.

Maude, P. 1998, De-escalating client aggression. In: J. Horsfall (ed.), *Violence and nursing*. Royal College of Nursing Australia, Canberra.

McLellan, B. 1992, *Overcoming anxiety*. Allen & Unwin, Sydney.

Melbourne Consumer Consultants' Group 1997, *Do you mind? . . . The ultimate exit survey. Survivors of psychiatric services speak out*. MCCG, Melbourne.

Morrison, M. 1997, *Foundations of mental health nursing*. Mosby, St Louis, Mo.

Peplau, H. 1989, In: A. O'Toole & S. Welt (eds), *Interpersonal theory in nursing practice. Selected works of Hildegard Peplau*. Springer, New York.

Perkins, R. & Repper, J. 1998, *Dilemmas in community mental health practice. Choice or control*. Radcliffe Medical Press, Abingdon, UK.

Poster, E. 1996, A multinational study of psychiatric nursing staff's beliefs and concerns about work safety and patient assault. *Archives of Psychiatric Nursing*, X(6): 365–73.

Ramos, F. 1996, Use of seclusion and restraints. In: S. Lego (ed.), *Psychiatric nursing. A comprehensive reference*, 2nd edn. Lippincott, Philadelphia.

Rickelman, B. 1997, Aggressive and violent behavior. In: B. Johnson (ed.), *Adaptation and growth. Psychiatric–mental health nursing*, 4th edn. Lippincott, Philadelphia.

Savage, L. & Salib, E. 1999, Seclusion in psychiatry. *Nursing Standard*, 13(50): 34–7.

Stuart, G. & Sundeen, S. 1991, *Principles and practice of psychiatric nursing*, 4th edn. Mosby, St Louis, Mo.

Turnbull, J., Aitken, I., Black, L. & Patterson, B. 1990, Turn it around. Short-term management for aggression and anger. *Journal of Psychosocial Nursing*, 28(6): 7–10.

Williams, M. & Taylor, J. 1995, Mental illness. Media perpetuation of stigma. *Contemporary Nurse*, 4(1): 41–6.

11

Complex upsetting behaviors: rejection and attraction*

Key concepts in this chapter:

- acting out
- borderline personality disorder
- consequences of child abuse and neglect
- externalization of inner pain ■ labeling
- mental health team and complex behaviors ■ self-mutilation
- suicide potential
- unconscious defense mechanisms

Introduction

Traumatic experiences in early childhood can have a negative impact on people's abilities and personal resources in later life. Sometimes the experiences are obviously tragic: these include being forcibly taken away from the mother, being a victim of incest, or experiencing other forms of violence. At other times, the child is damaged by more insidious experiences, such as emotional neglect, social deprivation or verbal and emotional abuse from family members. Such experiences can include family proscriptions against the expression of anger; living in a family where the children are actively cut off from mixing with others; or where a child is forced to take up adult responsibilities.

The building blocks of the self begin in infancy and continue throughout childhood. Communication, senses, behaviors and

* An earlier and shorter version of this chapter has been published previously: Horsfall, J. 1999, Towards understanding some borderline behaviors. *Journal of Psychiatric and Mental Health Nursing*, 6(6): 425–32.

feelings develop interactively between the infant and all family members. One of the developmental necessities for a young child is to feel secure in the love and reliability of primary carers to the extent that separating from them does not precipitate fear and anxiety. If a young child is damaged by violence, neglect or unpredictability, then these emotional building blocks can become impaired (Masterson, 1990). In this chapter, child abuse, incest and neglect are used as exemplars of childhood experiences that cause psychic damage and often have long-lasting, emotional, interpersonal or educational consequences. These are not the only early childhood traumas that interfere with emotional and social development. Being raised by one or both parents who have a substance abuse disorder, are emotionally immature, or who are depressed will also make growing up difficult.

Childhood abuse and neglect as a contribution to psychiatric vulnerability

There is research and clinical evidence from diverse sources indicating that physical abuse, emotional abuse, sexual assault and neglect in childhood are precursors to a range of psychiatric disorders, including (but not exclusively) depression, anxiety and some personality disorders. Long-term effects of childhood sexual abuse often emerge as post-traumatic symptoms, somatoform disorders, depression, anxiety, an impaired sense of self, dissociative symptoms, disturbed interpersonal relationships and self-destructive behaviors including self-mutilation, substance abuse and risky sexual behavior (Draucker, 1996).

Survivors of repeated childhood sexual assault commonly reveal severe disruptions of self such as 'an inability to regulate emotions, a lack of sense of [self] cohesion, a sense of alienation [from others], a deep distrust of others, failure to [healthily] attach to others' (Hartman & Burgess, 1998: 398). People with the diagnosis of borderline personality disorder are more likely than other mental health service users to be survivors of ongoing physical and/or sexual abuse as children (Melbourne Consumer Consultants' Group [MCCG], 1997). Herman et al. (1989) found, along with other small 1980s studies, that people with a borderline personality diagnosis were more than twice as likely to have been sexually assaulted, or to have witnessed violence by one parent against another, as a child. These survivors often have difficulties with impulse control, experience a profound sense of loss, are afraid of sexual intimacy, and have a hatred for, or a strong desire to protect, the perpetrator.

Acknowledging and understanding the consequences of childhood physical, emotional and sexual abuse, neglect and living within a family with a violent parent are necessary learning goals for RNs who specialize in mental health. Commonly, individuals and society at large deny, minimize or even dispute the prevalence of all forms of adult-perpetrated child assault. It is a responsibility for mental health professionals to commit themselves to understanding child abuse and neglect from the perspectives of survivors (Gardner, 1996).

Beyond that, it is necessary to develop, over time, the skills to recognize adult survivors of sexual, physical and emotional abuse, manage disclosure effectively and develop principles to guide practice whenever these issues emerge, as they inevitably will. If you find these issues too scary or reminiscent of your own experience, then undergoing medium-term counseling or psychotherapy are essential to enable you to process your own pain in order to provide competent nursing care to a vulnerable client group. Without such a personal journey, you will be highly likely to over-identify with the consumer or behave rejectingly—neither of which are therapeutic.

One of the reasons why working with adult survivors of ongoing child abuse is complex, is that sometimes they have identified with the perpetrator of the violence or neglect and internalized their own experiences and responses to the victimization and betrayal. Having unconsciously incorporated facets of both the violator and the victim during early childhood, survivors may act out aspects of these experiences in their relationships. *Their early life trauma is re-enacted in intense love–hate dynamics* with friends, lovers, acquaintances and fellow workers (Lego, 1996a), providing they have sufficient sense of self to actually have friends, partners or to hold down a job. They are afraid of living through yet again the experiences of being violated, taken advantage of, or being swamped by others. Unconsciously they hate their parent(s) or care providers for the abuse, neglect and pain; and this is often experienced as inexplicable anger directed towards anyone in their sphere of influence, especially intimates or people in authority.

Adult survivors of abuse or neglect have an unclear sense of self, because their basic emotional and safety needs were not met, especially during the first three years of life. Often their mother and father had been emotionally deprived, too, as children and they failed to care for their child because they still needed personal nurturance and sought it from the child. The child was used to fulfill the needs of the parent(s). Hence, the child has been unable to develop a sense of self as separate, for themselves, not for others. In other words, the child experiences people more powerful than them as being part of them and, at some level, they feel they are part of the mother, father or carer.

In people who have experienced childhood sexual assault, perhaps this *confusion of personal boundaries* is easiest to understand. Incest perpetrators seduce and/or coerce a child to give up some parts of their body and psyche to the adult for that adult's immature need for control, violence and gratification. (Research during recent decades has shown that men perpetrate more than 92 per cent of sexual assaults against both female and male children (Parker & Campbell, 1995)). It is not surprising that ongoing experience of incest would leave the child or adult feeling that they do not exist as a separate person and that their body is the occupied territory of an arbitrary and powerful father, stepfather, older brother, family friend or relative. A routine aspect of childhood sexual assault is that perpetrators endeavor to protect themselves by emotional blackmail; that is, they tell the child that they will harm someone or something important to the child if she or he tells anybody about the assaults. Another commonplace way of controlling the child victim is for perpetrators to tell the child that there is something special or bad about the child that has caused them to single the child out for the secret activities. A long-term result of these experiences is that the child or adult blames himself for the victimization and believes that they deserve to be taken advantage of; that they do not own their own body, do not have personal rights and are not sexually autonomous.

Survivors of childhood sexual assault and physical and emotional violence have frequently *internalized guilt and taken the blame for their own violation* (Gardner, 1996), experience shame and have repressed their anger. Guilt, shame and rage constitute a powder keg of unexpressed emotions. These powerful feelings, when superimposed on the boundary confusion and inadequate sense of self, add up to inflammatory, dramatic and chaotic interpersonal possibilities.

Working with abuse survivors

Adult survivors of childhood sexual assault in psychiatric settings may not have received counseling and support from specialized sexual assault services, may have been coerced into keeping the assaults secret, may feel responsible for the perpetrator's actions, and may minimize the consequences of the incest. Some survivors will benefit from a referral to a specialist service. Others (whose sexual assault may not be known, or which may have been covered up) will be hospitalized primarily for the treatment of psychiatric 'symptoms' and complex behaviors that may have arisen from assault or neglect and their ensuing long-term suffering. Consequently, RNs working in mental health settings need to develop appropriate and sensitive ways of working with these consumers. Some of these principles (Draucker, 1996: 318–22; Hartman & Burgess, 1998: 400–17) may include:

- comprehensive history-taking and holistic assessment
- development of interpersonal trust and safety within a therapeutic relationship
- acknowledging the seriousness of the assault experiences to break the minimization
- validating the disclosure calmly, seriously and supportively
- seeking agreement on therapy focus, as survivors should determine their own pace in processing the abuse and its effects, and others may have become fixated on the past during long-term 'therapy'
- planning social, practical and emergency support mechanisms at the outset
- maintaining usual daily activities such as work or studies
- working to resolve the trauma—which may heighten distress at times
- preparing the person for the mourning of past losses
- developing strategies to anchor the person in the present
- ensuring that the client has extra self-care strategies in place

- aiming to eventually re-frame childhood experiences from an adult perspective
- affirming gains, planning for the end of counseling, saying goodbye.

Survivors of sexual assault who experience intrusive thoughts, re-enactment of the assault, nightmares or flashbacks need to have these undermining sequelae treated. One method for doing so is EMDR (eye movement desensitization and reprocessing). EMDR involves a combination of brief hypnosis and cognitive re-framing and reduces intrusive thoughts and emotional hyper-arousal (Hartman & Burgess, 1998).

Setting the scene: expectations and boundaries

The ways in which the mental health team works with in-patients who exude anger and behave disruptively begin before any particular client is admitted. Gallop's (1988) research indicates that when mental health nurses respond to the description of a 'difficult patient', the majority have a person with a borderline personality disorder in mind. This means that early negative labeling of any consumer before, or just after, admission—especially if the description is colorful and negative—becomes part of generalized staff expectations of that person. Similarly, consumers with high levels of emotional dependency and chaotic lives often have unrealistic expectations regarding what can actually be achieved in hospital. This combination of negative staff expectations and unrealistic consumer expectations has to be addressed to prevent the hospital milieu from being anti-therapeutic from the outset.

Clear expectations of consumer behaviors and consequences for unacceptable behaviors need to be drawn to their attention as soon as possible after admission. Consumers must be clearly informed of their rights and their responsibilities. The consumer needs to understand the roles of all of the health professionals in the unit. At the team level, and at the level of each nurse, a balance between supportive empathy and adherence to rules and agreements has to be developed and maintained. Consumers with contradictory behaviors can be hostile towards people in positions of authority, especially if they are experienced as controlling. Given the ambivalence these consumers have regarding warmth and closeness (which they desire and fear), a therapeutic mixture of caring and not offering special privileges is much easier said than done. However, for the consumer to gain long-term benefit from serial hospitalization (often over years or decades), it is exactly this balance that needs to be aimed for.

Every member of the hospital mental health team has to manage their own professional boundaries, since inadequate boundaries between self and others and underdeveloped self-control characterize these consumers and contribute to their complex behaviors. Boundary clarification is required to balance the closeness and distance between the nurse and the consumer, for the medium-term benefit of the consumer. When working with consumers who behave in challenging ways, the primary nurse or special observation nurse role, should be circulated among a number of nurses (Townsend, 1988). This allows the consumer to develop trust with a variety of people and prevents nurses from slipping into a pseudo-friendship rather than a therapeutic relationship. Even in the face of a consumer questioning another staff member's competence (O'Brien & Flote, 1997), the nurse has to retain and role-model professional discretion. The amount of time spent with the consumer, what the aims of the therapy are, and the expectations of program participation all need to be made clear. Similarly, consumers need to realize that nurses can't read minds and if anything is troubling them, it is their responsibility to speak to a staff member.

Unconscious defense mechanisms: protection from early pain

The best way to begin developing the nursing skills to work effectively with consumers who are emotionally intense and complex, is to aim to teach yourself to understand the characteristic dynamics they activate, then develop a unique portrait of each particular person you work with. If other people's behaviors do not make sense, this is often confusing or intolerable for most members of our society. To learn about a consumer with more straightforward behaviors, the person themself is likely to provide the most useful information. For a consumer whose way of being in the world is confusing for you as a nurse, you will probably have to start your education campaign by reading explanations offered by experienced and thoughtful clinicians in their attempts to explain the contradictory and disturbing interactions and behaviors.

This inevitably means that unconscious defense mechanisms (UDMs) have to be grappled with intellectually and experientially. Acknowledging the unconscious is not fashionable at the present time, as the physical, cognitive and behavioral models that prevail ignore unconscious processes. However, 'the unconscious is with us on a daily basis, whether we know, or are interested, or not' (Horsfall, 1997: 188). Studying, observing and reflecting upon external evidence of unconscious dynamics is the only method available for mental health professionals to come to grips with strong feelings and ambivalence evoked by some consumers' disruptive behaviors.

UDMs are usually laid down in childhood under fearful or painful circumstances to protect the child from overwhelming anxiety and to allow the child to survive emotionally and 'get on with living'. These experiences and their unconscious consequences often have profound effects on that person's life even in adulthood. 'Early childhood abuse triggers the development of [unconscious] defensive behaviors and patterns that can become deeply ingrained personality and characterological traits' (Hartman & Burgess, 1998: 400).

Repression is the foundation of all UDMs. Repression effectively prevents conscious access to powerful and often negative feelings and thoughts that would cause overwhelming anxiety. Repression begins in childhood.

There are four main aspects of UDMs that need to be grasped at the outset.

1. UDMs are universal *unconscious* human capacities, which means that people *do not choose* to repress traumatic events, they just are repressed.
2. UDMs are inbuilt human *strategies for short-term survival* (Draucker, 1996). Survival is not merely a physical imperative; each of us has to survive practically and emotionally, and this is where UDMs step in.
3. UDMs, by definition, remove painful material from awareness, but the energy of repressed feelings strives for external expression.

4. Even though UDMs are emotional lifesavers in the first instance, by their nature they are unconsciously repeated and reinforced and perpetuate a self-defeating cycle that is interpersonally dysfunctional in the long term.

Once pain and distress is repressed, *denial* may be glimpsed at work in the external world. For example, some adult trauma victims carry on as usual afterwards as if nothing significant had happened at all. When denial comes into play and the nurse can recognize it as such, it needs to be understood as being protective in the first instance. If denial remains intact over a medium time frame and interferes with aspects of daily living, then the reality of the event can be broached carefully and firmly within a therapeutic relationship and supportive environment.

Denial can remain intact for years or decades. Hartman and Burgess (1998: 407–8) discuss Sam, a 29-year-old graduate student, who began to recall sexual abuse by men in authority during his teenage years at boarding school. A classroom movie about rape had triggered a disturbed emotional state and flickering memories of being raped by a teacher. When Sam sought counseling, he was highly anxious, felt that he was losing his mind and became aware that some segments of his school years were missing from his memory. The nurse and consumer worked on anxiety reduction, anger awareness and validation of the assaults and their consequences, as well as reinforcing the fact that they were not his fault. These themes and feelings are common in adult survivors of childhood sexual assault.

Projection is a UDM that can be evident in consumer or staff comments about other people. Projection is the attribution of one's own unacceptable (according to family beliefs, religion or behavioral standards) feelings or thoughts onto another. When a colleague describes other people in negative ways that are remarkably similar to how you and others see her or him, projection is likely to be at work. Projection gets the unacceptable ideas out in the open, but they seem to belong to someone other than the speaker. You can teach yourself to recognize other people's projections. When you are a recipient of projected feelings, you are likely to experience the emotions as alien to you, or inordinately intense. Witherspoon (1985), for example, speaks of a nurse's unease when 'Mary' was given day leave from a psychiatric unit: this resonated with Mary's feelings of being out of control at that time.

Splitting is a UDM that renders a person unable 'to deal with both positive and negative parts of self and others' (Marcus, 1998: 349). Parts of the self are experienced as 'bad' (and at times the abuser is rendered 'good') (Gardner, 1996). Similarly, others in the environment are perceived to be good or bad at any particular time. According to the consumer's recognition of 'good' or 'bad' in health workers, some are idealized (the good) and others are devalued (the bad). The person appears to live in a literal black and white movie of goodies and baddies, with different people inhabiting the exaggerated good or bad roles during different phases of the unwinding film. It is considered that this UDM originates during infancy when the child experiences one or more significant carers as both fearful and loving. Splitting unconsciously separates the good aspects of the parent from the bad aspects of the parent so that the child 'copes' with the parent by dealing with him or her as if they were two separate people, depending on their expression of affection or hostility at the time.

Projective identification is a complex UDM that involves the projection of one's own negative feelings (say, hate) onto another person. The object of the projection is now defined by the unacceptable disowned emotion, and becomes feared as the embodiment of the emotion itself (in this case, hate). The anxiety levels of the projecting person are heightened and she or he tries to control the object of the projection by behavior and/or words, which may feel like an attack to that person. If a consumer is feeling hate, projects it onto you, and becomes afraid of you, then he or she will behave towards you in ways that are likely to make you express anger or hate towards them. If you express the hate, you have confirmed the consumer's projection; but their hate is still unconscious and neither of you have been able to stop a vicious cycle that has been part of the consumer's life for years or decades.

Psychiatric diagnoses and negative labeling

Consumers whose early experience of abuse, neglect or other forms of violence has sown the seeds for the unconscious mechanisms of repression, denial, projection, splitting and projective identification are invariably described by mental health workers as 'difficult', 'aggressive' or 'manipulative'. At the present time in mental health settings, it appears that the phrase 'borderline personality disorder' is a coded label that means 'trouble' for many doctors, nurses and psychologists. Health professionals at times project their insecurity and fears onto people with a borderline diagnosis. This is not simply being unprofessional and victim blaming, but is also a gender issue. Since about 75 per cent of people with a borderline personality disorder are women, one consumer declares that, 'when they are dismissing PDs' [people with personality disorders] pain they are . . . dismissing the seriousness of women's suffering' (MCCG, 1997: 39).

Rosenhan's (1975) now classic research involved a small number of pseudo-patients gaining admission to a dozen psychiatric hospitals across the USA. All of the participants had difficulty convincing the psychiatrists that they were well and should be discharged: this took between 17 and 52 days to achieve. 'Once a person is designated abnormal, all of his [sic] other behaviors and characteristics are colored by that label' (Rosenhan, 1996: 75). In other words, negative labeling tends to stick to the labeled person, even in the face of contrary objective evidence observed by a number of people. Interestingly, in his study, the nursing notes did not document any psychiatric symptoms or difficulties, but described patient's note writing as 'writing behaviors' as if writing might be a special form of psychopathology.

Gallop (1988) explores labeling and stereotyping by nurses in relation to people with a borderline personality disorder diagnosis. Stereotyping is the attribution of characteristics to an individual by virtue of the belief that the person belongs to a specific group. In this instance, the group is defined by a medical diagnosis. Within psychiatric culture, this medical label frequently means that the person is going to be hard for mental health professionals to work with. The presence of such a diagnosis on an admission form, mentioning it during hand-over or describing a newly admitted person in vivid, colorful or strongly negative terms (Gallop, 1988) establishes a negative expectation in many, if not all, staff and this can easily be played out as a self-fulfilling prophesy. Borderline personality disorder is one of a few psychiatric diagnoses with negative connota-tions which are supplemented by a range of terms such as 'manipulative' or 'attention seeking' that are often used in clinical settings.

In the next sections of this chapter some common experiences and behaviors of consumers who have survived early childhood trauma or neglect will be discussed. The behaviors and experiences can be found among people with a range of psychiatric diagnoses including borderline personality disorder, depression, histrionic personality disorder, anorexia–bulimia and antisocial personality disorder. These are identity diffusion, distorted anger, self-mutilation and attempted suicide.

Identity diffusion as a consequence of trauma

The concept of identity diffusion means that the person has an unclear sense of self. People with very poorly developed self-esteem sometimes do not know 'who they are' or what they really believe. This inadequately developed self-esteem may result in identity diffusion, an unclear sense of personal boundaries and disruptive interactions with others. These characteristics are invariably the sequelae of early childhood trauma or neglect. The unclear sense of self is likely to emerge from emotional neglect or parental intrusiveness of an emotional, sexual and/or controlling nature. Similarly, a lack of recognition of own and others' boundaries can result from physical or sexual invasion of the child's body (Draucker, 1996).

A consequence of the insecurity arising from this constellation of personal characteristics, and from their interpersonal origins, is the development of behaviors to please, placate or engage with hostile or neglectful adults in their environment. Being overhelpful, offering excessive compliments, being charming, offering gifts to inappropriate people, or ingratiating oneself with people in positions of power are all behaviors that may be repeated in adulthood because they achieved some success in gaining attention and self-nurturance in an emotionally impoverished childhood. These interaction styles are just as evident among academic staff and students and hospital employees as they are among consumers of mental health services. Consequently, it may be useful to understand such dynamics as falling along a continuum, with the most damaged and vulnerable people receiving a psychiatric diagnosis. These, and other actions, such as behaving helplessly, touching others inappropriately, telling the nurse what the nurse wants to hear (Campbell & Poole, 1996) and being overdependent, replicate childhood ploys to gain assistance, affection or positive feedback from non-responsive adults.

It is important that students and RNs develop an understanding of these behaviors so that a therapeutic response is possible, rather than an unthinking reaction. Developing trust is an essential foundation for working constructively with consumers with identity diffusion, as they have commonly been emotionally betrayed within their family of origin and by others later on. The ongoing nursing challenge is to be empathic without disrespecting boundaries by succumbing to flattery or sharing your personal confidences. The second major challenge is to consistently not reward unacceptable behaviors without resorting to unprofessional controlling, anger or avoidance of the person. All of these negative responses—boundary invasion, inappropriate intimacy, controlling, anger and avoidance—repeat what adults in positions of power have done to these people over time. Hence, the nurse is required to develop a clarity about her or his own boundaries, not abuse professional power, manage her or his own anger and not seek personal gain from vulnerable and damaged people.

Distorted anger

One of the most common aspects of people with a borderline personality disorder diagnosis that is mentioned by others is their anger. Often the anger seeps through and is expressed indirectly, or acted out, towards a range of targets in their personal lives, their workplace or when they are hospitalized. The anger emerges in some of the following interpersonal ways: sarcasm, malicious gossiping, shouting, screaming, threatening, being overly critical, irritability, temper outbursts and scapegoating, (Campbell & Poole, 1996). Every nurse is bound to be the target of such anger when working in a mental health setting. The first principle when dealing with unexpected verbal hostility is: do not take it personally, although it can be hurtful. Even though you may feel a special barb directed at you, the anger is really about something inside the consumer. Understanding this allows nurses to step back from their personal indignation and step into more therapeutic and helpful shoes. If you feel that you have been emotionally attacked, then you can be sure that many others have in the past and they have reacted non-therapeutically.

'Understanding that their [consumers] intense anger is not caused by the current treatment relationship, but rather by what has happened in the past' (Platt-Koch, 1983: 1668) allows the consumer to make more sense of their roller-coaster emotions and slowly take control of their behavior. Their present target is a stand-in for people in their lives who caused loss and pain. Hence, the nurse should encourage consumers to recognize their anger, own it, normalize it and eventually understand it, as these skills will help the person to develop an adequate relationship with friends or a partner. Commonly, anger-bearing consumers want to have close relationships, but their lives are littered with interpersonal disasters, often going back to childhood. Consumers need to learn to express their anger with as little harm to themselves and to others as possible. Anger is frequently hidden beneath self-mutilation, depression and suicide attempts.

Self-mutilation behaviors

People with a borderline personality diagnosis, especially among those who were abused as children, often inflict injuries on themselves (Marcus, 1998). Self-mutilating behaviors are acts of physical self-disfigurement, and include cutting the skin of the wrist, penis or breast, self-hitting, head banging, deep scratching, excessive hair pulling, finger biting, piercing the skin with needles, hand bleaching, and burning self with cigarettes. These behaviors may go as far as self-amputation of body parts including genitalia, interference with post-surgical equipment and purposeful re-infection of wounds (Favazzo, 1989).

Obvious responses to the sight of such self-inflicted wounds would include disgust, disbelief, horror, fear and shock. Such strong and understandable reactions have to be acknowledged, processed and overcome—at least for a time—when working with the wounded person. Given the threatening feelings and thoughts associated with self-mutilating actions (O'Brien & Flote, 1997), along with the often dramatic and negative descriptions of these consumers, it is essential for nurses to aim to understand how such behaviors may come about. Without some sophisticated level of understanding of these behaviors, the nurse's actions are highly likely to be non-therapeutic. According to consumer feedback, in these situations inscribed with fear and anger, some nurses have been physically and verbally violent. One consumer states 'I had done something that was detrimental to myself, but I still didn't need to be treated like that' (McGuiness & Wadsworth, 1991: 53). Assault perpetrated by health employees is a criminal violation of human rights.

The consumer's bodily (somatic) manifestation of being in pain, wounded and disfigured mirrors their inner hurt, fear or chaos. At some level, our own strong emotional response to the sight of such *externalized* wounds expresses our own fear of bodily damage and internal pain. Guilt, self-loathing and self-punishment, especially in connection with childhood physical, emotional or sexual abuse, underpin much self-mutilation (Fontaine, 1996). Self-mutilation is not the only type of somatic expression of internal pain: eating disorders; violence directed towards others; and depression characterized by profound inertia, lack of appetite and disturbed sleep may be seen as non-verbalized distress externalized through the body. Physical hurt may be more bearable and more manageable than inner turmoil.

Marcus (1998: 363) says that the person who mutilates herself or himself 'acts out the [painful] feelings, due to the inability to express or process those feeling states'. *Acting out* 'occurs when the client relives or reproduces through actions, rather than words, the feelings, wishes or conflicts operating unconsciously' (Lego, 1996b: 33). These behaviors could be described as primitive because they work at a pre-verbal level and are therefore likely to have their origins in self-protective survival mechanisms of infancy and early childhood. Since acting out involves actions in the external world that bypass verbal self-expression, the aim of interpersonal nursing over time is to teach the consumer to recognize the type of distress experienced prior to the action and to express those feelings in words.

This unconscious, but learned (usually within the family of origin), displacement of internal conflict onto the external world may be seen in a range of behaviors. The following are three brief possibilities. Firstly, a consumer may act out aspects of his or her ambivalence towards a parent in behaviors towards the nurse that do not obviously relate to what the nurse has done or said: at 10.00 a.m. the nurse is wonderful, but an hour later the nurse is a hideous abomination. Secondly, if a nurse to whom a consumer with a borderline personality disorder has become attached is suddenly sick and does not arrive on the expected shift, the person may feel abandoned yet again when he or she realizes that the RN is not there, and may self-mutilate. The feelings that occurred prior to the self-harm need to be explored by a nurse who has a therapeutic relationship with the consumer.

A third form of acting out can occur in a psychiatric unit when nurse and consumer are processing intimate and painful aspects of the person's life and the consumer abruptly develops a close relationship with someone else in the milieu (Moscato, 1996). The consumer siphons off some of the emotions that have arisen in the counseling interactions onto the third person. This example is complex, but if the therapeutic connection is strong and the nurse is sure that the new relationship is sudden and intense, then they need to explore what feelings the consumer experienced as a consequence of counselling sessions immediately before diving into closeness with the third person.

When asked what is achieved by self-injurious behaviors, consumers offer a range of responses. If they can articulate the outcomes, then they are able to recognize the antecedents of the behaviors and therefore have the potential to learn alternative, constructive ways of dealing with their distress to gain positive ends. As with violence directed towards others, self-mutilation is often an externalization of pain, rage or emotions that the person cannot yet name.

Favazzo's (1989: 139–40) exploration of patients' understandings of their self-mutilating behaviors highlights tension release, returning to reality and regaining control. Other understandings include the following.

- To express anger that is forbidden by my family.
- I hate myself because a few years ago my father tried to have sex with me.
- It happens when I feel frantically and desperately alienated from my family.
- I cannot control what is happening in my married life, but I can control this.
- The sight of the blood relieves my feelings of being emotionally overwhelmed.
- The pain and the blood stop me from feeling empty (Favazzo, 1989).

These findings are supported and extended by more recent research by Harris (2000) with women who self-identified as having been self-harming for a number of years. The relief ensuing from self-injuring actions allowed the women to feel calmer, more relaxed and even comforted. They understood it to be an act of control which enabled them to cope with extreme emotional distress. Two of the women saw their self-harm as 'cutting out the bad' related to feelings of dirtiness or contamination arising from others' violence against them, such as incest or rape. One woman described the flowing of blood as a normalizing experience that stopped her from feeling dead inside (Harris, 2000).

It is important—in the face of disturbing self-injuries—that nurses develop an understanding of the distressing internal lives of consumers with borderline personality disorder and similar diagnoses. And, as a consequence of increased understanding and empathy, work with the person in genuine, caring and therapeutic ways. This can only occur in an environment where there are explicit limits to behaviors of nurses and consumers, and both consumers and nurses aim to be mutually respectful of each other's rights as people. Furthermore, the common medically prescribed practice of 'special observation' often serves organizational custodial interests, but does not guarantee the emotional security needs of self-harming consumers (Barker & Cutcliffe, 1999).

When working with people who continue to self-harm, nurses and consumers—within a therapeutic relationship—can explore alternative methods of distress relief that are less stigmatizing. These can be physical and/or cognitive, and may include vigorous exercise or strategies to gain control over compulsive or fearful thoughts (South, 1999). It is imperative that the nurse validates the person, patiently perseveres and teaches new methods of coping.

Suicidal potential

To assist in developing an understanding of self-mutilation and suicide—both of which are upsetting for nurses and others— these behaviors may be conceptualized as falling along a continuum (Stuart 1998). Many RNs draw a clear line between self-mutilating behaviors and suicide attempts; and a consequence of this is the belief that consumers who are considered to be intent on killing themselves are more 'worthy' as patients than those whose pain results in self-injury that is unlikely to be fatal. All hospitalized people should have support from nurses. There is not a hierarchy of worthiness or validity of patient status whereby some consumers are assumed to be 'not really suicidal.' The fact that a person has not killed her- or himself in a particular suicide attempt does not mean that she or he will not do so in the future. Likewise, because a person has self-slashed and been admitted to hospital for suturing, does not mean that next time the self-injury may be an attempted suicide.

It is believed that approximately eight per cent of people with a borderline personality disorder commit suicide. People who are suicidal or injure themselves often have a number of internal experiences in common, such as emotional distress, life difficulties and depression. Survivors of childhood abuse frequently experience psychic pain, feel alienated from self and disconnected from others in ways that may result in attempted suicide, self-injury or assaults on others (Hartman & Burgess, 1998). Not only are present levels of distress similar for hospitalized people who self-mutilate and those who are suicidal, but some of the events in their early lives have been traumatic or developmentally undermining.

Among people with a personality disorder who had contemplated suicide, one researcher found that they all had symptoms of depression or psychoactive substance abuse (Marcus, 1998). Hence, these matters are not clear-cut. Where do tattoos, hair removal by waxing and body piercing end and self-mutilation begin? Are not alcohol binging, playing dangerous sports, non-adherence to a medication regimen, using illicit drugs, driving a car at excessive speed and cigarette smoking, for example, potentially self-injurious? Many students and nurses are likely to be involved in these latter behaviors. Perhaps the characteristic of self-mutilating behaviors that we find so offensive is that there is vivid visual evidence of intentional physical self-harm and self-desecration. This also occurs in some suicide attempts, where emergency surgery saves the person's life but leaves them severely damaged and/or with disabilities.

Perhaps the most difficult aspect of working with a consumer who has suicidal ideas, has the means to kill themselves and is emotionally distraught, is the recognition that the person's life is full of pain, chaos and disrupted relationships. Such an actively suicidal person should be hospitalized. The first priority is the safety of the consumer. The second priority, which must be addressed simultaneously so that real safety is achievable, is to explore the person's feelings, actual events in their life and practical problems that are seen as insoluble. This is demanding work and at times feels like walking a tightrope. Ultimately, a nurse cannot stop a person from killing him-herself. But a nurse can work intensely with a suicidal person and emotionally accompany her or him through their pain and anguish. The aim is to uncover and support the 'I'm in deep trouble, but I might have hidden hopes and I don't want to be totally dead' parts of the person at the expense of the 'This pain is unbearable, my position is impossible and I can't face going on with living' parts of the person.

Interpersonal relationship disruptions in survivors of abuse and neglect

Low self-esteem, identity diffusion and unmet dependency needs constitute a constellation of emotional vulnerabilities. Emotionally needy people are egocentric because they are still unconsciously striving to get their basic needs met. When interacting with consumers who have complex and long-term reactions to these painful circumstances, other people do not have to just deal with the person's neediness, but with their understandable ambivalence about their emotional dependence on others. Ambivalence is the simultaneous experience of strong opposite emotions towards one person: for example, love and hate. The equivalent emotional pull of love and hate can keep some people in abusive relationships

Stormy relationships may repeat some aspects of childhood abuse that the person is unconsciously (and unsuccessfully) struggling to work his or her way out of. Re-enactments can include feeling anxious when someone is actually nice to them or if a potential sexual partner shows an interest in them. The person still needs nurturance that was lacking in childhood, but fears abandonment.

Sometimes this fear underpins intense attachments and clinging behavior in relationships (Campbell & Poole, 1996) that enhance the ego needs of the partner in the first instance, but eventually become suffocating. If a person with a borderline personality disorder is in a long-term relationship, it is important that the treating therapist work with both of them, or the family, at times. Often the emotional clinginess prevents the person from expressing ordinary anger or fear. Such people often associate feelings of anger with a building sense of panic that feeds on their inability to express suppressed anger at being abandoned earlier in life (Masterson, 1990). Not surprisingly, the outcome after some days, weeks or months is often an explosive separation and the re-experiencing of abandonment.

In the person's early childhood experience, it is likely that the adult who occasionally provided comfort was the same person who emotionally deserted the child at other times. Ambivalence, encapsulated by neediness and hostility, constitutes the essence of the personal challenges facing nurses when working with these consumers. Some nurses may like consumers who are dependent, compliant and agreeable, but the person being discussed here is both dependent upon, and rejecting of, those who provide emotional support. Hence, the nurse is required to be reliable, honest, non-egocentric and tolerant for the benefit of the consumer, self and others in the unit. This is not easy and requires authentic team collaboration and structured support and supervision for all health professionals working in such situations.

Inappropriate nursing behaviors

According to Lego (1996a), the unconscious dynamics played out by people with a borderline personality disorder diagnosis are likely to produce predictable non-therapeutic responses in unprepared hospital environments. Common reactions by nurses and others are outlined to help each reader gain an awareness of the negative possibilities, and to plan individual and group strategies to prevent or minimize inappropriate nursing behaviors and increase positive working relations with the consumer. Non-therapeutic responses include the following:

- feelings of overconcern for and attachment to the consumer (Witherspoon, 1985)
- urges to rescue the consumer from others who seem to mishandle him or her

- considering yourself privileged because the person has shared their pain with you
- wanting to take more responsibility than usual for the consumer
- feeling defensive about your 'weak spot' being struck (O'Brien & Flote, 1997)
- verbal or other retaliation when you feel that you have been 'attacked'
- questioning your competence, nursing specialty and your job
- feeling envious of this well-looking client who gets 'lots' of attention
- being emotionally drained for unusually long periods after work.

Given these possibilities, it is not surprising that, within a unit, some nurses will feel drawn to the client and some will feel defensive, contemptuous or rejecting of the consumer. One rationalization that the latter group may use to intellectualize their avoidance is to say that the consumer should be ignored to prevent 'secondary gain' associated with their behaviors. Secondary gain applies to excessive medical and nursing attention to physical injuries that have emotional causes (e.g., conversion disorders such as a paralysis with no organic basis). It is true that mental health nurses should not reinforce self-mutilation and other physical manifestations of distress because the whole treatment program should be aiming to encourage verbalization, rather than acting out. However, minimizing expressions of concern about a physical injury bears no resemblance to avoidance, antagonism, disdain or being over-controlling—none of which is therapeutic. The physical wound can be ignored once it has been dealt with effectively in a matter-of-fact way, but the consumer's feelings prior to self-wounding should be solicited, not ignored (Townsend, 1988).

Abandonment depression

Consumers displaying these types of complex behaviors usually lead difficult and painful lives. People with a borderline personality disorder diagnosis often experience a strong sense of personal emptiness, fear being alone, feel cut off from themselves and alienated from others (Campbell & Poole, 1996). These are troubling feelings and the person often feels very unsure and insecure. Such anxiety and personal insecurity is likely to have begun early in life.

The unconscious defense mechanisms of denial and dissociation result in the person being cut off from their feelings and at times inhabiting a world in which they just keep on doing routine work so that painful feelings are not recognized. Dissociation often arises from the necessity to cope with and survive childhood trauma (Gardner, 1996). *Dissociation* is the unconscious removal of thoughts, feelings and memories that would cause great anxiety if the person were aware of them.

Abandonment depression in people with a borderline personality disorder arises from identity diffusion, unsatisfied needs for personal validation and fear of separation (Masterson, 1990). Mood may vary noticeably during a given day—which is much more frequently than occurs in consumers with other psychiatric diagnoses. At times, the person experiences sudden depressions with suicidal thoughts (Campbell & Poole, 1996). Some people who live with this combination of emptiness, being cut off from others and unpredictable mood changes gain little pleasure from life. Despair is an understandable consequence of abandonment depression that is experienced over and over again by people with a borderline personality disorder diagnosis, sometimes for decades. The same nursing principles should be utilized when working with all depressed consumers, regardless of the present medical diagnosis.

Psychotic experiences

People with the diagnosis of borderline personality disorder are on the border between neurosis and psychosis. The term was coined in the 1930s, with 1940s analysts deeming derealization, depersonalization and déjà vu experiences to be part of the syndrome. People with this diagnosis lack an ongoing coherent sense of identity, behave in chameleon-like ways (reflect the people they are with) and have an 'as-if' personality or a 'false self' (Masterson, 1990). Under duress, these people can slip off the border into transient delusions or hallucinations.

Consumers with a borderline personality disorder may have depersonalization or derealization experiences. The former involves feeling strange or not like a person; and the latter is a feeling of disconnectedness from the surroundings, which seem strange or unreal (Lego, 1996a). It is essential to engage and connect with the consumer and reinforce reality to decrease anxiety and fear in response to these sensations, as you would with others who experience distorted perceptions, such as people with a schizophrenia diagnosis.

Mental health team difficulties and necessities

Psychiatric unit dynamics can become non-therapeutic—given the array of possible unhelpful individual responses to people who display complex and upsetting behaviors. Sometimes inappropriate responses can be acted out collectively by staff in the form of in-groups and out-groups (Lego, 1996a). Staff conflict can arise as a consequence of consumer splitting or projection, whereby the staff act out (thereby externalizing) the internal good-bad and blaming dynamics of the person with the borderline personality disorder. This can be destructive for the unit and it is scary for the consumer because these dynamics are likely to be a re-enactment of behaviors experienced earlier in her or his life.

To ensure that contradictory approaches to the consumer with a borderline personality disorder diagnosis do not occur, all members of staff have to be involved in developing protocols regarding behaviors, treatment and the rights of consumers and staff. This work begins before any individual consumer with disruptive behaviors is admitted to the unit. Health professionals need to develop respect for each other and have a repertoire of effective communication skills and the capacity to fairly manage power differences (which is especially important for sexual assault survivors) (Gardner, 1996). Without an appropriate level of whole unit professional development, the team is at risk for consumer recognition of both individual worker vulnerabilities and the weaknesses and deficiencies of the setting that is meant to place the safety and well-being of consumers first and foremost.

Given the unconscious defense mechanism underpinning complex negative behaviors, staff members have to prevent themselves from perpetuating 'primitive' interactions. As parents have to be caring, strong, and sure of themselves and each other in the face of a skilled child or teenager using diverse techniques to get the best advantage for herself or himself, so it is with the mental health team. The team needs to be cohesive, mutually respectful and supportive. All team members must be involved in the clarification of the aims of hospitalization and treatment (Marcus, 1998). Similarly, all members of staff must participate in respectful acknowledgment of each member's roles, rights and responsibilities. This sets the foundations for realistic limit setting, a bill of patient rights and responsibilities, and a viable and consistent approach to understanding consumers with complex self-defeating ways of interacting with others.

Individual staff have to understand the consequences of their actions on other team members. For example, doctors need to consider the ramifications of medical instructions (or lack of) in relation to consumers and nurses. The milieu necessary for the containment of unacceptable consumer behaviors and the development of constructive interpersonal relationships requires professionals to be able to manage their own impulses, feelings and capacity for behaving punitively. No single nurse or health professional can take responsibility for this, as it must involve all unit members working together in non-exploitative ways.

References

Barker, P. & Cutcliffe, J. 1999, Clinical risk. A need for engagement not observation. *Mental Health Practice*, 2(8): 8–12.

Campbell, J. B. & Poole, N. 1996, Clients with personality disorders. In: H. Wilson & C. Kneisl (eds), *Psychiatric nursing*, 5th edn. Addison-Wesley, Menlo Park, Calif.

Draucker, C. 1996, The client who was sexually abused. In: S. Lego (ed.), *Psychiatric nursing. A comprehensive reference*, 2nd edn. Lippincott, Philadelphia.

Favazzo, A. 1989, Why patients mutilate themselves. *Hospital and Community Psychiatry*, 40(2): 137–44.

Fontaine, K. 1996, Rape and intrafamily abuse. In: H. Wilson & C. Kneisl (eds), *Psychiatric nursing*, 5th edn. Addison-Wesley, Menlo Park, Calif.

Gallop, R. 1988, Escaping borderline stereotypes. *Journal of Psychosocial Nursing*, 26(2): 16–20.

Gardner, F. 1996, Working psychotherapeutically with adult survivors of child sexual abuse. In: T. Heller, J. Reynolds, R. Gomm, R. Muston & S. Pattison (eds), *Mental health matters. A reader*. Macmillan, Houndmills, UK.

Harris, J. 2000, Self-harm. Cutting the bad out of me: A qualitative exploration. *Qualitative Health Research*, 10(2): 164–73. Newcastle, NSW, April, 1999.

Hartman, C. & Burgess, A. 1998, Treatment of complex sexual assault. In: A. Burgess (ed.), *Advanced practice psychiatric nursing*. Appleton & Lange, Stamford, Conn.

Herman, J., Perry, C. & van der Kolk, B. 1989, Childhood trauma in borderline personality disorder. *American Journal of Psychiatry*, 146(4): 490–5.

Horsfall, J. 1997, Some consequences of the psychiatric dis-integration of the body, mind and soul. In: J. Lawler (ed.), *The body in nursing. A collection of views*. Churchill Livingstone, Melbourne.

Lego, S. 1996a, The client with borderline personality disorder. In: S. Lego (ed.), *Psychiatric nursing. A comprehensive reference*, 2nd edn. Lippincott, Philadelphia.

Lego, S. 1996b, Psychodynamic individual psychotherapy. In: S. Lego (ed.), *Psychiatric nursing. A comprehensive reference*, 2nd edn. Lippincott, Philadelphia.

Marcus, P. 1998, Personality disorders. In: A. Burgess (ed.) *Advanced practice psychiatric nursing*. Appleton & Lange, Stamford, Conn.

Masterson, J. 1990, *The search for the real self. Unmasking the personality disorders of our time*. The Free Press, New York.

McGuiness, M. & Wadsworth, Y. 1991, *Understanding and involvement. Consumer evaluation of acute psychiatric hospital practice*. VMIAC, Melbourne.

Melbourne Consumer Consultants' Group 1997, *Do you mind? . . . The ultimate exit survey. Survivors of psychiatric services speak out*. MCCG, Melbourne.

Moscato, B. 1996, The nurse–client relationship and individual therapy. In: H. Wilson & C. Kneisl (eds), *Psychiatric nursing*, 5th edn. Addison-Wesley, Menlo Park, Calif.

O'Brien, L. & Flote, J. 1997, Providing nursing care for a patient with borderline personality disorder in an acute inpatient unit. A phenomenological study. *Australian and New Zealand Journal of Mental Health Nursing*, 6(4): 137–47.

Parker, B. & Campbell, J. 1995, Care of survivors of abuse and violence. In: G. Stuart & S. Sundeen (eds), *Principles and practice of psychiatric nursing*, 5th edn. Mosby, St Louis, Mo.

Platt-Koch, L. 1983, Borderline personality disorder. A therapeutic approach. *American Journal of Nursing*, December: 1666–71.

Rosenhan, D. 1996 (orig. 1975), On being sane in insane places. In: T. Heller, J. Reynolds, R. Gomm, R. Muston & S. Pattison (eds), *Mental health matters. A reader*. Macmillan, Houndmills, UK.

South, R. 1999, *Adult survivors of child abuse/trauma project 1997–1999. Understanding and working with the long-term effects of childhood abuse and trauma in mental health patients/clients*. Central Coast Mental Health Service, Sydney.

Stuart, G. 1998, Self-protective responses and suicidal behavior. In: G. Stuart & M. Laraia (eds), *Stuart & Sundeen's principles and practice of psychiatric nursing*, 6th edn. Mosby, St Louis, Mo.

Townsend, M. 1988, *Nursing diagnoses in psychiatric nursing. A pocket guide for care plan construction*. F. A. Davis, Philadelphia.

Witherspoon, V. 1985, Using Lakovic's system of countertransference classifications. Focus. Borderline personality. *Journal of Psychosocial Nursing*,
23(4): 30–4.

12

Nursing people with altered perceptions and thoughts

Key concepts
in this
chapter:
■ anxiety ■ behavioral manifestations
■ emotional manifestations ■ expectations
■ meaningfulness
■ perceptual disturbances
■ psychosis and schizophrenia
■ relatedness ■ thought disturbances

Introduction

Mental health nurses work with people who experience problems related to perceptions, thoughts, feelings or behaviors. These people often have perceptions that do not correspond with consensus views of reality, communication that does not make sense, emotions that are extreme and debilitating, or behaviors that are harmful or troublesome. The work of the nurse is to decrease the anxiety associated with disrupted perceiving, thinking, feeling and behaving so that these can be understood and dealt with. This chapter explores how problems related to altered perceptions and thoughts—features prominent in psychosis, including schizophrenia—might arise and how the nurse can intervene therapeutically. Schizophrenia, the most prevalent type of psychosis, will be the focus of discussion.

What is schizophrenia?

Although thought and perceptual alterations are not exclusive to mental illness, they are the hallmark symptoms of psychosis and schizophrenia. Psychosis is an extreme response to stress, with or without organic damage, characterized by disturbed thinking and reality orientation and accompanied by affective, psychomotor and physical disturbances. Schizophrenia is a psychotic reaction marked by deterioration in social functioning with partial or complete withdrawal. The main disturbances in people with schizophrenia can be grouped as:

- disturbed perceptions (e.g., illusions and hallucinations)
- disturbed thinking (e.g., loose associations, delusions)
- disturbed feelings (e.g., apathy and inappropriate affect)
- disturbed behavior (e.g., bizarre behavior, autism, and withdrawal) (Carter 1981).

Approximately one to two per cent of the population will experience schizophrenia at some time in their lives (Keltner et al., 1991, Johnson, 1997). Although this figure might seem low, schizophrenia continues to be the most complex, disabling and costly type of mental illness. The onset of schizophrenia is most often in late adolescence or early adulthood.

The specific characteristics of schizophrenia have been categorized into positive and negative symptoms. Positive symptoms include distorted perceptions (hallucinations), distorted thinking (delusions), disorganized speech, grandiosity, suspiciousness, hostility and bizarre behavior. Negative symptoms include blunted emotional affect (affective flattening), social withdrawal, restricted initiation of goal-directed behavior (avolition), poor rapport, restricted thought and speech (alogia), loss of interest or pleasure (anhedonia), difficulty in abstract thinking (loosening of associations) (Johnson, 1997, Shives, 1998, Keltner et al., 1991).

As observed by Arieti (1974: vii–viii):

To study schizophrenia means to study more than half the field of psychiatry, because most of the problems pertaining to schizophrenia are connected to other psychiatric conditions as well. The study of schizophrenia transcends psychiatry. No other condition in human pathology permits us to delve so deeply into what is specific to human nature. Although the main objective of the therapist of the schizophrenic is to relieve suffering, he [sic] will have to deal with a panorama of the human condition, which includes the cardinal problems of truth and illusion, bizarreness and creativity, grandiosity and self-abnegation, loneliness and capacity for communion, interminable suspiciousness and absolute faith, petrifying immobility and freedom of action, capacity for projecting and blaming and self-accusation, surrender to love and hate and imperviousness to these feelings.

This passage outlines the challenge, fascination, distress and suffering that constitute the mystery of schizophrenia. While features of schizophrenia are indicative of a mental illness, they are not uncommon in other types of responses to extreme anxiety, spiritual encounters, or other human experiences. The actual frequency of these experiences remains unknown because of the stigma and fear that people associate with being mentally ill. An examination of the theoretical views that explain schizophrenia provides a background from which to interpret experiences and guide nursing responses.

Aetiological views of schizophrenia

Mainstream theories of schizophrenia causation can be organized into biological or psychodynamic categories. The biological views include genetic, biochemical and neuro-structural causes. The psychodynamic views include developmental, family and interpersonal influences. Despite years of research and theorizing, the specific aetiology of schizophrenia remains unknown and no cure has yet been discovered.

Biological models

Genetic views. Twin studies have produced the most convincing evidence to support the hereditary hypotheses. It has been shown that if one monozygotic (identical) twin becomes schizophrenic, the incidence for the other twin is significantly higher than it is for dizygotic (fraternal) twins (Johnson, 1997). If both parents have schizophrenia, 40 per cent of their children are likely to develop schizophrenia (Shives, 1998), regardless of being reared by biological or adoptive parents. If only one parent has schizophrenia, the likelihood drops to 10–16 per cent (Johnson, 1997).

Biochemical views. These hypotheses point to dysfunction of neurotransmitters that send messages from the synaptic receptors of the brain to various parts of the body. Substances such as dopamine, serotonin and norepinephrine play an important role in the transmission of sensory information in the nervous system. The most commonly accepted biochemical theory for schizophrenia concerns excessive production of dopamine or insufficiency of norepinephrine, which results in over-stimulation of the brain, creating symptoms such as hallucinations, delusions and alterations in thoughts. More recent research links hallucinations to the accelerated glucose metabolism in the left temporal lobe (Johnson, 1997). Other support for biochemical causation comes from the effective reduction of symptoms associated with the administration of anti-psychotic medications that block the excessive release of dopamine or restore balance to receptor sites.

Neuro-structural views. Technological advances such as the positron emission tomography (PET) scan, the computerized tomography (CT) scan, magnetic resonance imaging (MRI), regional cerebral brain flow (RCBF), and brain electrical activity mapping (BEAM) indicate structural changes of the brain that create increased ventricular brain ratios, brain atrophy and decreased cerebral blood flow. Brain imaging procedures also enable actual viewing of metabolic changes in blood flow, electrical activity, and neurochemistry that illustrates decreased frontal lobe activity, which is reversed with neuroleptic drugs (Johnson, 1997).

The results of these alterations include cognitive and social impairments (Keltner et al., 1991). Recent large-scale studies of abused and non-abused children demonstrate a possible link between abuse, underdeveloped frontal lobes, and subsequent episodes of aggression, violence and suicide attempts (Shin et al., 1997). While these studies are not directly related to schizophrenia, this kind of evidence supports the idea that brain abnormalities result from psychodynamic factors.

Psychodynamic models

Developmental views. These suggest a link between childhood deprivation of meaningful family relationships and the subsequent onset of schizophrenia. Freud and Myers in the early 1900s, and Erikson and Sullivan in the 1950s and 1960s proposed that early life events of stress and conflict leave the child vulnerable to later mental disturbances. According to Sullivan

(1959), anxious or disapproving primary carers transmit a state of tension to the child that eventuates into dysfunctional relating. For example, lack of a warm, nurturing and trusting environment during the early years blocks the expression of the same effective responses in later years (Keltner et al., 1991). People with schizophrenia who report that they felt unwanted, unloved or disregarded as children, find it difficult to adjust socially or intimately as adults (Barry, 1994).

The dysfunctional parental communication view. This is outlined in the double-bind hypothesis. Bateson (1956) first described double-bind communication as that of ambivalence, where the parents give the child a message with two opposing meanings, both of which must be obeyed. Because satisfying both requests at the same time is impossible, the child solves the dilemma by:

1. trying to figure out which message was intended
2. responding to one message and ignoring the other, or
3. withdrawing into fantasy and responding to neither message (Schwartzman, 1978).

Although this theory is considered outdated and unpopular because it appears to assign blame to poor parenting, it does highlight the impact that communication and interpersonal dynamics can have on family members. Families struggle to cope with a member affected by a mental illness and may develop ineffective ways of relating with each other that include overinvolvement, frustration and hostility, that create feelings of helplessness and hopelessness. In turn, these responses can lead to further negative consequences for the person with a mental illness as well as for the entire family system.

Interpersonal views. These explain symptoms of schizophrenia as attempts to cope with overwhelming anxiety that is generated between people. For example, isolation or withdrawal from others is seen as a means of protecting the self from feelings of vulnerability and anguish within relationships. Distorted communication, such as rapid unintelligible speech, can be understood to be a way to keep people at a distance. Interpersonal relations theory highlights the view that what goes on between people can be studied, explained, understood and, if detrimental, changed (Peplau, 1992).

Cameron (1963) identifies three sources of potentially overwhelming anxiety that may contribute to the aetiology of schizophrenia:

1. loss or threat of loss of gratification and security
2. sudden increase of hostility, guilt or erotic feelings, or
3. reduced effectiveness of ego defenses.

It is hypothesized that for some vulnerable individuals, the stress of transition from adolescence to adulthood can precipitate psychotic reactions. The transitional challenges of late adolescence often include leaving the family of origin; and the interpersonal demands of sex and new intimate relations can lead to troubling erotic feelings or extreme guilt that can render usual coping methods useless. The stress associated with other significant but less predictable life changes can also precipitate other psychotic reactions—for example, the experience of traumatic events such as war, rape or a motor vehicle accident involving the death of others. Overwhelming anxiety can mount to severe or panic proportions and interfere with the ability to make logical connections between events and lead to perceptual distortions (Schwartzman, 1978).

A combined model

A combination of the biological and psychodynamic views is contained in the stress-vulnerability framework for understanding schizophrenia. This model suggests that people have varying vulnerability to develop schizophrenia based on the stressors that they might have experienced (Brooker & Repper, 1998). The person's history may reveal a family background of mental illness, childhood experiences of loss or insecurity, exposure to extreme stress, brain injury, toxic drug and/or alcohol ingestion, or feelings of low self-esteem, guilt, loneliness, inadequacy, powerlessness and other sources of anxiety as predisposing stressors.

Despite the insights offered by embracing a combined model, it does not entirely solve the mystery of schizophrenia aetiology. Nonetheless, both perspectives are valuable and offer the nurse ideas for helpful involvement. Biological conditions alter psychodynamic relationships as much as dynamic factors affect physiology. For example, brain-imaging techniques show enlarged ventricles in some adults with schizophrenia and these may contribute to communication difficulty, which in turn can lead to frustration. Alternatively, psychosocial responses to stressful life events may alter neurochemical pathways, activating anxiety, depression, schizophrenia or somatic symptoms (Bendik, 1997).

In this chapter the focus is on the dynamic interplay between the person and how they experience their world, in order to provide a deeper understanding of the psychosis of schizophrenia. Most nursing textbooks provide a descriptive taxonomic approach where the symptoms of patients are recognized, described and labeled. That means that symptoms are observed as manifestations without any human meaning being attached to them. However, the nursing approach subscribed to here supports the view of Arieti (1974), who suggests that the symptoms can be interpreted as having meaning and that the symptomatology has a purpose, inasmuch as it can be related to the early life of the individual. 'It is impossible to overestimate the value of the dynamic approach to schizophrenia . . . nothing could be more important from a psychotherapeutic point of view' (Arieti 1974: 5).

Perceptions, thoughts, feelings and behaviors

Figure 12.1 illustrates the inter-relatedness between perceptions, thoughts, feelings and behaviors. It will be used to understand healthy and usual ways of responding to the world as well as those that are indicative of schizophrenia.

Personal background—or a person's total experience, education and knowledge—determines who we are and how we perceive the world. From the moment of birth, situational conditions and experiential interactions shape our lives.

A person's background includes culture, socioeconomic status, education, beliefs, religion, physical and mental attributes, health status and personality, as well as the accumulated everyday usual, unusual and traumatic experiences. Antonovsky (1979; 1987) claims that a person's background view of the world or sense of coherence (SOC) is influenced by the generalized resistance resources (GRRs) at their disposal (see chapter five). These are characteristics of the person or environment that determine how life is experienced. For

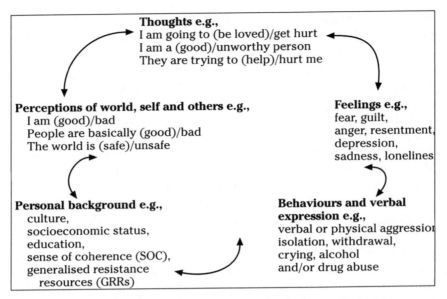

Figure 12.1 The inter-relatedness of perceptions, thoughts, feelings and behaviors

example, self-esteem, social support, high social class or cultural stability are GRRs, or properties of the person and his or her environment that, over time, lead to a strong SOC. Whereas, low self-esteem, isolation, low social class or cultural instability tend to diminish SOC (Antonovsky, 1990).

Perceptions. Perceptions of the self, others and the world are determined by a combination of the person's background and the sensory information that is presented and taken in through the body. Sensing includes sight, hearing, smell, touch and taste. Sensory information holds meaning based on memory and previous experience. Our perception of what is happening at the moment is highly personalized and interpreted from a background of accumulated knowledge and experience.

Thoughts. Perceptions are simultaneously translated into thoughts or cognitions, through a process that sorts out the information to determine if it is stressful, benign, positive or irrelevant (Lazarus & Folkman, 1984). There continues to be some debate regarding the degree to which sensory information is processed through cognition. Thoughts are private but may be accessible in the form of an inner dialogue in a person's conscious awareness. By tuning into your thoughts, you will notice that they tell you something about what is going on and how you feel about it (Burns, 1980).

Feelings. Cognitive theorists and therapists postulate that all feelings are created by cognition. The way that you look at things, your perceptions, attitudes, beliefs, thoughts, interpretations and what you say can have a significant impact on your feelings (Burns, 1980).

Behaviors. Behaviors, or actions, are influenced by feelings. How a person expresses himself or herself, or behaves, reflects an internal integration of perceptions, thoughts and feelings. Reflexive (automatic) actions are considered to be a means of coping with thoughts and feelings, or to provide relief from discomforting anxiety.

The connection between perceptions–thoughts–feelings–behaviors is interactive and not linear. That means that behaviors will influence feelings and generate new thoughts and perceptions of the world. In addition, some aspects of our perceptual world can become so ingrained that we might ignore or bypass thoughts and feelings and just react. For example, people who experience the world as a harmful and threatening place may interpret benign sensory information as dangerous, and automatically react by attacking or retreating without thinking or feeling. It can be argued, however, that thoughts and feelings generated the action, but the person did not notice them. If reflexive behavior successfully resulted in decreasing anxiety or getting needs met, it is likely that the same or similar automatic reactions that bypass thought or feelings will be used in the future. Thus, all behavior is meaningful.

We will use an example to illustrate this process. Sam has experienced a life of comfort, wealth, few health problems, abundant love and encouragement from family and friends, lives in a culture with strong kinship networks, and has a record of success and accomplishment. He views the world and people as basically good. When he meets a situation that he perceives as threatening or challenging, his thoughts, based on previous experience, most often tell him, 'I can manage this'. He feels secure and capable and will act in a way that affirms his capability. The success of the action he takes supports his feelings and thoughts of personal competence and confirms his perspective of the world as good.

Bill has lived in impoverished conditions, experienced mental and physical abuse, lack of love and acknowledgment, and has health problems. He perceives the world as a hostile place. When he encounters a situation of threat or challenge, he tells himself, 'I can't deal with this' and he feels insecure, worthless, sad, lonely, frustrated and resentful. He enacts his feelings by isolating himself and sometimes harms himself or attacks those he perceives to be a threat. Because he is successful in getting what he wants by withdrawing from, or attacking, others, he continues to do so even though his behavior gets him into trouble and confirms his sense of self-disdain.

The relative success a person has in negotiating the world also relates to how realistic their expectations are of what should happen and how they deal with unmet expectations. If expectations are impractical, the world will be experienced as disappointing and unpredictable. This will create a state of anxiety that may range from mild to extreme. The level and intensity of anxiety will coincide with the felt discrepancy between what was expected and what happened and will be based on what was at stake for the individual.

The role of expectations

The following five-step process illuminates the role that unmet expectations have in generating emotional and behavioral responses and how such behaviors might form a coping pattern if they provide relief from anxiety.

1. We all have *expectations*. For example, we believe that our bodies will function properly; that our belongings will be there when we go home; and that our friend who is coming for dinner will arrive as planned. Because these expectations seem reasonable, we will feel a sense of power and control over our life.

2. If we experience chest pain; go home and find that our house has been robbed; or our friend does not show up for dinner;

then our expectations are *unmet* and we may sense a lack of control or powerlessness.

3.   The loss of control is experienced as general anxiety that is transformed into some specific *feeling*. Following the examples, we might feel fear about the chest pain; we might be angry about the robbery; we might be worried about our friend's absence or feel rejected that they may have forgotten. The feelings are legitimate given the circumstances of the unmet expectation.

4.   The energy associated with the strong feelings is then connected to a *behavioral* response in an effort to regain a sense of power and control. Our fear of the chest pain may lead us to go and get help or alternatively engage in a distracting activity in an effort to ignore it. Anger about the robbery might initially result in yelling, crying or kicking. The friend's absence could lead us to telephone them, look along the road for an accident, or get drunk to attempt to drown feelings of disappointment or rejection.

5.   Then we justify the behavior of step 4. We say to ourselves, 'I had the right response given the situation'. 'Seeking help was the correct thing to do for my chest pain'; 'I was justified in my ranting and raving'; 'Getting drunk made me feel better at the time'.

As long as there is a justification for specific actions—that is, rationalizing why we behaved as we did—there is little reason or motivation to change responses next time we are met with a similar threat or challenge. If, however, the behavior becomes problematic or the emotional response disabling, the person may attempt to modify their feelings by altering their expectations or changing their response.

This model suggests that behaviors afford relief from anxiety as a means to cope. Since most people do not like feeling powerless or out of control, they consciously or unconsciously try to diminish negative feelings. It also explains how emotions result from unmet expectations or our perceptions and thoughts. Verbal and behavioral responses then can be understood to emerge from perceptions, thoughts and feelings which are shaped by our background and experiences.

Reflective exercise

The ability to work with others in applying information and educational techniques often requires first-hand experience and mastery. Using the five-step model for understanding the role of expectations and how personal background, perceptions, thoughts, feelings and behaviors interact, do the following:

■ Select an experience that you found difficult, upsetting, or that you would like to understand better.
■ On a piece of paper, write the numbers 1 through 5 in a column fashion with headings of: (1) expectations, (2) expectations unmet, (3) feelings, (4) behaviors, and (5) justification of behavior.
■ Under each heading, briefly describe: (1) what you expected to happen, (2) what happened, (3) how you felt, (4) what you did, and (5) how you defended your actions.
■ Examine your outline and determine if your expectations were realistic or understood by others on whom you were relying. Are there other ways that you could have ensured that your expectations were met? Analyze your behaviors. Were they reasonable or were there other more useful responses that you could have considered? Is your justification valid or should it be set aside to enable situations in the future to be dealt with differently?
■ Does the intensity of your feelings or behavioral response coincide with the level of importance of the issue or situation?
■ What have you learned by using this five-step procedure?
■ How can it be used in your work with patients?

Disrupted personal backgrounds

Aetiological views of schizophrenia point to a number of vulnerability factors that might predispose people to have psychotic reactions or develop schizophrenia. Genetic, biochemical and brain structure alterations are likely to affect neurological functioning and result in altered perceptions, thoughts, feelings and behaviors. Psychodynamic factors and experiences also set the stage for altered perceptions, thoughts and behaviors.

Early and ongoing life experiences include feedback from others that is incorporated into a sense of self. People who have not developed a solid sense of self feel vulnerable, insecure and inferior. They are too afraid to look at themselves realistically and see their limitations and shortcomings. They create an idealized self-image in order to feel secure, superior, unique and confident. This image furnishes them with a direction that shapes interactions with others (Janosik & Davies, 1991).

The idealized self-image can also create expectations that are so high that the person is constantly trying to fit into the image and, when unsuccessful, creates an illusory world where nothing is impossible. Whatever enhances the idealized self becomes important and whatever diminishes the idealized self becomes avoided. As a result, people with an altered sense of self do things that will maintain their idealized self-image (Janosik & Davies, 1991). A person with an extremely altered self-image and/or altered neurophysiological functioning may experience distorted perceptions and thinking.

Altered perceptions

Hallucinations are false sensory perceptions of objects or events in the absence of stimuli, with a compelling sense of their reality to the person who experiences them (Birckhead, 1989). Altered sensory perceptions can be auditory (hearing), visual (sight), olfactory (smell), tactile (touch) or gustatory (taste) hallucinations. Although hallucinations are most often associated with mental illness, they can be a response to drugs or other triggering events.

Hearing human voices that are not externally verifiable is not a rare human experience. It is estimated that at one time or another, a majority of people in the general population will have an inner voice experience that is not related to any kind of mental disorder (Barrett & Etheridge, 1992). Common occurrences include hearing a familiar voice upon falling asleep or waking up, the auditory aspects of dreams, and the voice of an imaginary childhood companion (Watkins, 1998). During bereavement and mourning, some people see, hear or feel the presence of the deceased person. People who undergo hypnosis or have a near-death experience often report vivid details of a conversation that they had with the voice of a friend, relative, spirit, god or angel. Other people claim creative inspiration and the call of vocation to be the result of an inner voice guiding them. There are also numerous medical conditions and traumatic stress reactions that precipitate hallucination-like experiences.

Sensory deprivation and isolation produce circumstances conducive to experiencing hallucinations. For example, people who are in isolated or constricted situations such as immobilization from injury, solo adventurers, prisoners, people with some physical handicaps such as deafness, or any situation that cuts off social, emotional or intellectual stimulation may experience hallucinations (Watkins, 1998). This fact raises the possibility that people with schizophrenia who have become isolated from the social world might hear voices as a result of their isolation alone.

The hallucinations associated with schizophrenia are considered by some theorists to be adaptive human maneuvre that transform inner emotional conflicts into external representations of the world in an attempt to gain control (Arieti, 1974). The content of the hallucination will reflect a highly personalized issue to the person who has the experience. Arieti (1974) explains this position with the use of several examples. If the person considers himself or herself a rotten person, he or she may hear voices that confirm this feeling and direct the person to harm herself or himself. Alternatively, the person may develop an olfactory hallucination—a bad odor emanates from their body. If a person feels that their partner is making their life miserable, they may develop a gustatory hallucination that the food being offered has a bad taste that must indicate poison.

Illusions are perceptions of actual external stimuli that are misinterpreted (Birckhead, 1989). For example, during periods of high anxiety people may mistake a moving curtain for a person coming through the window to harm them. The sound of an aeroplane flying overhead may be interpreted to be the voice of someone significant to the distressed person (Carter, 1981). An illusion is considered to be a less extreme experience in comparison with a hallucination because it is part of an externalized sensory experience rather than part of the internalized system, as hallucinations are. Nonetheless, they can be quite frightening and upsetting.

Altered thoughts

Impaired thinking in some people with schizophrenia is marked by thoughts that are seen by others to be irrational, scattered and incoherent. Distorted thinking may involve primitive or idiosyncratic symbols or fantasy (Murray & Huelskoetter, 1991). Disturbed thoughts are expressed in verbal communication and behaviors that indicate that the content of thinking is irrational and/or the way it is expressed is difficult to follow (Alchin & Weatherhead, 1976).

Disordered thought content

Delusions are fixed ideas based on a misinterpretation of facts. Delusions differ from illusions and hallucinations because they involve thought, not sensory perceptions (Carter, 1981). Some theorists consider that delusions develop through the stages of anxiety, denial, projection and rationalization (Benner, 1988). According to Peplau (1973, cited in Birckhead, 1989), a delusion is an idea involving an inadequate conclusion or explanation about an experience in which the person has experienced panic. The illogical conclusion serves to lessen the anxiety, even if it is false. Delusions may reflect an unconscious need to deny forbidden or unacceptable feelings. They can eventually become so strong that despite contrary evidence, rationalizations and projections emerge to support the delusion.

The various subtypes of delusions express the prominent theme of the person's anxiety. The most common delusions involve:

1. grandeur (the person believes themself to be immensely wealthy, famous, influential, or possessing superior talent or insight)
2. persecution (others are out to hurt them)
3. somatic changes (their body is changing or not functioning properly)
4. erotomania (the person believes that a prominent person is in love with them)
5. jealousy (partner or spouse is unfaithful) (Kennedy & Mitzeliotis, 1999).

According to Arieti (1974), the feelings of hostility or inadequacy that the person experienced before the onset of the psychosis become concrete to the point of becoming a delusion. The person's self-image is so terrible that they want to hide it, not only from the world, but also from themselves. Within this framework, delusions are desperate unconscious efforts to protect the self-image. Delusions of grandeur are a rejection of the inadequate self in favor of a powerful self. With persecutory delusions, a belief in the negative views and intentions of others is an unconscious re-enactment of one's fearful inner self-perceptions.

Ideas of reference are delusions in which the person believes that everyday events have special meaning to them. For example, the person sees two people talking and assumes that they are talking about him or that a red traffic light is a coded message to stop something important in their life.

Ideas of influence are delusions where the person is convinced that others are controlling or manipulating them. People with a psychotic illness might think that the television is transmitting messages directly to their brain.

Delusions are usually upsetting to the person, but it is important to consider that they are desperate unconscious attempts to provide relief or regain control of even more distressing feelings. It makes sense that the person who feels bad about himself or herself may claim to be Jesus, the Queen of England, or a famous movie star.

Disordered thought form

The way in which thoughts are expressed constitutes thought form. If the thinking processes are disrupted because of lack of stimulation, lack of opportunities to validate experiences, or repeated exposure to high anxiety, a primitive intrapersonal and autistic system of thought and communication develops (Bernstein, 1982). As a result, people will apply their own personal and private meanings to situations and use words that are not consensually validated (Arieti, 1974).

Concrete thinking is similar to underdeveloped or rudimentary levels of reasoning. There is a difficulty conceptualizing or clearly expressing meaning in thoughts and words. For example, people will mention some detailed differences between objects, but not recognize or articulate a more basic difference between categories. For example, when asked how do a coat and sweater differ, the person with concrete thinking might say 'one is green and one is brown' (Bernstein, 1982). The person attends to the specific appearance details, rather than the culturally defined abstract classification of things.

Magical thinking is another form of primitive thinking where the person believes that they can control the thoughts or wishes of others. This omnipotent view of the self enables the person to feel in control. The thoughts fulfill needs that are not otherwise met, such as the desire to be loved, important or needed.

Loose associations are apparently disconnected thoughts that become associated through some internal connection known only to the person (Vallone, 1997). This occurs because the person is unable to distinguish between ideas and organize them in a conventionally logical way. The person will string together several ideas that seem unrelated. For example, 'I like your hat and your hat likes me but your hat is red and your lips are red and I don't know how to read your lips.'

Disordered thought forms are most evident in altered speech and communication patterns. Speech may be so rapid that it sounds like a jumble of words or it may be so slow that the person will have to think desperately for the next word (Alchin & Weatherhead, 1976).

When expressing thoughts in words, the person may use unconnected words. This is called a *word salad*; for example, 'The worm yesterday laughed house person ate.' Some people with distorted thinking patterns make up new words called *neologisms* that have no meaning to the listener; for example, 'sitrocuim kabable yoit femeral' (Barry, 1994).

Echolalia is the repetition of a word or phrase and is often the last phrase spoken by another person; for example, 'See you later, see you later, see you later.' *Clang* associations are words that sound similar, or are word substitutions for those with a similar rhyme: 'The red fled bed said dead head.'

Distorted thinking and communicating is considered to be one of the most obvious markers of mental illness. However, even in the most profoundly disorganized forms, it is possible to trace some meaning to thinking and expressing (Arieti, 1974). Consider the following writing from a person with schizophrenia:

Do I see cake. Do I see the reverse of acting
Yes I do feel sensually deceived
thoughts in the mental suggestion in increase
of senses in suggestion
senses deceptive
in deception deception deception
deception
vanilla lemon as lemon vanilla as the beginning
of in in suggestion suggestion suggestion . . .

(cited in Arieti, 1974: 265)

Arieti (1974) interprets this as evidence of the person strug-gling to understand their own experiences—are they reliable or do they undergo mental suggestion? The world the writer is experiencing appears to be chaotic, fragmented and uncertain. 'Do I see the reverse of acting?'; that is, 'Do I do the opposite of what I would like to do?'. 'Do I see cake?'; that is, 'Do I see some-thing concrete and tangible?'

It is important for RNs in mental health to think about how expressions that seem nonsensical may actually convey poten-tially meaningful information about what the person is experi-encing. The interested nurse aims to understand symbolic communication and accept it as an expression of extreme inner distress.

Altered feelings

The emotional responses of a person with schizophrenia will correspond with their inner perceptions and thoughts. Conse-quently what is called—and appears to be—*inappropriate affect* in psychiatry is not necessarily 'inappropriate'. Even though it appears that the emotions are incongruent with what you observe, they will be connected to how the person is process-ing internal information. For example, a person may laugh hysterically when hearing the news of a tragic situation. This response is considered inappropriate; however, it is a means of self-protection that the person uses to help deny the painful emotional impact of the external world. Emotional changes in the person with schizophrenia evolve from a need to distance themselves from the intensity of feelings that becomes too over-whelming if dealt with directly (Bernstein, 1982).

The person may also display *flat affect*; that is, they may have an indifferent expression. The inability to show emotion or externalize feelings is common among people who are withdrawn. However, flat affect in people who live with schizophrenia is characterized by an unresponsive face, poor eye contact and no body language (Johnson, 1997). This indifference to environment and lack of commitment and involvement is a characteristic of apathy.

Depersonalization involves feelings and perceptions of an altered body image. Among people with schizophrenia, these experiences can include a sense of living in a dream; an inability to discriminate between inner and outer parts of one's body; feelings of being out of control; perceptions of merging into the environment; loss of orientation in space; and preoccupation with bodily sensations and functions. In attempts to deal with these feelings, the person may develop ideas that parts of themselves are strange and don't belong to them (Carter, 1981).

Ambivalence refers to experiencing opposing emotions simultaneously. Similar to the double-bind communication situation (which is a cognitive rather than an emotional quandary), the person is not sure what feeling should be acted on. As a result, often no decision or action is taken. On the one hand, indecision helps protect the person from positive or negative feelings about other people and situations. On the other hand, it contributes further to their already high level of anxiety in a no-win situation (Bernstein, 1982). The person experiencing ambivalence might allow others to make their decisions to attempt to decrease or avoid the distressing feelings.

A retreat from emotion is typical for people who interpret their world as threatening, harmful or unkind. Feelings of loneliness, emptiness, isolation, or alienation add to a person's overall sense of failure or inability to relate to other people. Attempts to avoid or cope with such extreme feelings lead to emotional and physical withdrawal and other behaviors that may seem peculiar.

Altered behaviors

The symptomatology of schizophrenia is a reflection of the person's inner reality (Arieti, 1974). The difficulty the person has in dealing with other people, and with the world in general, is the external counterpart of what goes on internally. According to this model of understanding psychotic distress, the human capacity to symbolize (verbally or behaviorally) transforms internal confusion into external and indirect communication.

Emotional withdrawal often results in *physical withdrawal*. In turn, physical withdrawal increases isolation, loneliness and introspection, and this affects one's ability to think, perceive and relate to others. The person may become reclusive and mistrustful of others, and judge them to be unauthentic, unreliable and dangerous.

If the loss of social contact is prolonged, deterioration of personal habits such as hygiene, nutrition, sleep and physical health results. As social constraints and reality become less important, so does the need to behave in what are considered socially acceptable ways (Alchin & Weatherhead, 1976). Being uninterested in others, appearing aloof, being preoccupied with fantasies, and displaying uninhibited behavior are all signs of social withdrawal (Johnson, 1997).

Mannerisms and gestures that seem *odd, bizarre or eccentric* are responses to disordered thoughts and feelings. Among people experiencing schizophrenia they often appear as disapproving gestures that indicate the person is censoring private thoughts (Bernstein, 1982). However, a person might mimic the movements and expressions of others in order to be like them.

A person who believes that the police are out to get them may gesture with their hands as if shooting a gun for protection. These types of behaviors are frightening and severely limit acceptance by others. In addition, they are embarrassing for the person who is aware of what they are doing but can't stop (Birckhead, 1989).

Impulsive behavior is acting without mediating thought, and can include apparently unpredictable verbal or physical aggression. Most often, violence occurs when the person feels trapped, compromised or threatened in some real or imagined way. On occasion, persons with auditory hallucinations will act impulsively on the command of the voice to either protect themself by attacking, or harming themselves.

In summary, hallucinations and delusions confirm or challenge the person's perception of himself or herself in the world. A person may hear a voice telling him/her that he or she is bad. Alternatively, the person may believe themself to be God. Emotional and behavioral responses to these perceptual and thought distortions are attempts to regain a sense of control over themself and to diminish anxiety or fear.

Approaches to working with people who experience psychosis

Reflective questions

Altered perceptions and thoughts lead to disturbed communications and behaviors. Mental health nurses are required to know the range of possible causes of such disturbances, as well as how to care for and comfort people who have such experiences. Assuming that all expressions and behaviors are meaningful, consider the following questions.

- If a person is convinced that they are no good, how might they communicate and act?
- If a person thinks that others are out to get them, what kinds of things might they say and do?
- If a person perceives the world as frightening and scary, how might they express themself and act?

From your answers above, think about someone you have come into contact with who was communicating or behaving in a bizarre manner. What did they actually say or do? How might their expressions or actions be an attempt to deal with altered perceptions of self, others or the world?

Arieti (1974) discovered that some hospitalized patients with severe long-term schizophrenia recovered or improved enough to be discharged after years or decades of hospitalization. He explains:

> These were considered to be cases of spontaneous recovery. I was not satisfied and looked more deeply into the matter. I soon discovered that these so-called spontaneous recoveries were not spontaneous at all but were the result of a relationship that had been established between the patient and an attendant or nurse.
>
> (Arieti, 1974: 545)

Arieti observed two stages of the relationship. In the first stage, the nurse was involved with the patient as a person and gave her or him special consideration. In the second stage, the patient became able to help the nurse with the work on the ward, which was welcomed due to the scarcity of personnel.

> The patient would then be praised, and an exchange of approval,
> affection, and reliability was established. In this climate of
> exchange of warmth and concern, the patient had improved to
> the point of being suitable for discharge.   (Arieti, 1974: 546)

This observation illustrates the favorable influence of human
contact. The nurse, through acknowledgment, acceptance and
empathetic understanding of the person's illness offered
'special' or personalized care that created a mutual connection
of trust and rapport. As the person's anxiety and isolation
decreased, self-esteem increased. Overall, the healthy and
capable aspects of the person were promoted and strengthened
by the nurse, thus helping to bring the person more out of their
psychosis and further into the world.

Specific nursing interventions cannot be prescribed exactly
because they are as much a consequence of the nurse's personality and creativity as they are of the patient's personality
and creativity and their contextual circumstances. Nursing principles that are often effective will be outlined in order for undergraduate students or RNs new to mental health to practice some
of these approaches.

The nurse's background, perceptions, thoughts, feelings and behaviors

Humanistic mental health nursing requires the nurse to have an
understanding of his or her own strengths and limitations in
working with others. Self-awareness is paramount in dealing
with individuals experiencing a psychotic illness. Because
people with perceptual and thought disturbances generate a
great deal of distress and anxiety, the nurse must acknowledge
and analyze reactive thoughts, feelings and behaviors that the
client arouses in them (Janosik & Davies, 1991).

The nurse's own background and experience will influence
how he or she interacts with the person with schizophrenia. It is
likely that a nurse has chosen the field of mental health because
of a personal fascination or interest in the area. Understanding
personal motivation is important because it will play a role in the
approach taken to care. For example, the nurse who was reared
by a parent with a mental illness brings an experiential perspective to practice that differs from the nurse who was not.

In addition, personal beliefs about mental illness and its causation will contribute to determining the emphasis of nursing interventions. If the nurse subscribes to the biological view, adherence to biochemical interventions such as medication are more likely to have top priority. The nurse who finds meaning in humanism and salutogenesis will be more likely to focus on interpersonal aspects of nursing and discerning the person's strengths and healthy attributes.

Arieti (1974) describes the personal characteristics necessary to work effectively with a patient with schizophrenia as being hopeful, straightforward and accepting, with unconditional positive regard for other people. These are the qualities espoused by humanist practitioners.

Interpersonal mental health nursing emphasizes the therapeutic potential of the exchange between the nurse and the person. The nurse will be challenged to comprehend the person's distorted communication. Understanding the possible causes and links between a person's background, perceptions, thoughts, feelings and behaviors will help the nurse realize that the unusual and bizarre expressions have meaning and are not necessarily directed toward the nurse. Because of their intense feelings of anxiety, loneliness, dependence or distrust, patients who are going through psychotic experiences can evoke 'intense, uncomfortable, and frightening emotions in all health care workers' (Varcarolis, 1994: 507). Consequently, clinical supervision is desirable for nurses who work with people who live with schizophrenia.

Reflexive (unthinking) nursing actions based on limited information can serve to perpetuate and reinforce negative patterns of response for both the patient and the nurse. People or environments intolerant of people with schizophrenia contribute to further emotional distress and compound the painful experience of the illness (Vallone, 1997). Consequently, the nurse is required to train her or his senses to observe a person well; make constructive exploratory and caring approaches; and think carefully before saying or doing anything that could be misconstrued as uncaring, insensitive or hostile.

People with schizophrenia are often acutely sensitive to the demeanor, body language and behavior of others. These strengths have been developed to help the person manage their own extreme sense of vulnerability. Therefore, some patients have what seems to be an uncanny ability to zero in on the vulnerabilities of others. Nurses may feel embarrassed, defensive or angry when patients comment on their peculiarities. Feelings of the nurse that go unrecognized or are not dealt with will create barriers to developing a therapeutic relationship (Schwartzman, 1978). It therefore becomes a professional nursing responsibility to reflect upon and process strong emotions that emerge from interactions with patients. In order to work with people with distorted perceptions, thoughts and feelings, it is not surprising that it is important for mental health nurses to continuously increase their awareness of their own perceiving, thinking and feeling styles, strengths and limitations.

Reflective questions

Have you ever heard that your strengths or assets can become weaknesses or liabilities and your weaknesses can become your strengths? For example, the ability to be tolerant of a person's behavior (strength) can become a liability (weakness) when that person's behavior requires immediate confrontation to avoid harm. Just as intolerance (strength) can become a liability (weakness) in situations where reflective consideration and compassionate understanding are called for. Think about your background experiences and personal strengths and weaknesses. Identify the following:

- What personal background experiences make you particularly effective in working with people experiencing a schizophrenic illness?
- What experiences have you had that make you ineffective in working with people manifesting symptoms of psychotic illness?
- Identify at least one area of concern (a liability, weakness, or blind spot) that you would seek help for when confronted with in clinical practice?
- How might you use your experiences, both positive and negative, to strengthen your approach to care?

Nursing care for people with perceptual and thought disturbances

The nurse begins by acknowledging and accepting that the patient's mental well-being is compromised and that the person is responding to their environment according to perceptions, thoughts and feelings that are valid for them at the time. Acceptance helps to reduce anxiety. Much of the distress of a person with schizophrenia is due to the inability to perform according to the expectations of others (Vallone, 1997). To accept persons as they are and provide support and understanding is the first step toward helping.

After establishing trust, conveying acceptance and developing a therapeutic relationship, the following principles can be drawn upon to work effectively with people who are experiencing auditory (the most common) hallucinations.

- Spend time with the person and be patient with them.
- Ask the person what is happening to them; you may need to repeat this.
- Remind the person that you are available to be with them if they are scared.
- If the person is unsure whether the voices are real or not, say clearly that you do not hear the voices.
- Do not touch the person without permission if they are suspicious.
- Do not agree with comments attributed to the voices.
- Explore with the person whether the hallucinations are related to increased stress or other precipitants in their immediate environment; if they are, these factors may be changeable or the person might choose to seek out a nurse when the voices intrude more.
- If the person starts a discussion about the voices or their content, listen to her or him.
- Focus on the likely human emotional response to what the voices are saying.
- Empathize with the person's distress if the voices are hostile or threatening.
- Doing something such as walking or talking with the person provides something to concentrate on and can distract them from their internal preoccupations.

■ Over time you may be able to assist the person to understand some personal reasons for voices starting again or escalating in intrusiveness (adapted from Varcarolis, 1994: 509).

The principles for working with people who hold delusional ideas are similar to those utilized to connect with people who are hallucinating. That is, the nurse conveys acceptance and interest, and because the nurse represents 'reality' in conversation it is important to discuss real events and people in the outside world.

The nurse can only explore possible meanings with the patient after a level of trust and relatedness has been established and maintained. Unless toxically induced, altered thought processes are generally related to low self-esteem, powerlessness, anger or fear. The nurse should listen carefully to what the person says about their delusions and attempt to understand how the themes may relate to them and their life experiences and aim to uncover some sort of meaning. If the intensity of the delusions waxes and wanes, explore with the person any interactions or events that increase anxiety or stress, heighten the feelings associated with the delusional beliefs, or strengthen those beliefs (Varcarolis, 1994; Townsend, 1988).

Reassuring the person that their delusion, while not shared by you, is valid and important given their current situation and feelings, will help to reduce anxiety and establish a connection. Disputing the content of delusions—for example, saying, 'You are not God' or 'There are no demons trying to get you'—will not work because the experience involving the delusion or hallucination is that person's reality. Disordered thoughts cannot be challenged or changed without some fundamental means of providing protection to the person's esteem.

The nurse can agree with the patient that his or her life has been confusing or painful. When the milieu is a safe haven and the nurse conveys respect and acceptance, the patient's feelings of being overwhelmed are likely to diminish. The self-saving value of delusions and hallucinations, while largely ignored, dismissed as a symptom, or medicated away, can offer a gateway for understanding the misery and suffering in a person's life. Experienced nurses can explore the symbolic meanings or emotional concomitants of delusions with the patient to help them make sense of some of their extreme experiences and reduce associated anxiety or fear.

Nursing care for people with disabling anxiety responses

Unless nurses can notice and control their own anxiety, it is likely to escalate in both the nurse and patient (Peplau, 1992). Working with patients who have severe communication problems or are withdrawn can be frustrating and discouraging because the goals are not easily achieved and the progress is slow.

The disturbing experiences of the person living with schizophrenia render people and the world at large as potentially frightening or threatening and this creates anxiety. One of the central aims of the nurse is to decrease or relieve the patient's anxiety, their difficulty in communicating, and the feeling of being disconnected from others (Carter, 1981).

The nurse must assess the person's level of anxiety and ensure that a safe and secure interpersonal environment is established and maintained. As anxiety increases, the person's ability to perceive people and events accurately and communicate effectively diminishes. People experiencing high levels of anxiety sometimes isolate themselves from others out of fear and in an attempt to exert some control over their lives (Townsend, 1988). It then becomes the nurse's responsibility to make a connection with the person, behave supportively and help the person make sense of the precursors of anxiety and the consequences, particularly those of retreating further into the hallucinatory or delusional world.

People who require mental health care usually have low self-esteem, particularly if the nature of their illness is misunderstood or ridiculed. Salutogenic nursing care aims to improve self-esteem by treating the person as a worthwhile human being. Opportunities to demonstrate capability should be created by the nurse. For a person with significant functional impairment, simple goals with a high probability of success have to be set. For example, almost anyone can create a painting of some kind if paper, watercolors, time, patience and support are available (Alchin & Weatherhead, 1976).

Nursing care for people with negative behavioral responses

As well as symbolizing 'reality', the nurse is a behavioral role model. This may not be apparent to undergraduate students or newly registered nurses; however, the following vignette makes the point much more obvious than is usual.

A student nurse reported that a patient kept mimicking his movements. This went on for some time until the student asked what she was doing. The patient responded, 'You must be sane because you're not a patient; and I thought that if I do what you do, perhaps they'll let me out!'. The nurse originally wondered whether the behavior was crazy, intended to attract attention or to be annoying. All of those interpretations are logical from an outsider's perspective, but they assume that the patient's behavior must be targeting other people. However, the patient's behavior was entirely egocentric in that it revolved around her own contracted world and her own desperate needs. By asking an obvious question, the student nurse created a connection, elicited meaning and prevented drawing stereotyping conclusions about madness, attention seeking and patients deliberately annoying nurses.

Nurses are human touchstones for people who are in chaos and distress. They are available to patients to provide reassurance and support as they work out their problems of living and relating. Nursing individuals whose worlds are deceptive, frightening and unreliable, require the nurse to be honest, con-sistent and dependable in their actions in order to create alternative experiences for the person. How the nurse relates to people and stress in the workplace is also a reflection of their own mental health and attitudes toward life.

Behavioral symptoms of schizophrenia such as physical and emotional withdrawal are responses to a lack of trust or the threat of harm. This means that therapeutic involvement must offer a relationship of security and safety. It is understandably difficult to establish trust with someone who is withdrawn. Murray and Huelskoetter (1991) recommend using the four As as a guide to fostering trust. They are:

1. acceptance—accept yourself and your shortcomings and the person's experience

2. awareness—listen to verbal, nonverbal and symbolic communication
3. acknowledgment—recognize fears and communication
4. authenticity—show honest human-to-human contact.

Other approaches can include brief but frequent contact, sitting
together quietly, or offering practical help such as making a
bed (Alchin & Weatherhead, 1976). These activities should
not be diminished because they seem to be simple. Such
actions demand personal confidence, risk taking, positive
expectations in the face of little or no positive feedback, hope,
and patience from the individual nurse. The patient's sense
of trust develops slowly over time as each contact builds on
the previous one and eventually the perseverance of the
nurse elicits improved patient accessibility, responsiveness and
communication.

People with schizophrenia may neglect hygiene and nutritional needs during an acute episode. In these circumstances,
the nurse aims to foster the person's independence and
provides positive feedback for even small improvements
(Townsend, 1988). The nurse may have to show the person
exactly what to do if their thinking is concrete or the person is
immersed in acute psychotic experiences, and at times the
nurse may have to directly assist with these activities. Adequate
rest, food and clothing are also required to maintain physical
stamina.

Other physical conditions can be mistaken for the behavioral
manifestations of psychosis. For example, vaginal yeast infec-
tions, dental pain and steroid medications can create high levels
of irritability and loss of judgment. Ongoing thorough physical,
psychological and social assessment are important processes
to clarify each patient's situation and determine appropriate
nursing plans.

Antipsychotic medications are commonly used to treat
the symptoms of schizophrenia. The nurse is required to be
up-to-date and well versed not only on the wide range of
available drugs but their actions, reactions, contraindications,
therapeutic levels and doses, allergic reactions and side-
effects. With experience, the nurse will learn to distinguish
behaviors of schizophrenia such as odd mannerisms and flat

affect from slowed movements and muscular rigidity caused by medications. It is especially important for the nurse to learn about adverse reactions such as akathisia (agitation or restless pacing) and tardive dyskinesia (involuntary muscle spasms) (Varcarolis, 1994). The unpleasant or dangerous side effects of antipsychotic medication contribute to patients' negative attitudes or non-adherence to the drug regimen. Open and honest discussion between the nurse and patient can lead to finding suitable alternatives and solutions that can help alleviate fears and promote a sense of personal control. Although the nurse may be responsible for administering medication and observing its effects while the person is in hospital, ultimately it is the person's responsibility to take charge of their own medication routine.

Health teaching and psychoeducation are essential nursing practices. The nurse is in a key position to offer the patient and their significant others information about their illness, symptoms, ways of coping, and available resources as relevant to the person's situation. There are myriad resources for the nurse to draw on and pass along to others that range from educational pamphlets, self-help books, information about legal rights and disability, support groups and organizations such as the Schizophrenia Fellowship, Association of Relatives and Friends of the Mentally Ill (ARAFMI), Clubhouse, kids support programs, educational videos, and web sites that provide the latest research findings, treatment programs, and medications. It is a good idea to keep at your fingertips a local resource book that includes a list of these materials, groups and organizations as well as names and phone numbers of general practitioners, help lines, and after hours care agencies that are responsive to people with schizophrenia.

In summary, nursing individuals with perceptual and thought disturbances calls for the nurse to be especially attentive to his or her own behavior, intentions, and the messages that they communicate to the patient, because it can be difficult to differentiate which fears and concerns belong to the nurse and which to the patient. In addition, while the nurse and patient may not share the same sense of reality, the nurse must acknowledge and validate the patient's experience and at the same time maintain his or her own reality.

Simon Champ: consumer story and reflection

In others' eyes

A nurse walks confidently and cheerfully into a ward to begin her shift. The nurse knows who she is and is confident in the role of nurse she has taken on. However to the 20 people living on the ward she may appear a very different figure. Different from the last time they saw her and with each person perceiving a different nurse to their fellows.

Once, during my first admission to a psychiatric ward, the nurse who was taking me to be showered became a guard leading me to the gas chambers in a concentration camp of my delusion's making. I was not being showered but led to my death, and my mind, under the influence of a delusion, saw no nurse but a guard working for a system that wanted me exterminated.

What is hardest to comprehend is that for that time, the guard who was leading me to my death was not a fantasy. That was my reality. The fear of that guard leading me to my death was the real fear of death's agent. It might have been kind of mistaken identity but the fear was real to me.

Delusions can take all kinds of forms, changing the perceived role of the nurse, their actions and behavior, weaving it into complex alternative scenarios in the consumer's own mind. Innocent everyday actions by the nurse might take on interpretations hard to comprehend. A particular movement might become a signal to aliens or hidden spies and again, the nurse is not the nurse but a key player in the consumer's delusional system, attempting to poison me.

Psychotic illness may alter a consumer's perceptions of the nurse in other ways. Perceptual distortions experienced by some consumers might actually alter the physical appearance of the nurse. For example, they may appear to be larger than they actually are and because of this appear more threatening to the consumer. Hallucinations might change the physical appearance of the actual face or body of the nurse, sometimes to the point where the nurse may become another being; an alien or devil, for example.

Again, auditory hallucinations may appear to make a nurse say things that are not being said to the consumer, who may come

—continued

—continued

to believe the nurse is not a nurse but another identity. Other forms of auditory hallucination may speak to the consumer from inside or outside their own head to tell them that the nurse is indeed someone other than a nurse.

Often, a nurse coming onto a ward receives very little indication from a consumer that they are perceiving them other than they are.

Beyond the more radical changes in perception of nurses that I have experienced because of psychotic symptoms, nurses have not always been seen by me as they intended because of my interpretation of their role. In the early years of my recovery, sometimes in the journals I kept nurses were referred to as 'soul fuckers' who dispensed what I would call 'mind death'. Nurses did indeed then seem to me to be interfering with my very soul with medications that significantly changed my emotions and sense of being in the world. I thought of my illness as a special sensitivity and often saw society as far more out of touch with reality than I was. At such times the healing role of nurses seemed secondary to a perceived role that they were indeed agents of social control, repressing original thought and enforcing a narrow conception of reality supported by the status quo. Sometimes such thoughts would actually develop into fully delusional forms that made me believe a powerful system was intent on repressing me.

For me a good nurse can recognize when a consumer has developed a strange belief about them and restore the consumer's perceptions of themselves as they truly are. Their practice as nurses is clear and straightforward but is likely to be misread into delusional systems by consumers who are experiencing psychosis.

Reflective questions

Effective mental health nursing is based on involvement and care that incorporates and is responsive to the person's specific understanding of their experience. If the person's interpretation

—continued

—continued

of their situation is not understood by the nurse, help can create further anxiety or be rendered useless. The narrative account provided by Simon is a powerful example of how one person's interpretation of the situation may differ from another's. The story begs the nurse to look through another's eyes.

Consider the following.

■ Describe a situation shared with someone else where your interpretation of the experience was different from the other person's. What was it like?
■ Imagine what it would be like to experience delusions and hallucinations and be hospitalized. How would you feel?
■ Generate an exhaustive list of how you as a nurse can attempt to see though others' eyes. How will gaining this perspective influence your care?

References

Alchin, S. & Weatherhead, R. 1976, *Psychiatric nursing. A practical approach.* McGraw-Hill, Sydney.

Antonovsky, A. 1979, *Health, stress, and coping.* Jossey-Bass, San Francisco.

Antonovsky, A. 1987, *Unraveling the mystery of health. How people manage stress and stay well.* Jossey-Bass, San Francisco.

Antonovsky, A. 1990, Personality and health. Testing the sense of coherence model. In: H. Friedman (ed.), *Personality and disease.* Wiley-Interscience, New York.

Arieti, S. 1974, *Interpretation of schizophrenia*, 2nd edn. Basic Books, New York.

Barrett, T. & Etheridge, J. 1992, Verbal hallucinations, I. People who hear 'voices'. *Applied Cognitive Psychology*, vol 6.

Barry, P. 1994, *Mental health and mental illness*, 5th edn. J. B. Lippincott, Philadelphia.

Bateson, G. 1956, Toward a theory of schizophrenia. *Behavioral Science*, vol 1, October: 251–64.

Bendik, M. 1997, Biological basis for care. In: B. Johnson (ed.), *Psychiatric–mental health nursing. Adaptation and growth*, 4th edn. J. B. Lippincott, Philadelphia.

Benner, M. 1988, *Mental health and psychiatric nursing. A study and learning tool.* Springhouse Notes, Springhouse, Penn.

Bernstein, L. 1982, Helplessness. In J. Haber, A. Leach, S. Schudy & B. Sideleau (eds), *Comprehensive psychiatric nursing*, 2nd edn. McGraw-Hill, New York (pp. 599–651).

Birckhead, L. 1989, *Psychiatric/mental health nursing. The therapeutic use of self*. J. B. Lippincott, Philadelphia.

Brooker, C. & Repper, J. (eds) 1998, *Serious mental health problems in the community. Policy, practice and research*. Balliere Tindall, London.

Burns, D. 1980, *Feeling good. The new mood therapy*. Signet, New York.

Cameron, N. 1963, *Personality development and psychopathology*. Houghton Mifflin, Boston.

Carter, F. 1981, *Psychosocial nursing. Theory and practice in hospital and community mental health*, 3rd edn. MacMillan, New York.

Janosik, E. & Davies, J. 1991, *Mental health and psychiatric nursing. A caring approach*. Jones and Bartlett, Boston.

Johnson, B. 1997, Schizophrenic disorders. In: B. Johnson (ed.), *Psychiatric–mental health nursing. Adaptation and growth*, 4th edn. J. B. Lippincott, Philadelphia.

Keltner, N., Schwecke, L. & Bostrom, C. 1991, *Psychiatric nursing. A psychotherapeutic management approach*. Mosby, St. Louis, Mo.

Kennedy, W. & Mitzeliotis, C. 1999, Schizophrenia and other psychotic disorders. In: P. O'Brien, W. Kennedy & K. Ballard (eds), *Psychiatric nursing. An integration of theory and practices*. McGraw-Hill, New York (pp. 277–301).

Lazarus, R. & Folkman, S. 1984, *Stress, appraisal, and coping*. Springer, New York.

Murray, R. & Huelskoetter, M. 1991, *Psychiatric mental health nursing. Giving emotional care*. Appleton and Lange, Stamford, Conn.

Peplau, H. 1992, Interpersonal relations. A theoretical framework for application in nursing practice. *Nursing Science Quarterly*, 5(1): 13–18.

Schwartzman, S. 1978, The client who generates anxiety. In: J. Haber, A. Leach, S. Schudy & B. Sideleau (eds), *Comprehensive psychiatric nursing*. McGraw-Hill, New York. (pp. 211–245)

Shin, L., Bremmer, D., van der Kolk, B. & McNally, R. 1997, Neuroimaging in PTSD. New findings invited symposium. International Society for Traumatic Stress Studies, Annual conference, Montreal, November 6–10.

Shives, L. 1998, *Basic concepts of psychiatric–mental health nursing*, 4th edn, J. B. Lippincott, Philadelphia.

Sullivan, H. S. 1959, *Clinical studies in psychiatry*. Norton, New York.

Townsend, M. 1988, *Nursing diagnoses in psychiatric nursing*. F. A. Davis, Philadelphia.

Vallone, D. 1997, Schizophrenia. In: A. Burgess (ed.), *Psychiatric nursing. Promoting mental health*. Appleton & Lange, Stamford, Conn.

Varcarolis, E. 1994, Schizophrenic disorders. In: E. Varcarolis (ed.), *Foundations of psychiatric mental health nursing*, 2nd edn. W. B. Saunders, Philadelphia.

Watkins, J. 1998, *Hearing voices. A common human experience*. Hill of Content, Melbourne.

Index

(Numbers in italics refer to consumer case studies.)